T5-CVT-166

Platelets and Thrombosis

Platelets and Thrombosis

Edited by
Sol Sherry, M.D.,
Professor and Chairman,
Department of Medicine,
Temple University Health Sciences Center
Alexander Scriabine, M.D.,
Senior Director,
Pharmacology,
Merck Institute for Therapeutic Research,
West Point, Pennsylvania

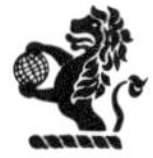

University Park Press
Baltimore · London · Tokyo

Proceedings of a symposium held in
Philadelphia on November 20–21, 1972

UNIVERSITY PARK PRESS
International Publishers in Science and Medicine
Chamber of Commerce Building
Baltimore, Maryland 21202

Printed in the United States of America

Library of Congress Cataloging in Publication Data
Main entry under title.

Platelets and thrombosis.

"Sponsored by the Physiological Society of Philadelphia."
1. Thrombosis—Congresses. 2. Blood platelets—Congresses. I. Sherry, Sol, 1916- ed. II. Scriabine, Alexander, ed. III. Physiological Society of Philadelphia. [DNLM: 1. Blood platelet disorders—Drug therapy—Congresses. 2. Blood platelets—Physiology—Congresses. 3. Thromboembolism—Drug therapy—Congresses. WH300 P718 1972]
RC694.3.P58 616.1'35 73-18179
ISBN 0-8391-0680-7

Contents

Contributors

Louis M. Aledort, M.D.
Division of Hematology
Department of Medicine
The Mount Sinai School of Medicine of the City University of New York
New York, New York 10029

William R. Bell, M.D.
Hematology Division
The Johns Hopkins Hospital
Baltimore, Maryland 21205

Sam Berger, M.D.
Division of Hematology
Department of Medicine
The Mount Sinai School of Medicine of the City University of New York
New York, New York 10029

Max E. Bierwagen, Ph.D.
Department of Pharmacology
Bristol Laboratories
Syracuse, New York 13201

Prof. Gustav V. R. Born
Chairman, Department of Pharmacology
Royal College of Surgeons of England
35/43 Lincoln's Inn Fields
London, WC2A 3PN, England

John O. Buchanan
Department of Pharmacology
Bristol Laboratories
Syracuse, New York 13201

Lewis Burrows, M.D.
Department of Surgery
The Mount Sinai School of Medicine of the City University of New York
New York, New York 10029

Beverly T. Cornish
Department of Pharmacology
Bristol Laboratories
Syracuse, New York 13201

H. James Day, M.D.
Specialized Center for Thrombosis Research
Temple University Health Sciences Center
3400 North Broad Street
Philadelphia, Pennsylvania 19140

Patricia R. Druzba
Sterling-Winthrop Research Institute
Rensselaer, New York 12144

Allan J. Erslev, M.D.
Cardeza Foundation
Jefferson Medical College
1015 Samsom Street
Philadelphia, Pennsylvania 19107

J. Stuart Fleming, Ph.D.
Department of Pharmacology
Bristol Laboratories
Syracuse, New York 13201

Zane N. Gaut, M.D., Ph.D.
Department of Biochemical Nutrition
Hoffmann-LaRoche, Inc.
340 Kingsland Street
Nutley, New Jersey 07110

Sheldon Glabman, M.D.
Department of Surgery
The Mount Sinai School of Medicine of the City University of New York
New York, New York 10029

Barbara Goldman, M.D.
Division of Hematology
Department of Medicine
The Mount Sinai School of Medicine of the City University of New York
New York, New York 10029

Moshe Haimov, M.D.
Department of Surgery
The Mount Sinai School of Medicine of the City University of New York
New York, New York 10029

John Hernandovich
Department of Pharmacology
Jefferson Medical College
Philadelphia, Pennsylvania 19107

Roy G. Herrmann, Ph.D.
Research Associate
The Lilly Research Laboratories
Eli Lilly and Company
Indianapolis, Indiana 46206

Ruth R. Holburn, Ph.D.
Assistant Professor of Physiology
Cardeza Foundation
Jefferson Medical College
1015 Sansom Street
Philadelphia, Pennsylvania 19107

Carol Ingerman
Department of Pharmacology
Jefferson Medical College
Philadelphia, Pennsylvania 19107

G. A. Jamieson, Ph.D.
The American National Red Cross
Blood Research Laboratory
9312 Old Georgetown Road
Bethesda, Maryland 20014

Phyllis T. Jordan
Department of Pharmacology
The Merck Institute for Therapeutic Research
West Point, Pennsylvania 19486

Suzanne P. King
Department of Pharmacology
Bristol Laboratories
Syracuse, New York 13201

James J. Kocsis, Ph.D.
Associate Professor of Pharmacology
Jefferson Medical College
Philadelphia, Pennsylvania 19107

William B. Lacefield, Ph.D.
The Lilly Research Laboratories
Eli Lilly and Company
Indianapolis, Indiana 46206

E. Leiter, M.D.
Department of Surgery
The Mount Sinai School of Medicine of the City University of New York
New York, New York 10029

Robert D. MacKenzie, Ph.D.
Merrell-National Research Laboratories
Division of Richardson-Merrell, Inc.
Cincinnati, Ohio 45215

Annette MacMillan
Department of Pharmacology
The Merck Institute for Therapeutic Research
West Point, Pennsylvania 19486

Jose Martinez, M.D.
Cardeza Foundation
Jefferson Medical College
1015 Sansom Street
Philadelphia, Pennsylvania 19107

David C. B. Mills, Ph.D.
Specialized Center for Thrombosis Research
Temple University Health Sciences Center
3400 North Broad Street
Philadelphia, Pennsylvania 19140

David H. Minsker, Ph.D.
Department of Pharmacology
The Merck Institute for Therapeutic Research
West Point, Pennsylvania 19486

Erik H. Mürer, Ph.D.
Specialized Center for Thrombosis Research
Temple University Health Sciences Center
3400 North Broad Street
Philadelphia, Pennsylvania 19140

Stefan Niewiarowski, M.D.
Blood Component Developmental Laboratory
Department of Pathology
McMaster University
Hamilton, Ontario, Canada
and
Specialized Center for Thrombosis Research
Temple University Health Sciences Center
3400 North Broad Street
Philadelphia, Pennsylvania 19140

Ganesh Nirmul, M.D.
The Mount Sinai School of Medicine of the City University of New York
New York, New York 10029

Patricia G. Phillips, Ph.D.
Sterling-Winthrop Research Institute
Rensselaer, New York 12144

Elena Puszkin, Ph.D.
Division of Hematology
Department of Medicine
The Mount Sinai School of Medicine of the City University of New York
New York, New York 10029

Franklin J. Rosenberg, Ph.D.
Director, Pharmacology
Sterling-Winthrop Research Institute
Rensselaer, New York 12144

Paul K. Schick, M.D.
Department of Medicine
The Medical College of Pennsylvania
3300 Henry Avenue
Philadelphia, Pennsylvania 19129

Sandor S. Shapiro, M.D.
Professor of Medicine
Cardeza Foundation
Jefferson Medical College
1015 Sansom Street
Philadelphia, Pennsylvania 19107

Sol Sherry, M.D.
Professor and Chairman
Department of Medicine
Temple University Health Sciences Center
3400 North Broad Street
Philadelphia, Pennsylvania 19140

Melvin J. Silver, D.Sc.
Cardeza Foundation
Jefferson Medical College
1015 Sansom Street
Philadelphia, Pennsylvania 19107

J. Brian Smith, Ph.D.
Cardeza Foundation
Jefferson Medical College
1015 Sansom Street
Philadelphia, Pennsylvania 19107

Robert N. Taub, M.D., Ph.D.
Assistant Professor of Medicine
The Mount Sinai School of Medicine of the City University of New York
New York, New York 10029

Peter N. Walsh, M.D., Ph.D.
Specialized Center for Thrombosis Research
Temple University Health Sciences Center
3400 North Broad Street
Philadelphia, Pennsylvania 19140

Byung P. Yu, Ph.D.
Department of Physiology
The Medical College of Pennsylvania
3300 Henry Avenue
Philadelphia, Pennsylvania 19129

Acknowledgment

The Physiological Society of Philadelphia gratefully acknowledges financial support of this Symposium from:

Ciba-Geigy Corporation

E. I. du Pont de Nemours & Co., Inc.

Hoffmann-LaRoche, Inc.

Eli Lilly and Company

McNeill Laboratories, Inc.

Merck Sharp & Dohme Research Laboratories

Merrell-National Laboratories

Pfizer, Inc.

Sandoz Pharmaceuticals

Schering Corporation

Sterling-Winthrop Research Institute

Introduction

Sol Sherry

This book represents an edited version of a symposium on "Platelets and Thrombosis" which was sponsored by The Physiological Society of Philadelphia. It was organized primarily through the personal efforts of the society's president, Dr. Alexander Scriabine.

The symposium is most timely because of the interesting and exciting developments in antithrombotic therapy that are now underway and that are likely to change radically our approach to the prevention and management of the thromboembolic disorders. Such a development is most fortunate; for, as a public health problem, thromboembolism is still increasing and currently represents a pathological event second to none as a cause of acute morbidity and mortality among the middle-aged and older population groups of the United States.

In these developments, the platelet has taken center stage: (*a*) it provides the critical link between the vascular wall and the subsequent activation of the clotting mechanism in the pathogenesis of most forms of arterial and perhaps venous thrombosis as well; (*b*) appropriate control of its function provides us with an important approach to the prevention of many of the thromboembolic disorders and perhaps other pathological lesions where platelet-fibrin deposition may be a critical step in the genesis of the lesion; and (*c*) it serves to bring together scientists of diverse interests and training who, focusing on a common problem, are advancing knowledge in this area at an extremely rapid pace.

The papers comprising this symposium by no means cover all the types of platelet research currently underway. More precisely, the symposium emphasizes such selected aspects as (*a*) the biological mechanisms controlling the function of the platelet as the body's primary hemostatic aide, (*b*) the inhibition of this function through a variety of pharmacological approaches, (*c*) the testing of the effect of pharmacological agents in appropriate experimental models of thromboembolism, and (*d*) an evaluation of the possible role of such agents in modifying the course of other types of lesions where platelet phenomena and fibrin deposition may play an important role.

To place the subject matter in perspective, it should be recalled that in response to an appropriate or thrombogenic stimulus, platelets stick to a vascular surface and then aggregate into a platelet mass. This mass becomes the white head of a thrombus and is the critical step in the formation of most arterial and some venous thrombi. The sequence of events which takes place in the platelet itself, in carrying out this functional role, is represented schematically in Figure 1.

As shown at the upper left of the scheme, the platelet normally circulates as a disc and contains within its structure several contractile fibrils and a number of light and dense granules. Upon stimulation, and as shown at the upper right, the platelet swells so as to assume a circular or rounded appearance.

If the stimulus is strong enough, as shown to the right of center, the actomyosin-like protein fibrils of the platelet, termed thrombosthenin, begin to contract, forcing the dense granules to the periphery of the platelet and the light granules to the center. At this point, platelets begin to stick and aggregate in what has been termed the primary wave of aggregation, a phase which is still reversible, depending upon the strength and duration of the stimulus. This primary wave of aggregation can be blocked by interfering with the cyclic AMP metabolism of the cell, either through activation of the adenyl cyclase, *e.g.* by prostaglandin E_1, or by inhibiting the phosphodiesterase, *e.g.* through the use of dipyridamole.

However, in the presence of a potent or protracted stimulus, further contraction of the thrombosthenin occurs, and this results in the extrusion of the dense granules and the liberation of their high concentration of adenine nucleotides, serotonin and platelet activators of the coagulation mechanism. The release of these

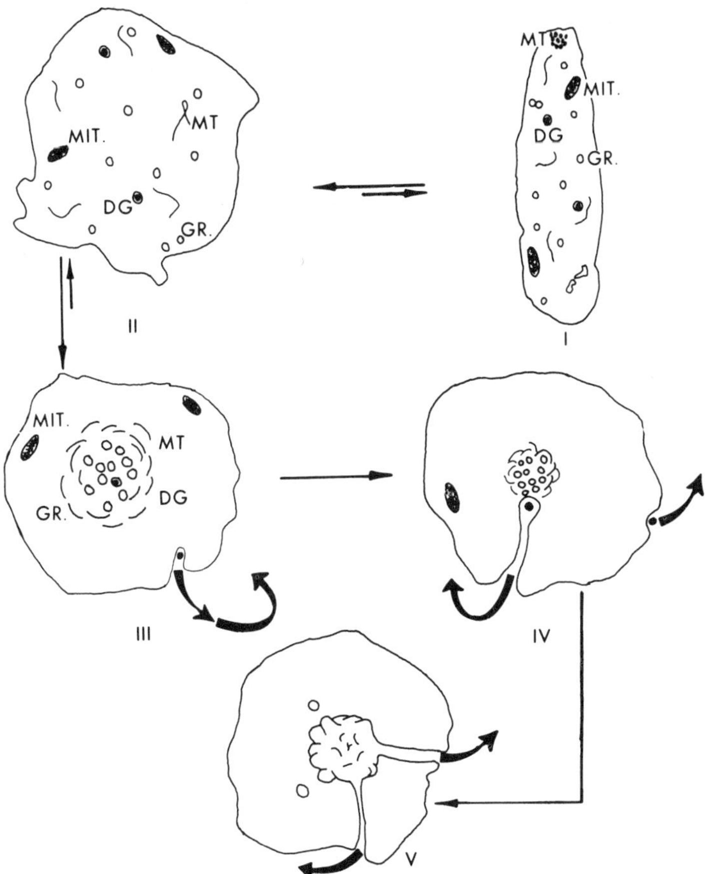

Figure 1. See text. Reprinted with permission from Day, H. J., and Holmsen, H. 1971. Concepts of the platelet release reaction. Ser. Haematol. 4: 3.

dense granules is termed the platelet release reaction and, unless blocked by such pharmacologically active compounds as aspirin and sulfinpyrazone, results in a secondary, more extensive and irreversible wave of aggregation. Then, as shown to the left of center of Figure 1, the platelet extrudes its light granules which, like lysosomes, contain a number of acid hydrolases and other factors. Ultimately, as shown in the bottom center of Figure 1, the platelet is reduced to an empty sac, a process formerly referred to as viscous metamorphosis.

The anatomical features and associated biochemical events involved in this fascinating sequence are now being mapped out in great detail, since they provide the opportunity to explain the action of certain inhibitors and to uncover others which may prove useful for therapeutic purposes. It is against this background that many of the papers comprising this symposium are best viewed.

SOL SHERRY, M.D.
Temple University School of Medicine

Observations on the Platelet Release Reaction

Erik H. Mürer and H. James Day

The blood platelet represents an interesting cell type, for it may be viewed in its function as a hemostatic cell or as an experimental model for cellular biochemistry and physiology.

A functioning platelet can stick to surfaces or to other platelets, aggregate, support retraction of a blood clot, and specifically release stored compounds into the blood stream. The platelet's biological function in the blood stream may or may not include all of these activities. Platelet aggregation depends partly on adenosine diphosphate (ADP) and calcium ions (Ca^{++}), both of which are released from the platelet. The events leading to aggregation, or the release reaction, or both, also seem to be a prerequisite for the adhesion to foreign surfaces.

We have, so far, been able to delegate only one function of physiological importance to the platelet, namely that of hemostasis. This is accomplished by a *primary event*, the formation of a platelet plug which may itself halt the flow of blood when the lesion is minor, or the vessel wall is small, and a *later event*, the stabilization of a fibrin clot via activation of the coagulation mechanism following vessel wall injury. In the absence of platelets the clot will be fragile with little ability to resist the pressure of the flowing blood. Owing to the embedded platelets, the clot initially becomes more solid, then retracts to form a firm plug. With certain hemorrhagic diseases the platelet's ability to form a hemostatic plug is lost or reduced, presumably by a defect in the binding of platelets to fibrin strands or to each other. Other abnormalities result from the platelet's failure to release compounds into the environment caused by a lack of releasable adenine nucleotides or a failure of the release process (Holmsen and Weiss, 1970, 1972). The fact that these platelet defects result in bleeding disorders is one of the indications of the important role the platelet release reaction plays in hemostasis.

The platelet also takes part in the initiation of thrombosis either through the formation of a platelet-platelet (white thrombus) or a platelet-fibrin clot (red thrombus) in circulating blood. A white thrombus occurs in arterial blood flow when the platelet receives an impulse from a damaged vessel wall, resulting in the alteration of the platelet membrane so that it will adhere to the subendothelial structures, releasing its contents and thereby causing other platelets to adhere. The other type of clot, the red thrombus, containing fibrin and red cells as well as platelets, may occur secondarily to the platelet plug, but is usually formed by the activation of the coagulation factors of blood plasma in veins. Such a clot would be less likely to stick to a surface, but might occlude the vessel by its sheer bulk and continue to grow. When a fibrin-platelet clot has stopped a major hemorrhage from a disrupted vessel, retraction might result in a secondary hemorrhage at this spot (Niewiarowski, 1973).

For its physiological function as a cell, the platelet has the ability to function in specific ways which are partly unique, partly shared by other cells. Stormorken (1969) has demonstrated the similarity between the activities of secretory cells, including the platelet, in which the secretory process has been called the *release reaction.* The role of calcium in promoting secretion is of interest in this regard. The platelet (at least in some species) does not seem to have an absolute requirement for extracellular Ca^{++} for its secretory activity, whereas calcium is required in most other cell systems. This finding is not unique since the release of catecholamines from nerve endings also can take place in the absence of added Ca^{++} when the impulse is of sufficient strength. The storage of secretory substances in granules is a widespread phenomenon among secretory cells and is characteristic of platelets. Only a few specialized cells (*e.g.* salivary glands and gastric mucosa) seem able to release compounds which are not stored in separate compartments.

A unique property of platelets, and one which is currently the subject of widespread investigation, is the ability to aggregate in the presence of ADP. Thrombin- or collagen-induced reactions seem also to be unique for these cells. There are some indications that the lipoglycoprotein nature of the membrane or the extramembranous "fluffy coat" and the glycosyltransferase-activating formation of gluconeoglucan bonds may be the key to the understanding of the platelets' ability to aggregate and to adhere to collagen (Jamieson, 1973). Presently it is unknown if the ADP-induced aggregation can be explained along the same lines.

The ability of platelets to support retraction of fibrin clots may be the result of a less unique ability to adhere to fibrin strands at some stage of the conversion from fibrinogen to cross-linked fibrin. Niewiarowski (1973) has shown that mouse L cells and fibroblasts, and to a lesser degree leukocytes, share this property with the platelets.

Much of the popularity of platelets as a research object rests on their role in hemostasis and thrombosis. For the biochemist or cell physiologist, however, they are very practical tools, as they are easily isolated and can be studied in their native state, in blood plasma, without interference from other cells, or placed into an artificial medium without any previous disruption of tissue which might cause damage to the cell. Although the cell is very reactive to the proper impulses, it is at the same time resistant to controlled changes over a long period of time.

THE PLATELET RELEASE REACTION

The secretion process of platelets called the *platelet release reaction* by Grette (1962) has gone through several stages of redefinition. This author, studying thrombin- or trypsin-induced release of adenine nucleotides and serotonin, suggested that the released material was extruded selectively from the cytoplasm through the

Table 1. Definition of the platelet release reaction

1. The substances released are (as far as it has been established) located in platelet granules, both the "usual" α-granules and "dense" α-granules with "Bull's eye" as well as "very dense bodies."
2. Substances located in either cytoplasm, mitochondria, or membranes are retained during release.
3. Maximal release is reached within 60 sec at 37°C.
4. The process is dependent on energy derived from both glycolysis and oxidative phosphorylation.
5. After release, the platelet participates almost normally in several of its known functions.
6. Extracellular Ca^{++} promotes the process in many cases.

platelet membrane following a Ca^{++}-induced contraction of the cell (Grette, 1963). He proposed that thrombin might condition the platelet for release by making the cell membrane permeable to Ca^{++} (Grette, 1962).

Later research demonstrated a number of other releasing agents (see Holmsen *et al.*, 1969, for review), at the same time casting doubt on the crucial role of Ca^{++} as the trigger for release (Mürer, 1968; Holmsen and Day, 1968).

The definition of the platelet release reaction proposed by Holmsen *et al.* (1969) presented the points summarized in Table 1.

This definition is generally still valid except for point 3. It is probably more correct to include in the platelet release reaction all types of release where the released material can be shown to come from a pool assumed to be localized in the platelet granules, even if the releasing process is slower. This review will elaborate on points 3, 4, and 6, and on one subject not covered in the definition, namely the release induction and what is known about this process.

RELEASED MATERIAL

That platelets have the ability to liberate intracellular constituents was first demonstrated with serotonin. Bigelow (1954) showed that blood coagulation was followed by an increase in serotonin in the serum. Both Humphrey and Jacques (1955) and Zucker and Borelli (1955) demonstrated that blood platelets were the source of this increase. Grette (1959) demonstrated that the release process was fast, although his experimental procedure did not permit an accurate estimation of the original velocity.

The release of serotonin seems to be the same whether it is derived from the original platelet storage pool or newly absorbed by the platelet *in vitro*, which indicates that storage granules are in both cases the site from which the release takes place (Day *et al.*, 1972). This seems to represent the only situation in which the contents of the storage pool in human platelets are exchangeable with extracellular material; the situation in rabbit platelets may be different (DaPrada and Pletscher, 1970).

Born (1958) first noted the intracellular disappearance of ATP and "ten-minute phosphorus" from platelets during clotting, but Grette (1962) originally demonstrated that part of the disappearing intracellular material appeared as adenine nucleotides outside the platelets. Holmsen (1965) showed that there were at least two pools of adenine nucleotides taking part in the release reaction: one cytoplasmic, which provides energy for the release reaction and quantitatively changes, and another, the *storage pool*, directly extruded during the reaction, yet not in contact with the cytoplasmic material.

Potassium also seems to be released partly from a granulum-located storage pool (Buckingham and Maynert, 1964; Zieve *et al.*, 1964). Magnesium release has been demonstrated from human platelets (Day *et al.*, 1973) and from other species (Kinlough-Rathbone and Chahil, 1972). The previous report of release of Zn^{++} (Foley *et al.*, 1968) has not been confirmed (Zucker, 1972).

A number of lysosomal acid hydrolases seem to need a somewhat stronger releasing impulse than the adenine nucleotide-serotonin group. Calcium, under conditions where it has little effect on the release of adenine nucleotides, increases the acid hydrolase release up to four times (Holmsen and Day, 1968, 1969). This, plus kinetic data, probably reflects a different granular location from that of serotonin and nucleotides.

Robert *et al.* (1970) demonstrated that collagen releases elastase which can attack the arterial wall. One coagulation factor, heparin-neutralizing activity (platelet factor 4, PF_4), is released together with adenine nucleotides (Niewiarowski and Thomas, 1969). Nachman *et al.* (1970) describe release of a heat-resistant

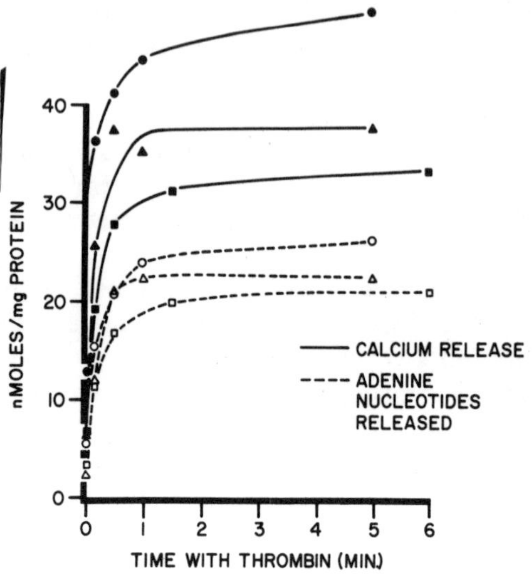

Figure 1. The concomitant release of calcium and adenine nucleotides from washed human platelets at 37°C in buffered saline in the presence of 0.3 m*M* EDTA is followed in three separate experiments: 1, ● and ○; 2, ▲ and △; and 3, ■ and □. The open symbols and dotted lines represent adenine nucleotides; the black symbols and solid lines represent calcium found in supernatant after release with 0.6 NIH unit of thrombin per ml of platelet suspension. (Reproduced from: Mürer and Holme, 1970. Biochim. Biophys. Acta 222: 201 (Fig. 1).)

polypeptide which increases the permeability of vessel walls. The release of fibrinogen was one of the early discoveries in the field of platelet release (Grette, 1962; Solum and Stormorken, 1965).

Calcium (Mürer, 1969a; Mürer and Holme, 1970; Wolfe and Shulman, 1970) is released with a time course exactly paralleling the release of adenine nucleotides (Fig. 1). This suggests that the released metal ion is stored in the same granules as are the adenine nucleotides, and White (personal communication) has postulated that the decrease in electron density seen in the dense granules during the release reaction reflects a loss of calcium.

RELEASING AGENTS

The releasing agents are numerous and varied. The classical type is the proteolytic enzyme thrombin, which can be used interchangeably with trypsin, as was shown by Grette (1962). A great deal of work has also been done with collagen fibers which were shown by Hovig (1963) to be releasing agents. Immunocomplexes were later established as releasing agents (see Mueller-Eckhardt and Lüscher, 1968). While all of these agents act on platelets in plasma as well as on washed platelets, studies from different laboratories are not always in agreement. Glynn *et al.* (1965) have shown that latex particles are capable of causing release from washed platelets if they were coated with γ-globulin. Mürer (1968) was able to demonstrate release from washed platelets using uncoated latex particles, although the condition of washing and the size of the latex particles were not the same. Other studies (Mustard and Packham, 1970; Mürer, 1972b) have shown that some plasma proteins are capable of inhibiting release induced by latex particles. The same inhibition may be true for inorganic cations (Mürer, unpublished observation). It is possible that the platelet is protected from release in its physiological surrounding by plasma proteins other than those which may actually potentiate release.

The other commonly used release inducers, ADP, adrenaline, serotonin, and some pharmacological agents, will not be discussed here (see review, Day and Holmsen, 1971). It is still premature to say whether ADP and adrenaline work directly as release inducers or through their effect as inducers of aggregation, although recent evidence would seem to favor the former explanation (Holmsen *et al.*, 1972).

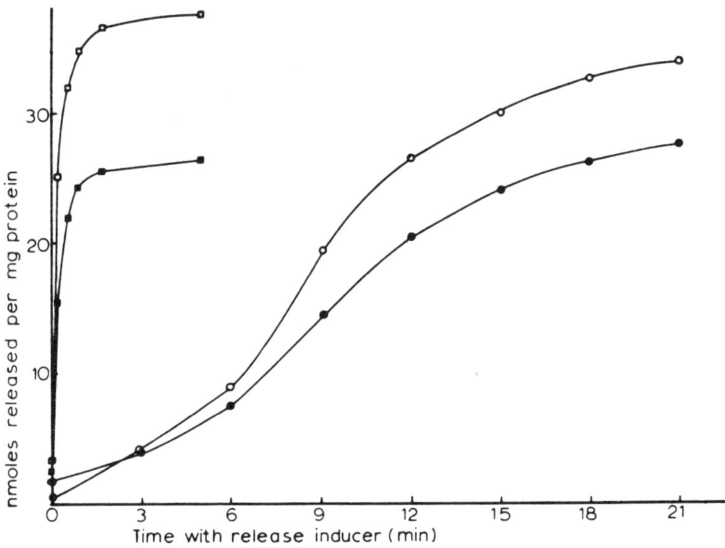

Figure 2. Time course of thrombin- and fluoride-induced release of adenine nucleotides with two separate platelet preparations (preparation 1, open symbols, preparation 2, black symbols). □ and ■, adenine nucleotides found in supernatant after release with thrombin; ○ and ●, same after fluoride-induced release. (Reproduced from: Mürer, 1968. Biochim. Biophys. Acta 162: 323 (Fig. 1).)

We are currently interested in the role of inorganic ions as release inducers. Sodium fluoride (NaF) at 10 m*M* concentration acts as a platelet release inducer. The release process is very slow, as can be seen from Fig. 2 where the steep slope of the thrombin-induced release is compared with that of the fluoride-induced release (Mürer, 1968). The mode of action of fluoride, as to whether the release is induced from the outside of the membrane or through a possible transport into the cell, is unknown. This unique type of release inducer may hold important clues to the nature of induction of platelet function.

Grette's (1962) finding that Ca^{++} was absolutely necessary for release induced by thrombin or trypsin at 15°C in the presence of EDTA, but less necessary at 37°C, was interpreted by him as indicating that, at 15° C, EDTA penetrated the platelet membrane and chelated all available Ca^{++}. Another interpretation results from

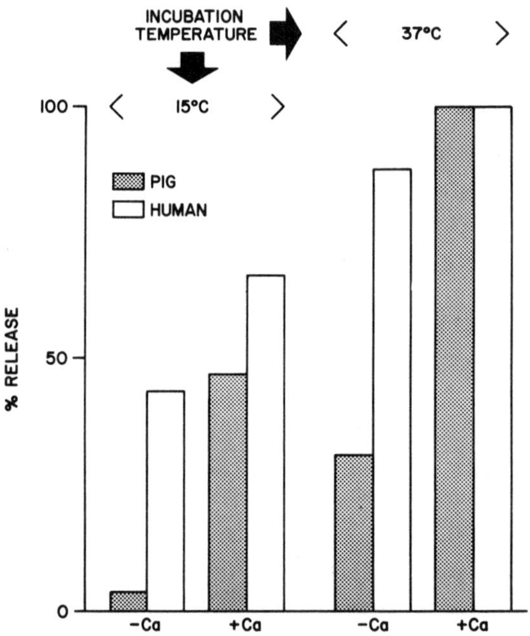

Figure 3. Release of adenine nucleotides from washed human and pig platelets in the presence and absence of Ca^{++} and at 15°C and 37°C. 0.3 m*M* EDTA was present in all samples. $CaCl_2$-addition was 1.25 m*M*. The experimental conditions have been described in Table 1 of Mürer (1972a).

the finding that the thrombin-induced release from human or rat platelets becomes independent of Ca^{++} when the thrombin concentration is increased (Mustard and Packham, 1970; Wolfe and Shulman, 1970; Mürer, 1972a; Sneddon, 1972). It is possible that at lower temperatures, where the enzymatic action of thrombin is slowed, there is an increased need for Ca^{++}. There is a great difference in the need for Ca^{++} as a release promoter according to whether human or other species of platelets were used. Figure 3 compares pig and human platelets with respect to their ability to release adenine nucleotides (Mürer, 1972a).

The release from pig platelets seems to be much slower than that following the action of thrombin on human platelets, indicating that the rapidity of the thrombin-induced release is species-dependent. There is a possibility, however, that the method of blood collection for the pig, done either by cardiac puncture or jugular section, was sufficiently different from the human that the quality and reactivity of the platelets were affected. Such a possi-

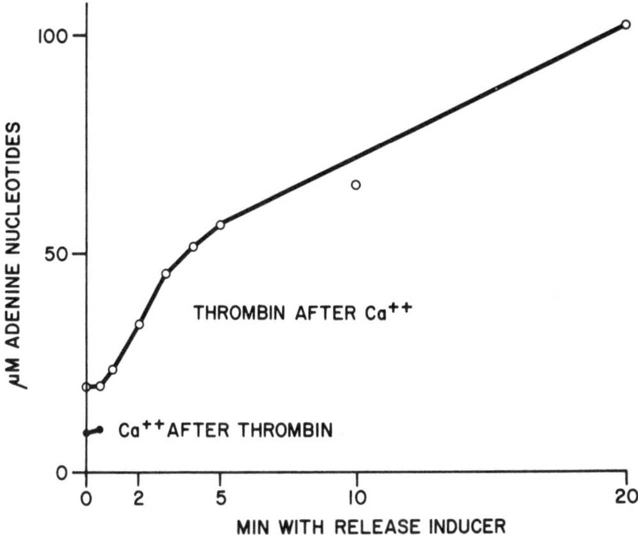

Figure 4. Adenine nucleotides found in supernatant after incubation of a washed pig platelet suspension in buffered saline with 0.6–1.2 NIH units thrombin/ml and 1.25 m*M* $CaCl_2$, in the presence of 0.2 m*M* EDTA. All samples were incubated for 20 min at 37°C, open circles with Ca^{++} present during entire incubation, black circles with thrombin; thrombin or $CaCl_2$, respectively, was added at the indicated time before end of incubation.

bility is supported by the finding that the amount of supernatant nucleotides obtained by incubation of pig platelets with Ca^{++} in the absence of thrombin was greater than that obtained by incubation with thrombin in the absence of Ca^{++} (Fig. 4). This suggests that the cells have already been "initiated" during blood collection, but that release was arrested by the presence of anticoagulants.

It seems reasonable to assume that the difference between species is a relative rather than a fundamental one and that by decreasing the temperature below the 15°C where Grette (1962) found the striking Ca^{++} requirement for pig platelets, a similar requirement could be demonstrated for human platelets. This was accomplished by incubating the platelets with varying concentrations of thrombin at 0°C (Mürer, 1972a), then inactivating the thrombin with hirudin and removing it by subsequent washing.

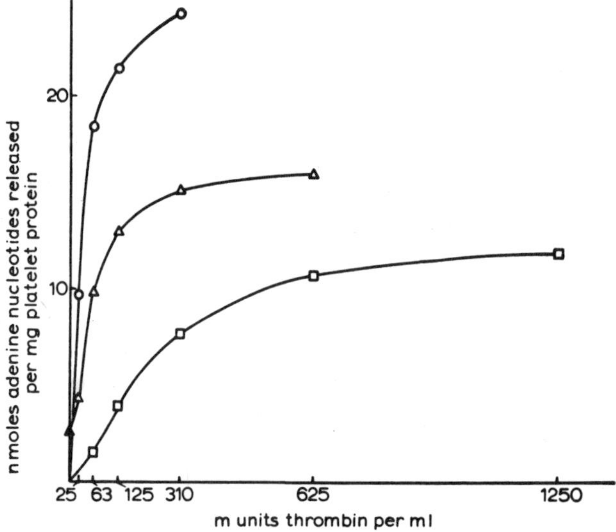

Figure 5. Release of adenine nucleotides after "cold initiation," compared with release from same washed platelet preparation when thrombin was added at 37° C. ○—○, varying amounts of thrombin were added to an EDTA-containing suspension of washed human platelets at 37° C and release measured after 5-min incubation at 37° C. △—△, thrombin was added to the buffered platelet suspension at 0° C, after 15 min hirudin was added and platelets washed, and the washed platelets incubated 5 min at 37° C in buffered saline in the presence of 1.25 m*M* Ca^{++}. □—□, same procedure, but with EDTA instead of Ca^{++} during the 37° C incubation. (Reproduced from: Mürer, 1972a. Biochim. Biophys. Acta 261: 439 (Fig. 2).)

The published findings demonstrated that at 0°C the thrombin had altered the platelet in such a way that a subsequent increase in the temperature to 37°C after thrombin inactivation and removal resulted in release of adenine nucleotides. The treatment with thrombin at 0°C was named "cold initiation," the release at 37°C "extrusion." Ca^{++} added during "cold initiation" depressed rather than activated the releasing process, while calcium added during extrusion had a moderate to great activating effect depending on the amount of thrombin added during "initiation" (Fig. 5). It appears that the lower the thrombin impulse the greater the relative activation (Mürer, 1972a).

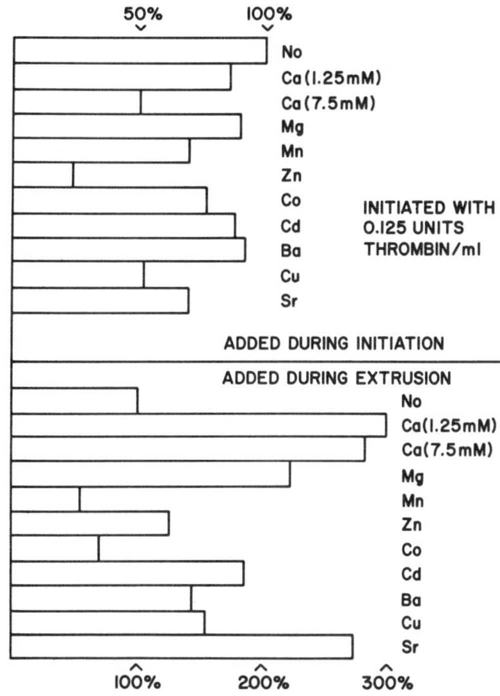

Figure 6. Upper part of figure, cold initiation (see text) in the presence of 5 m*M* concentration of different cations, then extrusion at 37°C in the presence of 1.25 m*M* $CaCl_2$. Lower part of figure, initiation in the presence of 0.2 m*M* EDTA, extrusion in the presence of different cations at 1.25 m*M* concentrations. All results as percentage of base release (no addition) during the stage at which the different cations were added. Experiments performed with washed human platelets.

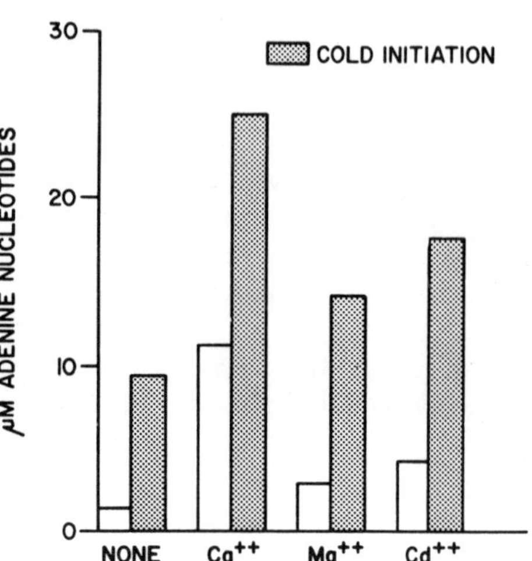

Figure 7. Release from cold-initiated human platelets with cations added during extrusion phase, compared with release from platelets which had not been treated with thrombin in the cold. All cation additions were 1.25 m*M*, thrombin 0.125 unit/ml during cold initiation (experiments performed as described in legend of Fig. 6).

Of a number of other divalent cations tested, only Mg^{++}, Sr^{++}, and to some degree Cd^{++} exerted any appreciable activation of the release induced by a low concentration of thrombin (Fig. 6). Calcium by itself activated release at 37°C. Neither Cd^{++} nor Mg^{++} initiated significant release at 37°C (Fig. 7) but Sr^{++} was frequently a stronger inducer than Ca^{++} causing a release which was almost the same as that caused by a low concentration of thrombin alone (Table 2). The table also demonstrates that the release with Ca^{++} is reduced by 60 per cent by preincubation at 37°C, the release with Sr^{++} by 30 per cent, and that both reactions are inhibited by metabolic inhibitors.

It is possible that the effect of Ca^{++} in inducing a low degree of release in the absence of thrombin is an activation of platelets which have received a very weak releasing impulse. Niewiarowski and Thomas (1966) described an additive effect of ADP and thrombin on platelet aggregation. A similar explanation for the Sr^{++} induction seems less likely, since the activation of cold-initiated platelets is weaker than for Ca^{++} (Table 2) (Mürer, 1972a,c).

PLATELET ADENINE NUCLEOTIDES

Organophosphates (mainly ATP and ADP) can be labeled by preincubation of platelet-rich EDTA-plasma at 37°C for 2 hr with $^{32}PO_4$. The preincubation reduces the releasing capacity of the

Table 2. Release induced by divalent cations

Preincubation	With antimycin and deoxyglucose	Added	Release (%)*
0	0	Thrombin	100
0	0	$CaCl_2$	55.4
0	0	$SrCl_2$	73.3
+	0	$CaCl_2$	22.6
+	+	$CaCl_2$	16.7
+	0	$SrCl_2$	51.3
+	+	$SrCl_2$	15.2

* Mean of two experiments.

The release of adenine nucleotides from washed human platelets effected by 0.125 NIH unit of thrombin, 1.25 m*M* $CaCl_2$, or 1.25 m*M* $SrCl_2$ after 5-min incubation at 37°C and affected by metabolic inhibitors (100 ng of antimycin/ml or 12.5 m*M* 2-deoxy-D-glucose). Preincubation for 10 min at 37°C was included for some of the samples in order to bring about metabolic inhibition. Release is given as a percentage of the release induced by thrombin.

platelets to a certain degree, and changing the anticoagulant from EDTA to citrate does not prevent this reduction in releasing capacity. After the preincubated platelets are washed twice in the cold with buffered EDTA-saline they may be used experimentally for most platelet function testings (Mürer, 1969a, 1969b,c). Holmsen (1971) has discussed the different labeling methods.

Through the use of platelets labeled in this manner, we have shown that the adenine nucleotides released by latex particles or by NaF (Fig. 8) belonged to the nonlabeled storage pool demonstrated by Holmsen (1965, 1967) and Ireland (1966, 1967). By chromatography or electrophoresis (Holmsen and Day, 1971) of a trichloroacetic acid or ethanol extract of the isolated platelets one can also demonstrate that the fast release induced by thrombin or latex particles with human platelets is followed by a sharp drop of the radioactive ATP which is up to 60 per cent with washed platelets. With experiments performed at 37°C most of the decrease takes place within the first 10 sec (Fig. 9).

The initial sharp fall in ATP indicates that the energy for the fast release reaction is provided by the metabolically available ATP

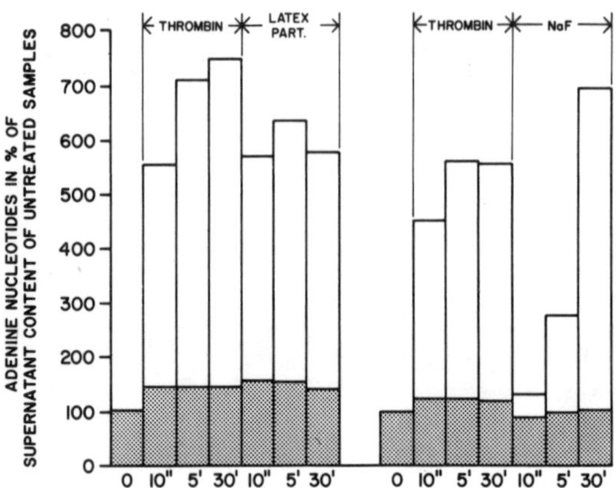

Figure 8. Two different experiments comparing release induced by 0.6 unit of thrombin with that induced by 0.25 per cent polystyrene latex particles (diameter 0.234 μ) or 10 m*M* NaF. The hatched area of the columns shows the amount of ^{32}P-labeled adenine nucleotides found in supernatant after chromatographic separation with isopropyl ether and 90 per cent formic acid (9:6 by volume). The white area of the columns represents the released, nonradioactive nucleotides. Material was washed human platelets.

already present in the platelet. This is in contrast to the energy necessary for clot retraction, which event takes place after the thrombin-induced release. Here the metabolically active ATP is at the lower postrelease level owing to the irreversible conversion to hypoxanthine of the ATP used for the release reaction (Holmsen and Day, 1971). Thus, the energy for clot retraction must be provided by a continuous resynthesis of ATP, probably from the remaining adenine nucleotides. ATP itself seems to be the immediate source of energy for platelet reactions in all cases studied (Mürer, 1969b).

When fluoride is the release inducer, the fall in radioactive ATP is as fast as with thrombin (Fig. 9) but the release reaction does not take place until several minutes later. In this case the fall seems to be of the same type as that caused by deoxyglucose (Fig. 9), which inhibits platelet reactions without having a release inducing effect (Mürer, 1969c). It seems that either the energy for the fluoride-induced release is provided by the continuous production of ATP, or the low level of residual metabolic ATP is sufficient to provide the energy for the release reaction. This might explain the slow course of the reaction. With the metabolic inhibitor deoxy-

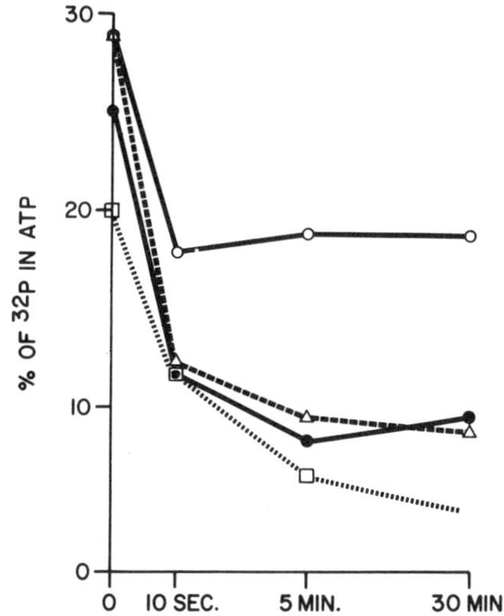

Figure 9. Decrease in the ATP part of total trichloroacetic acid-extractable ^{32}P in platelets after incubation with different agents: ○—○, with polystyrene latex particles; ●—●, with thrombin; △- - -△, with 2-deoxy-D-glucose (6m*M*); and □ · · · · □, with 10 m*M* NaF.

glucose, however, the reduction in metabolic ATP leads not to a release with a slower course, but to a reduction in amount of released material, the time course being as rapid as for the nonimpaired reaction. Conversely, the release induced by fluoride is as complete as that induced by any of the other agents (Figs. 2 and 8) (Mürer, 1968, 1969c).

PLATELET ENERGETICS

Judicious use of metabolic inhibitors which block either glycolysis or mitochondrial respiration has demonstrated that the energy for platelet functions can be provided by either oxidative phosphorylation or anaerobic glycolysis (Mürer, 1968, 1969b). It seems reasonable to believe that, *in vivo*, platelet energy is mainly provided by breakdown of glucose to lactic acid, while the mitochondrial function may be to regulate the energy production, as has been suggested by Salganicoff and Fukami (1972). The energy for the release reaction may be provided by a special ATP pool. Holmsen and Day (1971) have shown that there is a difference between the metabolically active ATP extracted with ethanol and that extracted with trichloroacetic acid, and that ethanol-extractable ATP shows a greater fall when the platelets undergo the release reaction.

Figure 10. Effect of incubation of platelets with large concentrations of aspirin. The amount of calcium and of radioactive ATP in the ^{32}P-labeled platelets was determined before and after incubation with thrombin in the presence of varying amounts of aspirin. The figure demonstrates the following effects when the aspirin concentration is increased: 1, increased retention of calcium after incubation with thrombin; 2, decrease in ^{32}P-ATP before incubation with thrombin; 3, reduction of thrombin-induced decrease in ^{32}P-ATP.

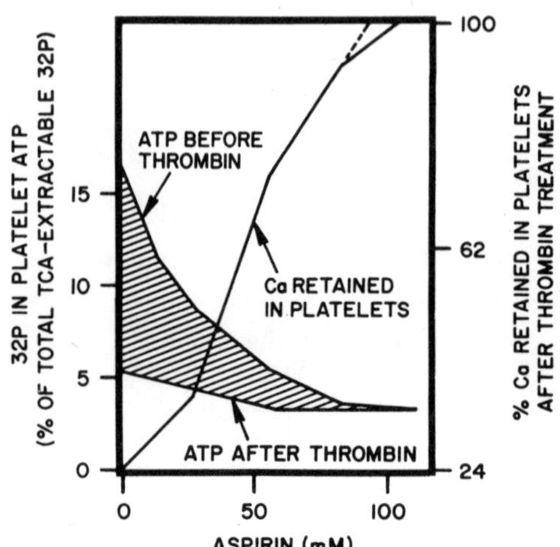

Experiments to test the effect of aspirin on the inhibition of the thrombin-induced release of calcium from washed platelets were not successful in demonstrating an effect at low concentration, but with high concentrations of aspirin which had been shown elsewhere (Miyahara and Karler, 1965) to interfere with mitochondrial functions, there was a simultaneous drop in releasing ability and in the amount of metabolically active ATP which disappeared during release (Fig. 10). However, there was a threshold value below which there was no further drop in labeled ATP, and this was associated with complete inhibition of the release reaction (Mürer and Holme, 1970). It is unknown whether the residual labeled ATP participates in other energy-requiring platelet functions.

CONCLUDING REMARKS

The release reaction can be divided into three steps (Fig. 11): Initiation or Induction, Transmission, and Extrusion (Holmsen *et al.*, 1969). It might be valuable to make a further distinction between initiation and induction, limiting the term initiation to that step following induction in which no further reaction takes place without an additional activating impulse. Of these processes the transmission and the extrusion steps are energy-dependent, while initiation does not seem to require energy. Studies of plate-

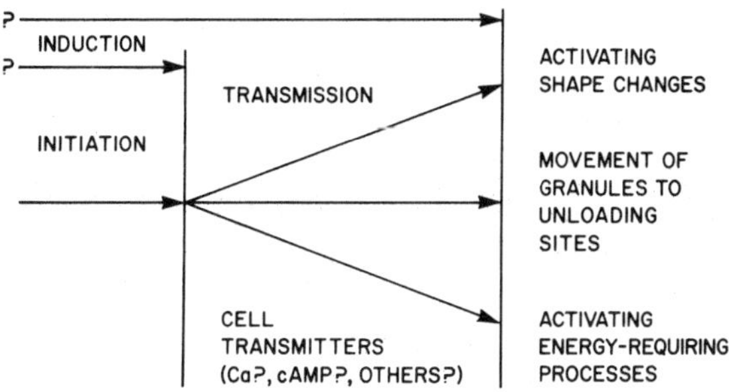

Figure 11. The separation of platelet activity into *initiation*, *transmission*, and platelet *action* is illustrated. Induction may be only the initiation phase, or may include part or all of the transmission phase, with transmission impulses activating different processes resulting in, among others, the extrusion of releasable material.

let energetics by several groups (Gross and Schneider, 1971; Holmsen, 1972), of cyclic AMP (see Mills, 1972), of the possible intracellular transmitter Ca^{++} (Mürer, 1972b,c; Robblee *et al.*, 1972; Detwiler and Feinman, 1972; Kinlough-Rathbone and Chahil, 1972) as well as those with cytocholasins and Vinca alkaloids (see White, 1971) all seem to be promising approaches to the understanding of the transmission and extrusion processes. At present the induction step is not as easily studied, possibly because fewer comparisons can be made with conditions in other cells. A mere cataloguing of promoters and inhibitors of induction has failed to develop a common pattern helpful to understanding the process. Several of the inhibitors of the release reaction seem to work on stages following initiation (*e.g.* prostaglandins, adrenergic blockers, metabolic inhibitors (Mürer, 1971, 1972a; Mills, 1972)). Aspirin may act on the initial step, but so far we have no clue as to the exact mechanism (Mills, 1972). The demonstration that thrombin initiates platelet action at 0°C (Mürer, 1972a) may be a promising lead as may the interaction between collagen and platelet membrane preparations described by Jamieson and collaborators (Barber and Jamieson, 1971, 1971a).

Recently Baenziger *et al.* have demonstrated a change in a protein during the specific action of thrombin on the intact platelet (Baenziger *et al.*, 1971, 1972), although this change has not been proved to take place during initiation. On the contrary, I. Hagen (personal communication) does not find that thrombin treatment of intact platelets induces changes in the protein content of subsequently isolated and purified platelet membranes.

Studies on the action of metal ions may demonstrate whether this action is on the initiation or the transmission phase of the release reaction. It is possible that the action of Sr^{++} bypasses the initiation; this would suggest that induction is a combined process of initiation and transmission (Fig. 11), but further elaboration of this point is not justified at present.

There has been some question as to the possible physiological significance of the release of Ca^{++} into a calcium-rich medium such as blood plasma (Mürer and Holme, 1970). If Ca^{++} is needed for the release reaction, its locus of action may be inside the canniculi leading from the interior of the platelets to the surface. If these canniculi are the channels for transportation of released material to the platelet surface, the release would cause a great increase in Ca^{++} concentration within the canniculi, which might activate further release and cause the release reaction to go to completion. This might also explain what seems most probable, that the release reaction is an all-or-none phenomenon, resulting in each platelet being either totally emptied or unaffected.

One might speculate that a weak "initiation" of platelet function could make the platelet more reactive to other weak impulses so that "initiated" platelets would increase the danger of thrombosis. It would be of importance to clarify whether platelets can build up their reactivity successively until they overcome the action barrier. Such an action barrier might be the inhibition of platelet action by prostaglandin (Mürer, 1971) or the lack of free Ca^{++} (Mürer, 1972a), or it could be the as yet undefined minimum strength of impulse (amplified or not) needed for onset of platelet action (Detwiler and Feinman, 1973).

REFERENCES

Baenziger, N. L., Brodie, G. N., and Majerus, P. W. 1971. A thrombin-sensitive protein of human platelet membranes. Proc. Nat. Acad. Sci. U.S.A. 68: 240.

Baenziger, N. L., Brodie, G. N., and Majerus, P. W. 1972. Isolation and properties of a thrombin-sensitive protein of human platelets. J. Biol. Chem. 247: 2723.

Barber, A. J., and Jamieson, G. A. 1971. Platelet collagen adhesion characterization of collagen glucosyltransferase of plasma membranes of human blood platelets. Biochim. Biophys. Acta 252: 533.

Barber, A. J., and Jamieson, G. A. 1971a. Characterization of membrane-bound collagen galactosyl transferase of human blood platelets. Biochim. Biophys. Acta 252: 546.

Bigelow, F. S. 1954. Serotonin activity in blood. J. Lab. Clin. Med. 43: 759.

Born, G. V. R. 1958. Changes in the distribution of phosphorus in platelet-rich plasma during clotting. Biochem. J. 68: 695.

Buckingham, S., and Maynert, E. W. 1964. The release of 5-hydroxytryptamine, potassium and amino acids from platelets. J. Pharmacol. Exp. Ther. 143: 332.

DaPrada, M., and Pletscher, A. 1970. Synthesis and storage of nucleotides in blood platelets. Life Sci. 9: 1271.

Day, H. J., and Holmsen, H. 1971. Concepts of the blood platelet release reaction. Ser. Haematol. 4: 3.

Day, H. J., Holmsen, H., Østvold, A., and Sjaastad, Å. 1972. Behaviour of endogenous and absorbed serotonin in the platelet release reaction, p. 184. Abstract, Third Congress of International Society on Thrombosis and Haemostasis, Washington D.C.

Day, H. J., Scrutton, M. C., and Holmsen, H. 1973. Metal ions in human platelets: Evidence for populations having differing contents of calcium and magnesium. Fed. Proc., Abstract 3523.

Detwiler, T. C., and Feinman, R. D. 1972. Thrombin-induced release of calcium from platelets, p. 186. Abstract, Third Congress of International Society on Thrombosis and Haemostasis, Washington, D.C.

Detwiler, T. C., and Feinman, R. D. 1973. Kinetics of the thrombin-induced release of Ca^{++} by platelets. Biochemistry 12: 282.

Foley, B., Johnson, S. A., Hackley, B., Smith, J. C., Jr., and Halsted, J. A. 1968. Zinc content of human platelets. Proc. Soc. Exp. Biol. Med. 128: 265.

Glynn, M. F., Movat, H. Z., Murphy, E. A., and Mustard, J. F. 1965. Study of platelet adhesiveness and aggregation, with latex particles. J. Lab. Clin. Med. 65: 179.

Grette, K. 1959. The release of 5-hydroxytryptamine (serotonin) from blood platelets during coagulation. Scand. J. Clin. Lab. Invest. 11: 50.

Grette, K. 1962. Studies on the mechanism of thrombin-catalyzed hemostatic reactions in blood platelets. Acta Physiol. Scand. 56 (suppl. 195). See Holmsen, Day and Stormorken, 1969.

Grette, K. 1963. Relaxing factor in extracts of blood platelets and its function in the cells. Nature 198: 488.

Gross, R., and Schneider, W. 1971. Energy metabolism, pp. 122–188. *In* S. Johnson (ed.) The circulating platelet. Academic Press, New York.

Holmsen, H. 1965. Collagen-induced release of adenosine diphosphate from blood platelets incubated with radioactive phosphate *in vitro*. Scand. J. Clin. Lab. Invest. 17: 239.

Holmsen, H. 1967. Adenine nucleotide metabolism in platelets and plasma, pp. 81–90. *In* E. Kowalski and S. Niewiarowski (eds.) Blood platelet biochemistry. Academic Press, New York.

Holmsen, H. 1971. Platelet adenine nucleotide metabolism and platelet malfunction, pp. 109–124. *In* J. Caen (ed.) Platelet aggregation. Masson, Paris.

Holmsen, H. 1972. The platelet: Its membrane, physiology and biochemistry. Clin. Haematol. 1: 235.

Holmsen, H., and Day, H. J. 1968. Thrombin-induced platelet release reaction and platelet lysosomes. Nature 219: 760.

Holmsen, H., and Day, H. J. 1970. The selectivity of the thrombin-induced platelet release reaction: Subcellular localization of released and retained constituents. J. Lab. Clin. Med. 75: 840.

Holmsen, H., and Day, H. J. 1971. Adenine nucleotides and platelet function. Ser. Haematol. 4: 28.

Holmsen, H., Day, H. J., and Setkowsky, C. A. 1972. Secretory mechanisms. Behaviour of adenine nucleotides during the platelet release reaction induced by adenosine diphosphate and adrenaline. Biochem. J. 129: 67.

Holmsen, H., Day, H. J., and Stormorken, H. 1969. The blood platelet release reaction. Scand. J. Haematol. (suppl. 8).

Holmsen, H., and Weiss, H. J. 1970. Hereditary defect in the platelet release reaction caused by a deficiency in the storage pool of platelet adenine nucleotides. Brit. J. Haematol. 19: 643.

Holmsen, H., and Weiss, H. J. 1972. Further evidence for a deficient storage pool of adenine nucleotides in platelets from some patients with thrombocytopathia–"storage pool disease." Blood 39: 197.

Hovig, T. 1963. Release of platelet-aggregation substance (adenosine diphosphate) from rabbit blood platelets induced by saline "extract" of tendons. Thromb. Diath. Haemorrh. 9: 264.

Humphrey, J. H., and Jacques, R. 1955. The release of histamine and 5-hydroxytryptamine (serotonin) from platelets by antigen-antibody reactions (*in vitro*). J. Physiol. 128: 9.

Ireland, D. M. 1966. The liberation of adenosine diphosphate from blood platelets by thrombin. Biochem. J. 100: 72P.

Ireland, D. M. 1967. Effect of thrombin on the radioactive nucleotides of human washed platelets. Biochem. J. 105: 857.

Jamieson, G. A. 1973. Biochemical events in platelet-collagen adhesion. These proceedings.

Kinlough-Rathbone, R. L., and Chahil, A. 1972. The role of calcium and magnesium in the platelet release reaction, p. 212. Third Congress of International Society on Thrombosis and Haemostasis, Washington, D.C.

Mills, D. C. B. 1972. Drugs that affect platelet behavior. Clin. Haematol. 1: 295.

Miyahara, J. T., and Karler, R. 1965. Effect of salicylate on oxidative phosphorylation by liver mitochondria. Biochem. J. 97: 194.

Mueller-Eckhardt, C., and Lüscher, E. F. 1968. Immune reactions of human blood platelets. II. The effect of latex particles coated with gammaglobulin in relation to complement activation. Thromb. Diath. Haemorrh. 20: 168.

Mürer, E. H. 1968. Release reaction and energy metabolism in blood platelets with special reference to the burst in oxygen uptake. Biochim. Biophys. Acta 162: 320.

Mürer, E. H. 1969a. Thrombin-induced release of calcium from blood platelets. Science 166: 623.

Mürer, E. H. 1969b. Clot retraction and energy metabolism of platelets. Effect and mechanism of inhibitors. Biochim. Biophys. Acta 172: 266.

Mürer, E. H. 1969c. A comparative study of the action of release inducers upon platelet release and phosphorus metabolism. Biochim. Biophys. Acta 192: 138.

Mürer, E. H. 1971. Compounds known to affect the cyclic adenosine monophosphate level in blood platelets: Effect on thrombin-induced clot retraction and platelet release. Biochim. Biophys. Acta 237: 310.

Mürer, E. H. 1972a. Factors influencing the initiation and the extrusion phase of the platelet release reaction. Biochim. Biophys. Acta 261: 435.

Mürer, E. H. 1972b. Biochemical aspects of clot retraction and the platelet release reaction. Doctoral thesis. Universitetsforlaget, Oslo.

Mürer, E. H. 1972c. Divalent cations as release inducers, p. 226. Abstract, Third Congress of International Society on Thrombosis and Haemostasis, Washington, D.C.

Mürer, E. H., and Holme, R. 1970. A study of the release of calcium from human blood platelets and its inhibition by metabolic inhibitors, N-ethylmaleimide and aspirin. Biochim. Biophys. Acta 222: 197.

Mustard, J. F., and Packham, M. A. 1970. Factors influencing platelet function: adhesion, release, and aggregation. Pharmacol. Rev. 22: 97.

Nachman, R. L., Weksler, B., and Ferris, B. 1970. Increased vascular permeability produced by human platelet granule cationic extracts. J. Clin. Invest. 49: 274.

Niewiarowski, S. 1973. Interaction of fibrin with various cells. International Symposium Intravascular Coagulation and Fibrinolysis. Sherbrooke, Canada; Fibrin retraction induced by platelets and fibroblasts. These proceedings.

Niewiarowski, S., and Thomas, D. P. 1966. Platelet aggregation by ADP and thrombin. Nature 212: 1544.

Niewiarowski, S., and Thomas, D. P. 1969. Platelet factor 4 and adenosine diphosphate release during human platelet aggregation. Nature 222: 1269.

Robblee, L., Towle, C., Belamarich, F. A., and Shepro, D. 1972. Calcium flux and platelet membranes, p. 240. Abstract, Third Congress of International Society on Thrombosis and Haemostasis, Washington, D.C.

Robert, B., Szigeti, M., Robert, L., Legrand, G., Pignaud, G., and Caen, J. 1970. Release of elastolytic activity from blood platelets. Nature 227: 1248.

Salganicoff, L., and Fukami, M. H. 1972. Energy metabolism of blood platelets. I. Isolation and properties of pig platelet mitochondria. Arch. Biochem. 153: 726.

Sneddon, J. M. 1972. Divalent cations and the blood platelet release reaction. Nature New Biol. 236: 103.

Solum, N. O., and Stormorken, H. 1965. Influence of fibrinogen on the aggregation of washed human blood platelets induced by adenosine diphosphate, thrombin, collagen and adrenaline. Scand. J. Clin. Lab. Invest. 17 (suppl. 84).

Stormorken, H. 1969. The release reaction of secretion. Scand. J. Haematol. (suppl. 9).

White, J. G. 1971. Platelet morphology, pp. 46–121. *In* S. Johnson (ed.) The circulating platelet. Academic Press, New York.

Wolfe, S., and Shulman, N. R. 1970. Inhibition of platelet energy production and release reaction by PGE_1, theophylline and cAMP. Biochem. Biophys. Res. Commun. 41: 128.

Zieve, P. D., Gamble, J. L., Jr., and Jackson, D. P. 1964. Effect of thrombin on the potassium and ATP content of platelets. J. Clin. Invest. 43: 2063.

Zucker, M. B. 1972. Proteolytic inhibitors, contact and other variables in the release reaction of human platelets. Thromb. Diath. Haemorrh. 28: 383.

Zucker, M. B., and Borelli, J. 1955. Relationship of some clotting factors to serotonin release from washed platelets. J. Appl. Physiol. 7: 432.

Platelets, Blood Coagulation, and Hemostasis

Peter N. Walsh

The purpose of the experiments reported here was to study the role of platelets in blood coagulation and hemostasis. Freshly collected intact platelets were shown to initiate intrinsic coagulation by two distinct alternative mechanisms. The first mechanism concerns contact product-forming activity, a metabolic or physicochemical property of the platelet surface which may be altered by exposure to adenosine diphosphate to activate factor XII and subsequently form contact activation product on the platelet surface when factor XI is present. By an alternative mechanism, collagen-stimulated platelets were shown to initiate intrinsic coagulation in the absence of factor XII provided factor XI was present. Subsequently, platelets provide intrinsic factor Xa-forming activity, *i.e.* the capacity of platelets to enhance the reactions of factors XIa, VIII, IX, and X to form factor Xa activity on the platelet surface in the presence of natural inhibitors to active clotting factors. Finally, platelets provide platelet factor 3 activity, the well known capacity of platelets to catalyze the reaction of factors Xa and V to activate prothrombin in the presence of calcium.

Some possible interrelationships between platelet plug formation and blood coagulation, based on evidence presented here and by other investigators, are presented as an hypothesis which may account for the events of hemostasis. The events leading to platelet plug and fibrin formation are seen as proceeding concurrently, initiated in common by the events of vascular injury and closely linked by autocatalytic or "positive feedback" interrelationships.

"Hemostasis may be defined as the spontaneous arrest of bleeding from ruptured blood vessels" (Macfarlane, 1972). It has been inferred through experimentation and observation of patients with hemostatic disorders that hemostasis comprises a complex chain of events including vascular reactions to injury, platelet adhesion to extravascular surfaces, platelet aggregation, platelet plug formation, and subsequent blood coagulation and "consolidation" of the hemostatic plug. When any of the links in the chain is weak, bleeding may not be arrested spontaneously. What is perhaps more astonishing than arrest of bleeding is the fact that control mechanisms, including fibrinolysis and the natural inhibitors to active clotting factors, are apparently so efficient that the vascular tree does not normally contain fibrin deposits or adhesive platelet clumps.

Paradoxically, although much is known about the individual components of the hemostatic mechanism, little is known about how it is started in life or about the relationship between formation of platelet plugs and fibrin clots, both of which are needed for normal hemostasis. Primary hemostasis may be defined as the composite of events including platelet adhesion and aggregation leading to platelet plug formation. Blood coagulation is the complex interaction of clotting factors which results in fibrin formation. Primary hemostasis and blood coagulation have been studied as if they were totally separate phenomena, but the fact remains that they invariably occur together during normal hemostasis. Any consideration of the tenuous links which may join these two phenomena is conjectural and gives rise to many examples of circular reasoning, which comprise some of the major enigmas of hemostasis. The purpose of this communication is to identify some of these enigmas and to present observations which may explain how hemostasis is initiated, how platelet plug formation and blood coagulation are linked, and how control mechanisms can maintain blood in a fluid state.

MATERIALS AND METHODS

Methods employed for collecting blood, preparing high spun platelet-poor plasma (HSPPP) and albumin density gradient separation (ADGS) and washing of platelets were previously described (Walsh, 1972a,b). Platelet counts and assessment of platelet morphology were done by phase contrast microscopy (Brecher and Cronkite, 1950). The basis for and validation of test systems used to assess platelet coagulant activities, including reagents and glassware used, have been presented elsewhere (Walsh, 1972a,b,c,d; Walsh and Biggs, 1972).

RESULTS

Interrelationships between Primary Hemostasis and Blood Coagulation: Possibilities and Objections

Some of the possible interrelationships between primary hemostasis and blood coagulation, emphasizing the activation of both mechanisms *in vivo*, are presented in simplified form in Fig. 1. The fundamental question is whether platelet plug formation and fibrin formation are initiated by a common cause or by separate and independent causes or whether one triggers the other. Any serious consideration of the logical alternatives gives rise to more objections than answers. Some of the arguments are briefly summarized below and in Fig. 1.

Following vascular injury and exposure of the subendothelial component of the vessel wall to which platelets adhere, the coagulation mechanism is activated, possibly by something released or exposed by the injury. One possibility is that collagen or some other contact-activating surface is exposed and activates clotting through factors XII and XI. The most serious objection to this answer is that it requires a necessary and crucial function of the one clotting factor whose apparent absence is not associated with a hemostatic defect (*i.e.* factor XII). This mechanism may operate in life to activate clotting in normal people, but another mechanism must suffice for those who lack factor XII.

Another possible trigger mechanism for platelet plug and fibrin formation is the release of substances from injured tissue which promote platelet adhesion and aggregation on the one hand and

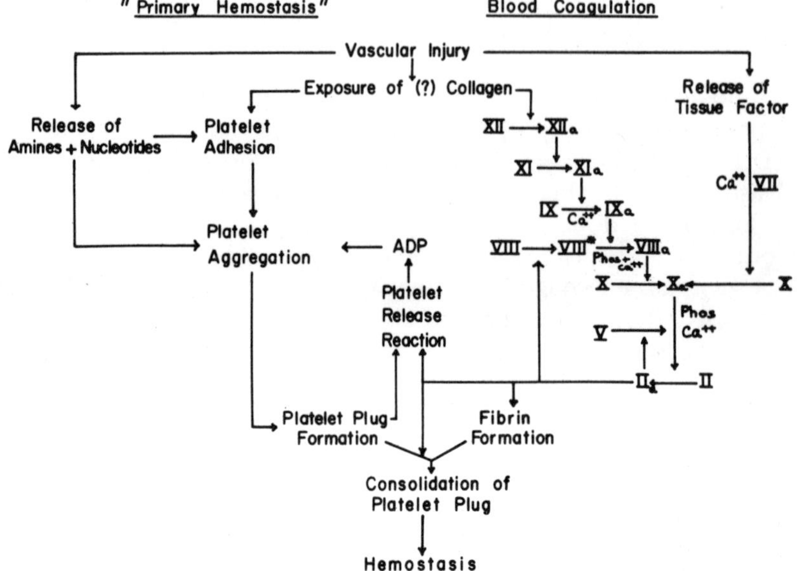

Figure 1. Some possible interrelationships between primary hemostasis and blood coagulation, based on existing evidence.

blood coagulation on the other. Released tissue factor might initiate extrinsic clotting by reacting with factor VII and activating factor X, thus by-passing intrinsic coagulation. However, if this were the major clot-promoting mechanism, one would expect a mild hemostatic defect in patients with hemophilia and Christmas disease, and a severe hemostatic defect in patients with factor VII deficiency. Generally, the converse is true.

A third possibility is that blood coagulation is promoted by the events of primary hemostasis. It seems very likely that platelet membrane, or granular lipoprotein, or both, are somehow made available during platelet plug formation. Available evidence suggests that this lipoprotein functions to accelerate coagulation reactions known to occur after the initiation of clotting. The agent which many investigators believe is responsible for making PF3 available (*i.e.* thrombin) is formed only after reactions accelerated by PF3 have occurred. This proposed action of thrombin may be the basis for an autocatalytic mechanism involving platelets and clotting similar to that proposed for the activation by thrombin of factors VIII and V (Rapaport *et al.*, 1963; Biggs *et al.*, 1965).

However, the available evidence, which suggests that the events of primary hemostasis accelerate intrinsic coagulation, provides no explanation for how clotting is initiated.

A final possibility to be considered concerns the effects of coagulation upon platelet plug formation. So far as is known these effects seem to be mediated by thrombin, which causes release of platelet constituents including ADP, which in turn causes platelet aggregation. Thrombin is also considered to produce the morphological alterations in the platelet plug referred to as "viscous metamorphosis." Thereby it promotes consolidation of the platelet plug by a direct effect on platelets in addition to reinforcing the platelet plug by promoting fibrin formation within it. In view of the observations of Marr *et al.* (1965) that fibrin formation, which implies prior thrombin formation, occurs within 15 to 30 sec of injury to vessels in guinea pig mesentery, it might be considered possible that the events of blood coagulation are primary and those of platelet aggregation and plug formation secondary to the generation of small amounts of thrombin. The obvious objections to this explanation are, first, that it fails to account for the initial activation of the clotting mechanism, and, second, that it ignores the fact that platelet plug formation can occur normally when the coagulation mechanism is blocked and fibrin formation prevented.

Platelets and the Initiation of Intrinsic Coagulation

A series of experimental observations has suggested the possibility that platelets possess coagulant activities separate and distinct from platelet factor 3 (PF3) activity (Walsh, 1972b). The data which define the mode of action of one of these coagulant activities can be summarized briefly as follows.

1. A progressive reaction can be shown to occur in the absence of calcium between normal or factor XII-deficient platelets and normal plasma which does not occur if factor XII is absent (Fig. 2).
2. This progressive reaction is enhanced by adenosine diphosphate (ADP), which has no effect on clotting times of platelet-plasma mixtures when factor XII is absent.
3. In the absence of platelets, even with ample phospholipid and factor XII present, ADP has no effect on clotting times.
4. When platelets to which factor XII is adsorbed are incubated with ADP, a progressive reaction occurs, but no such response to

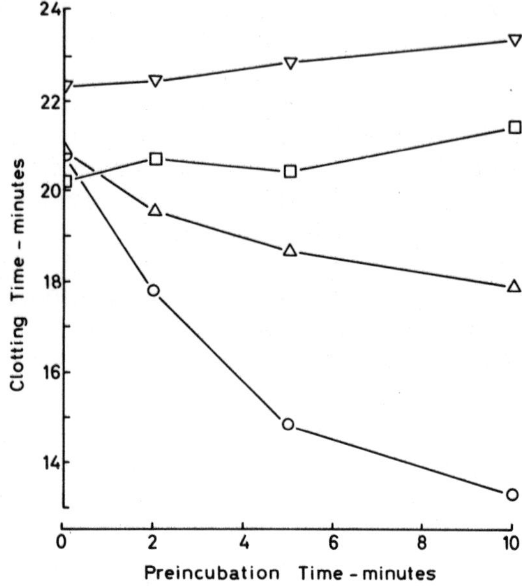

Figure 2. Effect of preincubating washed normal or factor XII-deficient platelets with normal or factor XII-deficient HSPPP upon plasma recalcification times in a noncontact system. Nine-tenths milliliter of factor XII-deficient or normal HSPPP was placed in a plastic tube at 37°C. One-tenth milliliter of normal or factor XII-deficient platelets washed twice by ADGS and resuspended in calcium-free Tyrode's solution was added. After preincubation times indicated, 0.1 ml of the mixture was subsampled into 0.1 ml of normal or factor XII-deficient HSPPP in a plastic tube at 37°C, 0.05 ml of 0.1 *M* $CaCl_2$ was added, and the clotting times recorded.

	Preincubation mixture		HSPPP in indicator system
	HSPPP	Platelet suspension	
○	Normal	Normal	Factor XII-def.
△	Normal	Factor XII-def.	Factor XII-def.
□	Factor XII-def.	Normal	Normal
▽	Factor XII-def.	Factor XII-def.	Normal

ADP occurs if factor XII is either removed from the platelets by washing or if factor XII is congenitally absent (Fig. 3).

From these observations and many others (Walsh, 1972c) it has been concluded that intact platelets can enhance the reactions of factors XII and XI to form contact activation product in the absence of calcium. This platelet coagulant activity, termed con-

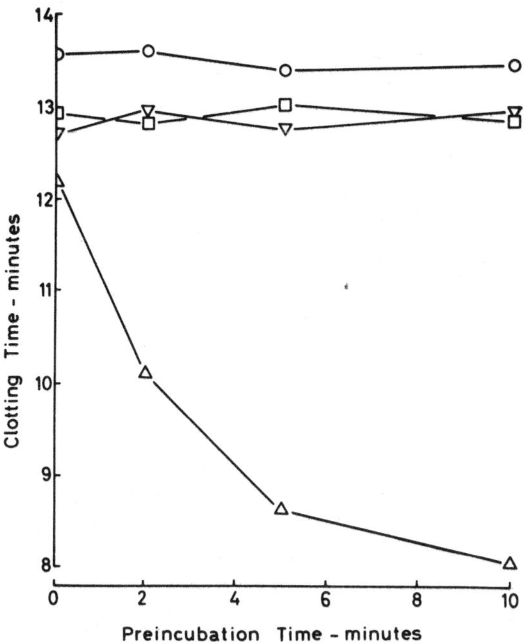

Figure 3. Effect of ADP upon separated normal and factor XII-deficient platelets tested in normal HSPPP. Normal and factor XII-deficient platelets were separated once from plasma by ADGS and suspended in calcium-free Tyrode's solution. Two milliliters of a platelet suspension were prewarmed for 2 min in a plastic tube at 37°C and 0.2 ml of 0.85 per cent NaCl or ADP, 100 μM, was added. At intervals 0.1 ml of the mixture was subsampled into 0.2 ml of normal HSPPP in a plastic tube at 37°C, 0.05 ml of 0.1 M $CaCl_2$ added, and the clotting time recorded.

	Test platelets	Addition
○	Normal	NaCl
△	Normal	ADP
□	Factor XII-deficient	NaCl
▽	Factor XII-deficient	ADP

tact product-forming activity, is specifically and rapidly stimulated by "physiological" concentrations of ADP in platelet suspensions not stirred and not undergoing platelet aggregation. The stimulation of contact product-forming activity by ADP is reversible, directly related to the concentration of ADP employed and not

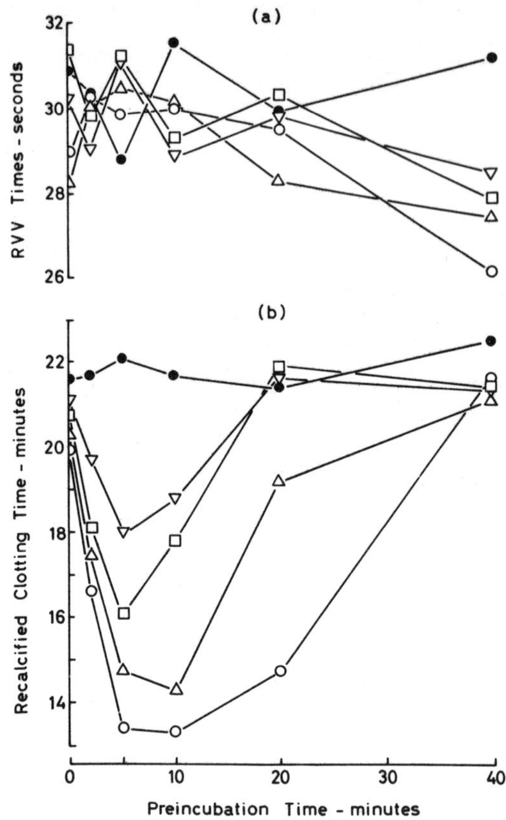

Figure 4. Effect of ADP upon CPFA and PF3. Normal platelets were separated from plasma by ADGS and resuspended in calcium-free Tyrode's solution. One-milliliter aliquots were pipetted into plastic tubes and stored at room temperature until tested, at which time they were prewarmed at 37°C for exactly 2 min before testing. At this time, 0.1 ml of 0.85 per cent NaCl or ADP, 10, 40, 100, or 400 μM, was added and the mixture was tested immediately or after 2, 5, 10, 20, or 40 min of incubation. (a) Russell's viper venom (RVV) times: an aliquot 0.1 ml of the preincubation mixture was subsampled into 0.1 ml of normal HSPPP, 0.1 ml of a 1:100,000 dilution of RVV and 0.1 ml of 0.025 M $CaCl_2$ added and the clotting time recorded. (b) Recalcification times: an aliquot, 0.1 ml, of the preincubation mixture was subsampled into 0.4 ml of normal HSPPP in a plastic tube at 37°C, 0.05 ml of 0.2 M $CaCl_2$ added, and the clotting time recorded.

	Addition	Final concentration
○	ADP	40 μM
△	ADP	10 μM
□	ADP	4 μM
▽	ADP	1 μM
●	NaCl	0.85%

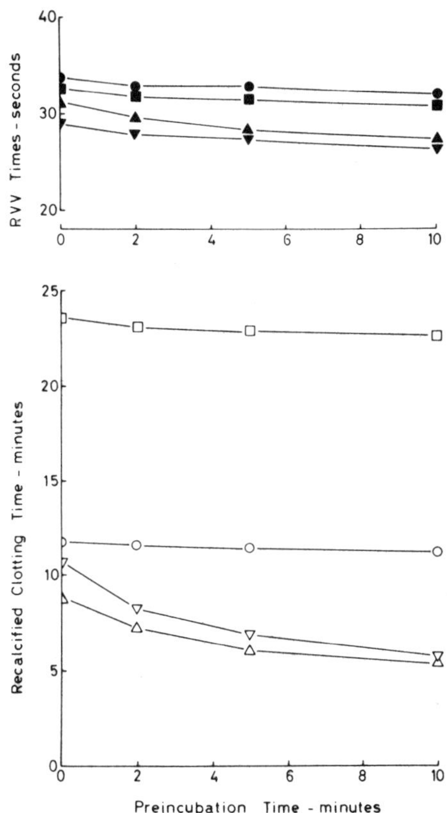

Figure 5. Effect of collagen upon normal and factor XII-deficient platelets in two test systems. One milliliter of normal or factor XII-deficient platelets, separated once by ADGS and suspended in calcium-free Tyrode's solution, was placed in a plastic tube at 37°C and 0.1 ml of 0.85 per cent NaCl or a saline suspension of human collagen was added. After initial mixing the samples were left undisturbed and were not stirred. The mixture was subsampled at intervals and tested as follows. *Recalcification times:* an aliquot, 0.1 ml, of the preincubation mixture was subsampled into 0.2 ml of factor XII-deficient HSPPP in a plastic tube, 0.05 ml of 0.1 *M* $CaCl_2$ added, and the clotting time recorded. *RVV times:* an aliquot, 0.1 ml, of the preincubation mixture was subsampled into 0.1 ml of factor XII-deficient HSPPP in a glass tube, 0.1 ml of RVV at a 1:100,000 dilution and 0.1 ml of 0.025 *M* $CaCl_2$ added, and the clotting time recorded.

Recalcification time	RVV time	Test platelets	Preincubation addition
○	●	Normal	NaCl
△	▲	Normal	Collagen
□	■	Factor XII-def.	NaCl
▽	▼	Factor XII-def.	Collagen

accompanied by any significant increase in the availability of platelet factor 3 (Fig. 4).

The observations concerning contact product-forming activity suggest a possible mechanism by which blood coagulation might be triggered *in vivo* by platelets in normal individuals, but they do little more than add to the enigma of the absence of a hemostatic defect in individuals with the Hageman trait. In contrast, the reactions of platelets with collagen have been studied (Walsh, 1972d), and the results may provide an explanation for normal hemostasis in patients lacking factor XII. These results may be summarized briefly as follows.

1. When platelets from a normal or factor XII-deficient donor are washed four times by albumin density gradient separation and incubated with collagen for 10 min without stirring, very little platelet factor 3 activity develops, as assessed by Russell's viper venom (RVV) time determinations (Fig. 5, top).
2. When these same normal or factor XII-deficient washed platelets are tested in plastic tubes in factor XII-deficient substrate plasma the large difference in clotting times after incubation with saline is abolished when collagen-incubated platelets are tested (Fig. 5, bottom).
3. When factor VIII-, IX-, XI-, and XII-deficient and normal platelets are washed four times by albumin density gradient separation and subsampled after preincubation with collagen or saline into the same plasma from which they were originally separated, the only platelet-plasma mixture completely normalized by preincubation of platelets with collagen is the factor XII-deficient system, and not the factor VIII-, IX-, or XI-deficient platelet-plasma mixtures (Fig. 6).
4. When normal platelets are washed four times by albumin density gradient separation they retain factor XI activity, but factor XII activity is removed, whereas washed platelets from a factor XI-deficient donor lack both factor XI and XII activity (Walsh, 1972a). When normal or factor XI-deficient washed platelets are incubated with saline or collagen and tested for their capacity to catalyze the reactions of factors VIII, IX, and X in the generation of factor Xa, it can be seen that collagen has a pronounced effect on factor XI-containing platelets, but no effect on factor XI-deficient platelets (Fig. 7).

These results are consistent with the hypothesis that an alternative pathway, independent of factor XII and dependent on factor

Preincubated Platelets	Substrate Plasma	Clotting Time (min) after Preincubation with:	
		NaCl	Collagen
F-VIII def.	F-VIII def.	87	59
F-IX def.	F-IX def.	93	62
F-XI def.	F-XI def.	81	56
F-XII def.	F-XII def.	49	8.8
Normal	Normal	10.4	8.2

Figure 6. Effect of collagen on platelets in the absence of factors VIII, IX, XI, and XII. Platelets from a normal donor and from subjects deficient in factors VIII, IX, XI, and XII were washed four times by ADGS and resuspended in calcium-free Tyrode's solution at platelet concentrations of 450,000–500,000/μl. To 1.0 ml of the platelet suspension in a plastic tube was added 0.1 ml of 0.85 per cent NaCl or saline suspension of human collagen. After a 10-min incubation, a 0.1-ml aliquot was subsampled into 0.2 ml of the plasma from which the platelets were originally separated in a plastic tube, 0.05 ml of 0.1 *M* $CaCl_2$ added, and the clotting time recorded in quadruplicate.

XI, may be operative in the initiation of intrinsic coagulation, provided platelets and collagen are present. To assess the time course of development of the collagen-induced coagulant activity, washed normal platelets were preincubated with collagen or saline for varying times and tested for their capacity to promote intrinsic factor Xa formation. The results (Fig. 8) showed a rapid development of collagen-induced coagulant activity followed by a rapid decay of activity and a slower return to control levels after 60 min of preincubation. This reversibility contrasts with the slower and irreversible development of platelet factor 3 activity of platelet suspensions incubated with collagen. The reaction by which the collagen-induced coagulant activity develops is independent of platelet aggregation and platelet factor 3 release.

Platelets and Intrinsic Factor Xa Formation

It was originally shown by Lundblad and Davie (1964) that phospholipids catalyze the reactions of factors VIII, IX, and X, an activity which can also be demonstrated for platelets washed by

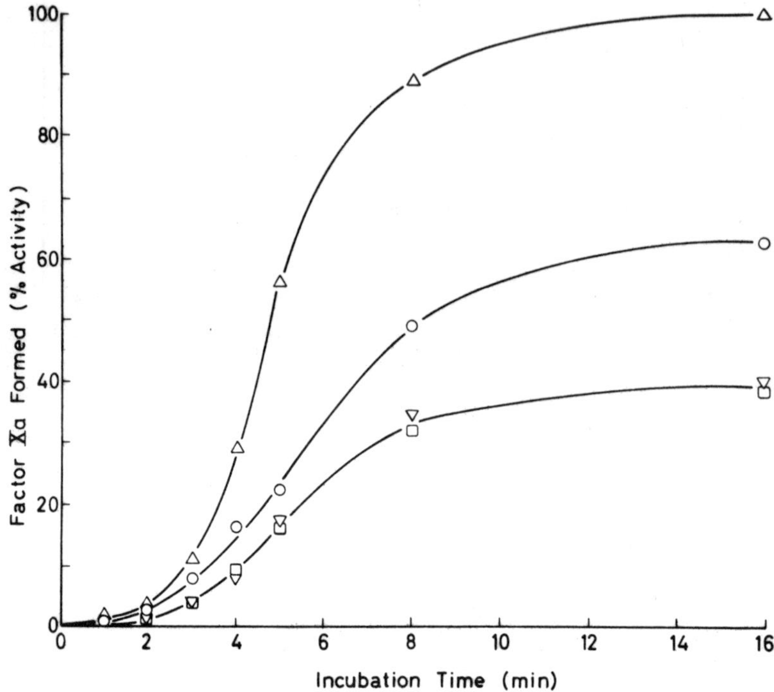

Figure 7. Effect of collagen on normal and factor XI-deficient platelets in factor Xa formation. Platelets from a normal or a factor XI-deficient donor, washed four times by albumin density gradient separation were preincubated with collagen or saline and the following additions made: citrate-saline, factor VIII, thrombin, serum eluate, and calcium chloride. The development of factor Xa activity was followed. The points represent the means of four similar experiments. Additions were:

	Test platelets	Preincubation addition
○	Normal	Saline
△	Normal	Collagen
□	Factor XI-def.	Saline
▽	Factor XI-def.	Collagen

albumin density gradient separation (Walsh and Biggs, 1972). In addition to catalyzing intrinsic coagulation reactions, platelets would also appear to provide a protective nidus for factor Xa formation in the presence of the natural inhibitors to active clotting factors (Fig. 9). Washed normal platelets or phospholipid

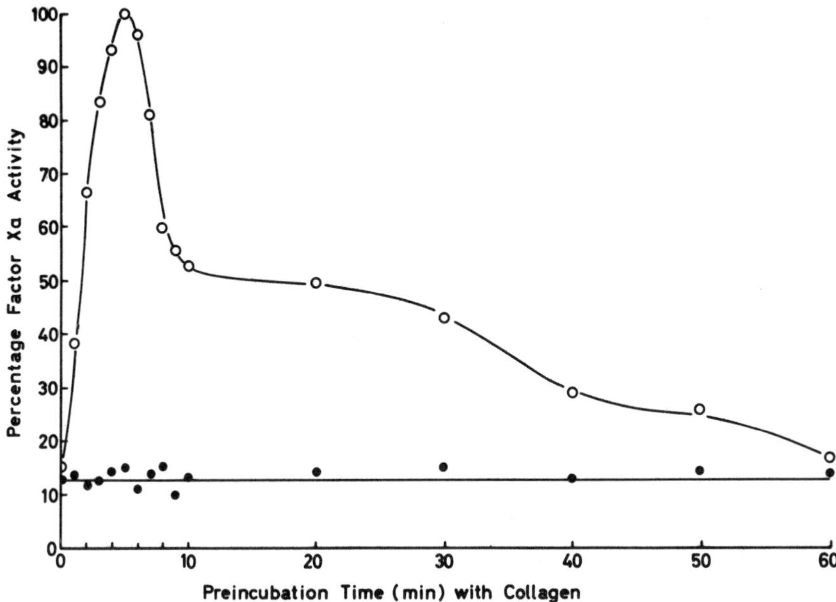

Figure 8. Time course of development and decay of platelet CICA. Normal platelets were washed four times by ADGS and resuspended in calcium-free Tyrode's solution. A 0.2-ml aliquot of washed platelets was preincubated for various times with 0.1 ml of saline suspension of human collagen (○) or with 0.85 per cent NaCl (●), at which time additions of citrate-saline, factor VIII, thrombin, serum eluate, contact product, and calcium chloride were made. After a 5-min incubation the mixture was tested for factor Xa activity.

were incubated with factor VIII, thrombin in trace amounts, a barium sulfate eluate of human serum containing the activities of factors IX and X, contact product, and calcium chloride. When this incubation was carried out in the presence of citrate-saline 100 per cent factor Xa activity developed in both phospholipid and platelet samples, but when heat-inactivated plasma containing natural inhibitors to active clotting factors was present instead of citrate-saline factor Xa activity developed only in the sample containing platelets and not in the phospholipid sample. Furthermore, when the platelets were separated by centrifugation and tested in comparison with the supernatant, the factor Xa activity was found in association with the platelets and not with the surrounding plasma.

Addition	Sample: Portion Tested	Percent Factor-Xa Formed in Presence of:	
		Platelets	Phospholipid
Citrate-saline	Uncentrifuged	100	100
	Centrifuged: Supernatant	54	97
	Centrifuged: Sediment	96	12
Heated Plasma	Uncentrifuged	100	3.2
	Centrifuged: Supernatant	27	2.9
	Centrifuged: Sediment	100	0.7

Figure 9. The incubation mixture consisted of washed normal platelets (ADGS X 4) or phospholipid (1:1000 dilution), citrate-saline, or alumina-adsorbed normal plasma heated at 60°C for 30 min, factor VIII, thrombin, human serum eluate, contact product, and calcium chloride. The centrifuged sample was allowed to incubate for 4 min and was centrifuged at room temperature for 8 min at 3000 X *g*. The supernatant was removed with a Pasteur pipette and tested after a total elapsed incubation time of 16 min. The sediment was reconstituted in a mixture of 0.4 ml of citrate-saline, 0.2 ml of 0.05 *M* CaCl, and 0.4 ml of 0.85 per cent NaCl and similarly tested for factor Xa activity after a total elapsed incubation time of 16 min. The "sediment" in the case of phospholipid consisted of approximately 0.2 ml left in the bottom of the tube and reconstituted as indicated. The centrifugal forces employed were sufficient to sediment platelets but not phospholipid. Platelets are not a limiting factor in this particular experiment; for example doubling the platelet number would not double the observed factor Xa activity. For this reason the amounts of factor Xa developed in the supernatant and deposit would not necessarily be expected to be additive.

The "protective" effect of platelets in contrast to phospholipid, which allows formation of factor Xa activity in the presence of inhibitors, might have one of several alternative explanations. One of these is that platelets protect factor Xa from destruction by antifactor Xa. This possibility was examined by allowing full factor Xa activity to develop in the presence of platelets or phospholipid, adding either citrate-saline or antifactors IIa, Xa, and XIa and determining the decay of factor Xa activity.

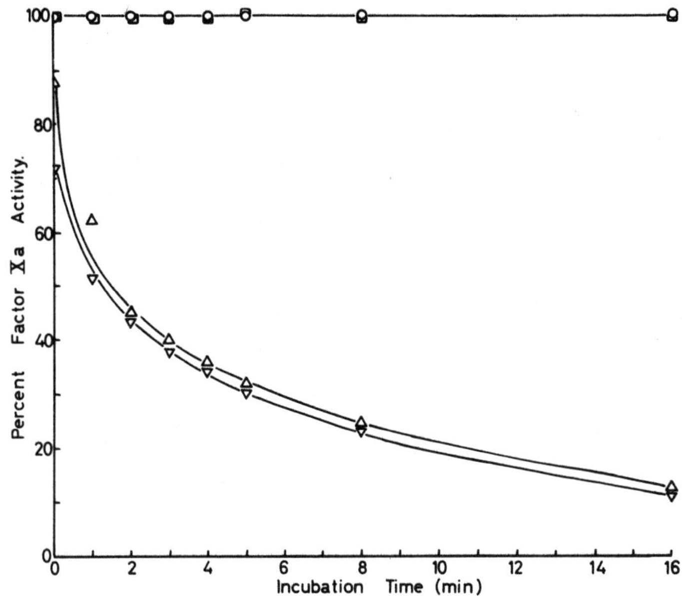

Figure 10. Decay of factor Xa activity in the presence of platelets and phospholipid. The following components were preincubated for 5 min to allow full development of factor Xa activity: washed normal platelets (ADGS X 4) or phospholipid, factor VIII, thrombin, human serum eluate, contact product, and calcium chloride. After 5 min either citrate-saline or alumina-adsorbed normal plasma heated at 56°C for 30 min was added and percentage of factor Xa activity determined at the times indicated. The additions were as follows: ○, platelets and citrate-saline; △, platelets and heated plasma; □, phospholipid and citrate-saline; ▽, phospholipid and heated plasma.

From the results (Fig. 10) it is evident that, once formed, the destruction of factor Xa by antifactor Xa is nearly as rapid in the presence of platelets as in the presence of phospholipid.

Another possible explanation for the platelet "protective" effect is that contact product is protected from destruction by antifactor XIa. To test this hypothesis, either washed normal platelets or phospholipid was mixed with contact product, and either citrate-saline or antifactor XIa was added. At intervals the mixture was tested for contact product activity (Fig. 11). An immediate and rapid decay in contact product activity occurred in the phospholipid sample to which inhibitory plasma was added. In contrast, when inhibitory plasma was added to the sample containing platelets, a 3–4 min delay was observed after which contact

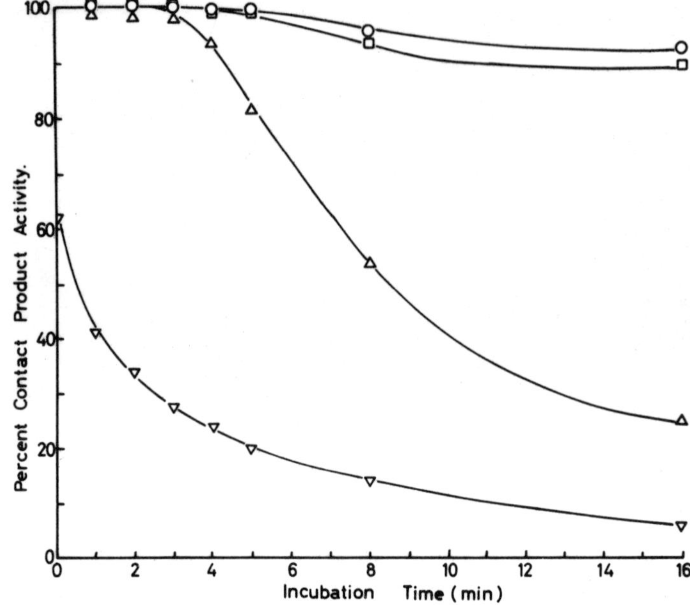

Figure 11. Decay of contact product activity in the presence of platelets and phospholipid. When 0.85 per cent NaCl instead of contact product was added and the contact product activity determined, less than 0.5 per cent of maximum contact product activity was detected in both platelet and phospholipid mixtures. Additions were as follows: ○, platelets and citrate-saline; △, platelets and alumina-adsorbed normal plasma heated at 60°C for 30 min; □, phospholipid and citrate-saline; ▽, phospholipid and heated plasma.

product decay proceeded at a rate less than that observed in the phospholipid sample. It is concluded that platelets can protect factor XIa from destruction by antifactor XIa.

DISCUSSION

A number of basic observations concerning the hemostatic mechanism would appear to be sufficiently valid and important that any theory of hemostasis should be consistent with them. These are the following.

1. Following *in vivo* vascular injury with bleeding the events leading to platelet plug formation on the one hand and blood coagulation on the other occur rapidly and concurrently.
2. The full hemostatic sequence requires: (*a*) platelets capable of

forming hemostatic plugs, (*b*) an intact coagulation mechanism (excepting factor XII), and (*c*) sufficiently extensive injury to hemostatically normal blood vessels.

3. Minimal vascular injury without rupture of the vessel wall is not sufficient to evoke the full hemostatic sequence, but only the temporary formation of platelet clumps which form repeatedly and embolize.

4. The full hemostatic sequence probably consists of the following events: (*a*) exposure of a subendothelial component of the vessel wall (possibly collagen) to which platelets adhere, (*b*) release of substances (possibly including ADP) from cells (possibly endothelial cells, platelets, or red cells, or both) which promote platelet adhesion and aggregation, (*c*) fibrin formation within and around platelet plugs, first appearing close to the site of vascular injury, and (*d*) morphological changes in platelets with degranulation and "consolidation" of the platelet plug.

5. Factor XII, in contrast to the other plasma-clotting factors, is not needed for normal hemostasis.

6. Platelet degranulation, probably mediated by thrombin and possibly by other substances, is accompanied by release from platelets of substances which may enhance platelet plug and fibrin formation.

Some possible interrelationships between platelet plug formation and blood coagulation, based on evidence presented here and by other investigators, are presented in Fig. 12 as an hypothesis which may account for the events of hemostasis. Excluded from this simplified diagram are important hemostatic factors such as fibrinolysis, vasoconstriction (Zucker, 1947), and stasis (Wessler, 1969). The events leading to platelet plug and fibrin formation are seen as proceeding concurrently, initiated in common by the events of vascular injury and closely linked by complex autocatalytic or "positive feedback" interrelationships.

Vascular injury results in exposure of a subendothelial substance, such as collagen (Hugues, 1960; Zucker and Borrelli, 1962), to which platelets can adhere and simultaneously initiate intrinsic clotting through collagen-induced coagulant activity (CICA). Since these events can occur in the absence of factor XII, they might explain the observation of normal hemostasis in patients with Hageman trait. At the same time substances, such as ADP, are released from injured cells present in blood vessels (Honour and Mitchell, 1964) and promote platelet adhesion,

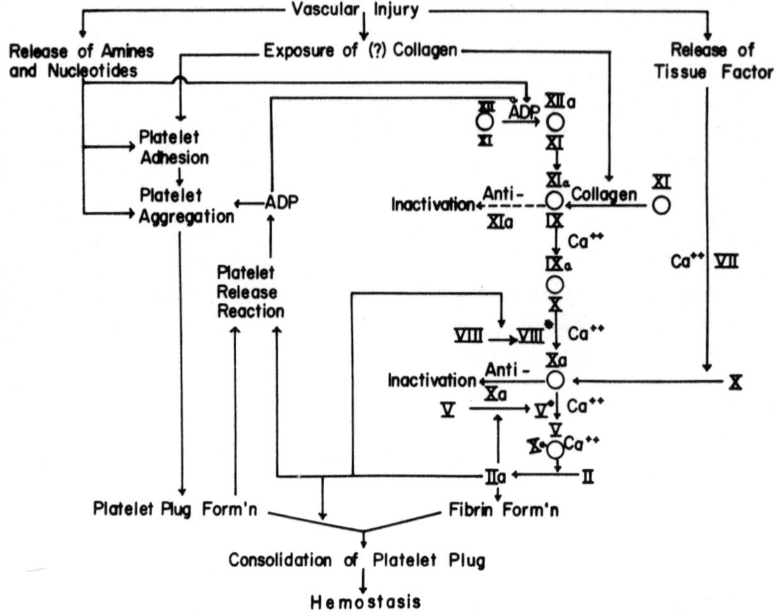

Figure 12. Some possible interrelationships between platelet plug formation and blood coagulation: an hypothesis concerning the hemostatic mechanism.

aggregation, and plug formation (Hellem, 1960; Gaarder *et al.*, 1961; Spaet and Zucker, 1964; Packham *et al.*, 1969; Begent and Born, 1970), and simultaneously initiate intrinsic coagulation through platelet contact product-forming activity (CPFA). Both the CPFA and CICA reactions are reversible, which might be viewed as a control mechanism preventing too extensive clotting in response to suboptimal stimuli. Vascular injury also leads to release of tissue factor which can lead to fibrin formation via the extrinsic clotting system.

After the initiation of intrinsic clotting by ADP- or collagen-stimulated platelets, the subsequent clotting reactions are seen as occurring on the surface of platelets (Roskam, 1923) as they aggregate to form a hemostatic plug. The platelets provide a protective nidus where coagulation factors can interact in the presence of naturally occurring inhibitors. Factor XIa formed on the platelet surface is protected from inactivation by antifactor XIa. Factor Xa forms on the platelet surface but not in plasma because its formation is prevented in the absence of platelets by natural inhibitors. Once formed, platelet-associated factor Xa is susceptible to inactivation by antifactor Xa and is also involved with factor V, calcium, and platelet lipoprotein in prothrombin activation. Thereby the balance of hemostasis is determined by the strength of the initial stimulus. When the stimulus is suboptimal, factor Xa is inactivated as rapidly as it is formed and is not available to promote thrombin generation. This is seen as a control mechanism which helps to maintain the blood in a fluid state and to prevent generalized intravascular clotting. If the initial stimulus is adequate, the balance between formation and inactivation of factor Xa shifts toward formation of sufficient factor Xa that thrombin generation occurs.

As the first traces of thrombin are formed, powerful autocatalytic effects occur including activation of factors V and VIII (Rapaport *et al.*, 1963; Biggs *et al.*, 1965) and the platelet release reaction (Zucker and Borrelli, 1955; Grette, 1962; Day *et al.*, 1969). ADP released from platelets can stimulate both platelet aggregation (which potentiates platelet plug formation) and platelet CPFA (which potentiates blood coagulation). Platelet lipoproteins may also be made available to potentiate clotting by enhancing the interaction of factors XIa, VIII, IX, and X (intrinsic factor Xa-forming activity) and factors Xa, V, and II (platelet factor 3 activity). These autocatalytic effects of thrombin are viewed as "positive feedback" mechanisms whereby thrombin in minute amounts can potentiate platelet plug formation and simultaneously potentiate the generation of sufficient quantities of thrombin to catalyze fibrin formation. The hemostatic process is completed when the platelet plug is "consolidated" and fibrin formed within and around it.

ACKNOWLEDGMENTS

I am most grateful to Dr. Rosemary Biggs for advice, support, and criticism, and to Professor E. A. Loeliger, in whose laboratory investigations involving patients with Hageman trait were carried out.

The work was supported in part by special postdoctoral fellowship No. 5 FO3 HE 39031 03 from the National Heart and Lung Institute, National Institutes of Health, United States Public Health Service.

Figures 2, 3, 4, 7, 10, and 11 are reprinted with permission from the British Journal of Haematology.

Figures 5 and 8 are reprinted with permission from Medicina.

REFERENCES

Begent, N., and Born, G. V. R. 1970. Growth rate *in vivo* of platelet thrombi, produced by iontophoresis of ADP, as a function of mean blood flow velocity. Nature 227: 926.

Biggs, R., Macfarlane, R. G., Denson, K. W. E., and Ash, B. J. 1965. Thrombin and the interaction of factors VIII and IX. Brit. J. Haematol. 11: 276.

Brecher, G., and Cronkite, E. P. 1950. Morphology and enumeration of human blood platelets. J. Appl. Physiol. 3: 365.

Day, H. J., Holmsen, H., and Hovig, T. 1969. Subcellular particles of human platelets. Scand. J. Haematol. Suppl. 7: 1.

Gaarder, A. M., Jonsen, J., Laland, S., Hellem, A., and Owren, P. A. 1961. Adenosine diphosphate in red cells as a factor in the adhesiveness of human blood platelets. Nature 192: 531.

Grette, K. 1962. Studies on the mechanism of thrombin-catalyzed hemostatic reactions in blood platelets. Acta Physiol. Scand. 56 (suppl. 195): 5.

Hellem, A. J. 1960. The adhesiveness of human blood platelets *in vitro*. Scand. J. Clin. Lab. Invest. 12 (suppl. 51): 1.

Honour, A. J., and Mitchell, J. R. A. 1964. Platelet clumping in injured vessels. Brit. J. Exp. Pathol. 45: 75.

Hugues, J. 1960. Accolement des plaquettes au collagène. C. R. Séances Soc. Biol. 154: 866.

Lundblad. R. L., and Davie, E. W. 1964. The activation of antihemophilic factor (factor VIII) by activated Christmas factor (activated factor IX). Biochemistry 3: 1720.

Macfarlane, R. G. 1972. Haemostasis, pp. 543–585. *In* R. Biggs (ed.) Human blood coagulation, haemostasis and thrombosis. Blackwell Scientific Publications, Oxford.

Marr, J., Barboriak, J. J., and Johnson, S. A. 1965. Relationship of appearance of adenosine diphosphate, fibrin formation and platelet aggregation in the haemostatic plug, *in vivo.* Nature 205: 259.

Packham, M. A., Ardlie, N. G., and Mustard, J. F. 1969. The effect of adenine compounds on platelet aggregation. Amer. J. Physiol. 217: 1009.

Rapaport, S. I., Schiffman, S., Patch, M. J., and Ames, S. B. 1963. The importance of activation of antihaemophilic globulin and proaccelerin by traces of thrombin in the generation of intrinsic prothrombinase activity. Blood 21: 221.

Roskam, J. 1923. Contribution a l'étude de la physiologie normale et pathologique du globulin. Arch. Int. Physiol. 20: 241.

Spaet, T. H., and Zucker, M. B. 1964. Mechanism of platelet plug formation and role of adenosine diphosphate. Amer. J. Physiol. 206: 1267.

Walsh, P. N. 1972a. Albumin density gradient separation and washing of platelets and the study of platelet coagulant activities. Brit. J. Haematol. 22: 205.

Walsh, P. N. 1972b. The effect of dilution of plasma on coagulation. The significance of the dilution-activation phenomenon for the study of platelet coagulant activities. Brit. J. Haematol. 22: 219.

Walsh, P. N. 1972c. The role of platelets in the contact phase of blood coagulation. Brit. J. Haematol. 22: 237.

Walsh, P. N. 1972d. The effects of collagen and kaolin on the intrinsic coagulant activity of platelets. Evidence for an alternative pathway in intrinsic coagulation not requiring factor XII. Brit. J. Haematol. 22: 393.

Walsh, P. N., and Biggs, R. 1972. The role of platelets in intrinsic factor-Xa formation. Brit. J. Haematol. 22: 743.

Wessler, S. 1969. The role of stasis in thrombosis, pp. 461–468. *In* S. Sherry, K. M. Brinkhous, E. Genton, and J. M. Stengle (eds.) Thrombosis. National Academy of Sciences, Washington, D.C.

Zucker, M. B. 1947. Platelet agglutination and vasoconstriction as factors in spontaneous hemostasis in normal, thrombocytopenic, heparinized and hypoprothrombinemic rabbits. Amer. J. Physiol. 148: 275.

Zucker, M. B., and Borrelli, J. 1962. Platelet clumping produced by connective tissue suspensions and by collagen. Proc. Soc. Exp. Biol. Med. 109: 779.

Factors Influencing the Adenylate Cyclase System in Human Blood Platelets

David C. B. Mills

Human blood platelets in citrated platelet-rich plasma have been studied by allowing them to incorporate ^{14}C-adenine into their metabolically active nucleotide pool, and following the incorporation of radioactivity into adenosine cyclic 3′:5′-monophosphate (cyclic AMP). Cyclic AMP accumulation measured by this technique is increased by a number of inhibitors of platelet aggregation. These can be distinguished as those that activate adenylate cyclase (including prostaglandin E_1, isoprenaline, and adenosine) and those that inhibit cyclic AMP phosphodiesterase (including methyl xanthines, papaverine, and pyrimidopyrimidine derivatives). The aggregating agents, ADP and adrenaline, antagonize the stimulation of cyclic AMP formation induced by prostaglandin E_1 (PGE_1). The effect of ADP is greater when ADP addition precedes the addition of PGE_1, and is greater in the absence of phosphodiesterase inhibitors than in their presence. The sulfhydryl reagent N-ethylmaleimide (NEM), also an inhibitor of platelet aggregation, enhances the stimulation of cyclic AMP accumulation by PGE_1, with an optimal concentration in platelet-rich plasma near 0.4 m*M*. The same effect is observed in

platelets suspended in synthetic media, only at 10-fold lower concentrations of NEM. The action of NEM is due neither to the activation of adenylate cyclase nor to the inhibition of phosphodiesterase. The presence of an endogenous intracellular regulator of platelet adenylate cyclase is postulated, and it is suggested that NEM acts by relieving the inhibition due to this moderator.

The concentrations of NEM that maximally enhance the action of PGE_1 also abolish the inhibition of cyclic AMP formation that occurs with ADP. The effect of adrenaline, however, is not inhibited. This supports the view that, whereas adrenaline acts directly on the cyclase through the hormone-receptive modulator in the membrane, ADP acts indirectly through an intracellular mechanism, possibly by activating the postulated inhibitor that is inactivated by NEM.

Aggregation of human blood platelets by adenosine diphosphate (ADP) is inhibited by adenosine (Born, 1962), by prostaglandin E_1 (Kloeze, 1967), and by isoprenaline (Mills and Roberts, 1967); all of these agents have been shown to increase the accumulation of cyclic AMP in other tissues (Sattin and Rall, 1972; Butcher, 1970; Robison *et al.*, 1971). Methyl xanthines, including theophylline and caffeine, which are known as inhibitors of cyclic AMP phosphodiesterase in other tissues (Robison *et al.*, 1971), also inhibit platelet aggregation when present at high concentrations (Ardlie *et al.*, 1967), and this observation led these authors to suggest the existence of an adenylate cyclase mechanism in platelets involved in the inhibition of aggregation. The existence of a hormonally responsive adenylate cyclase in platelets has been reported by a number of observers (for review see Salzman, 1971), and it has been shown that the inhibitory effects of adenosine, prostaglandin E_1 (PGE_1), and isoprenaline are attendant on an increase in the intracellular formation of cyclic AMP (Ball *et al.*, 1970; Mills and Smith, 1971) and that they are strongly enhanced by drugs that inhibit cyclic AMP phosphodiesterase. A number of these are now known that are considerably more active than the methyl xanthines (see below).

A highly simplified view of the cyclic AMP system in platelets is shown in Fig. 1. The concentration of cyclic AMP in the cell is controlled by the activity of two enzymes, adenylate cyclase and phosphodiesterase. A number of complicating factors have been purposely omitted. There is good evidence that platelets contain more than one phosphodiesterase, characterized by different substrate affinities and different susceptibilities to inhibition by drugs

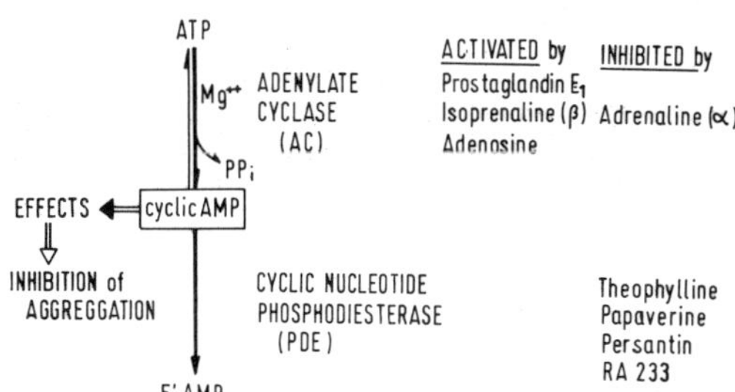

Figure 1. Simplified scheme of cyclic AMP metabolism in platelets.

(Mills and Smith, 1971); the adenylate cyclase may likewise be heterogeneous. Furthermore, the distribution of cyclic AMP in the cell may not be uniform. These and other factors may well affect the detailed mechanisms that regulate cyclic AMP metabolism. The simple scheme shown in Fig. 1 forms the theoretical base from which we have examined the action of aggregating agents and of sulfhydryl reagents on cyclic AMP metabolism.

Several of the experiments to be described were performed with Dr. J. B. Smith in the Medical Research Council's Thrombosis Research Group at the Royal College of Surgeons in London, England.

METHODS

We have developed a technique of investigating platelet cyclic AMP metabolism that relies upon the ability of platelets to take up adenine from plasma and incorporate it into the metabolically active fraction of their adenine nucleotides (Ball *et al.*, 1969). The method has been described in detail (Mills and Smith, 1971) and has in general given results that agree well with measurements based upon the direct estimation of cyclic AMP by the protein-binding assay (Harwood *et al.*, 1972). Cyclic AMP is measured by the incorporation of radioactive carbon into a cyclic AMP fraction isolated from other radioactive nucleotides by the method of Krishna *et al.* (1968) and controlled for recovery by the inclusion of tritiated cyclic AMP of known purity. The authenticity of the cyclic AMP has been checked by incubation with phosphodiesterase and by parallel isolation by a chromatographic procedure.

Because the increases in radioactive cyclic AMP formation induced by isoprenaline and adenosine are small in comparison with those brought about by PGE_1 and consequently difficult to measure accurately, we have used PGE_1 to activate adenylate cyclase in the experiments to be described.

INHIBITION OF PLATELET CYCLIC AMP PHOSPHODIESTERASE

As a number of the following experiments involve the use of an inhibitor of phosphodiesterase (PDE), the reasons for using the particular compound (RA233) should be given. RA233 is a structural analogue of dipyridamole, a coronary vasodilator that also inhibits the PDE of ox heart (Poch *et al.*, 1969). We have shown that the activities of dipyridamole and its analogues as inhibitors of platelet PDE depend on the concentration of cyclic AMP that is used in the assay (Mills and Smith, 1971). At high concentrations dipyridamole is most effective, but at the low concentrations (less than 10 μM) of cyclic AMP that actually occur in platelets under the conditions of our experiments, papaverine and RA233 are more powerful inhibitors. The results given in Fig. 2 show that when measurements are made at an initial cyclic AMP concentration of 3 μM, RA233 and papaverine are much more powerful inhibitors than are caffeine or theophylline, or even dipyridamole (Smith and Mills, 1970).

KINETICS OF ADENYLATE CYCLASE STIMULATION BY PGE_1

When platelets are exposed to PGE_1 there is a very rapid increase in the incorporation of radioactive ATP into cyclic AMP that reaches a peak within 20–40 sec. The radioactivity of cyclic AMP then declines to a steady state at a level dependent on the concentration of PGE_1 used (Fig. 3a). In the presence of RA 233 the incorporation is enhanced, and the peak level is maintained (Fig. 3b). No satisfactory explanation has yet been found for the characteristic shape of the curves seen in Fig. 3a; adenylate cyclase in broken cell preparations of platelets prepared by ultrasonic homogenization is activated by PGE_1 in a linear manner for at least 15 min (Fig. 4). A possible explanation is that cyclic AMP is formed from a specific pool of ATP at the membrane that is only slowly replenished from the general cytoplasmic pool. This does

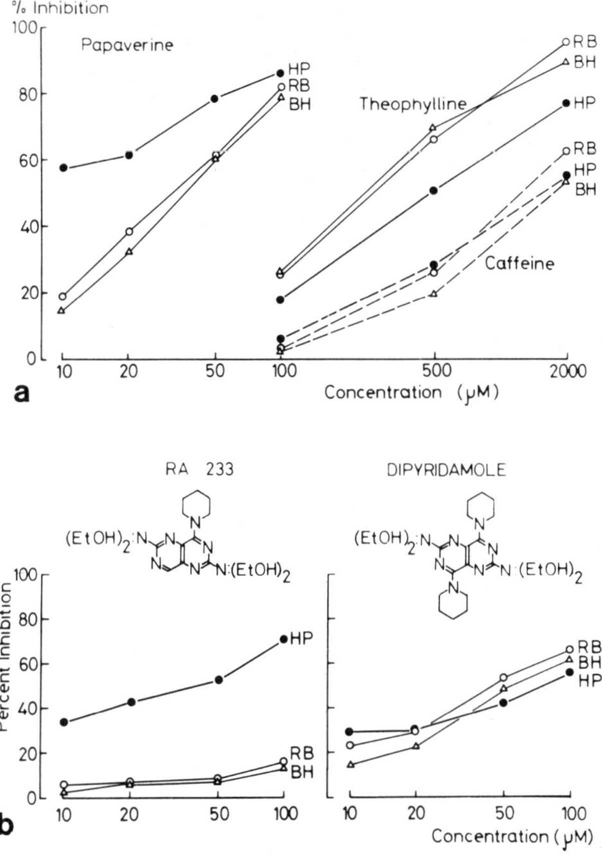

Figure 2. Inhibition of cyclic AMP phosphodiesterase from human platelets (●——●, HP), from rabbit brain (○——○, RB), and from ox heart (△——△, BH) plotted against concentration on a logarithmic scale. (a) Papaverine, theophylline, and caffeine. (b) RA233 and dipyridamole. The initial concentration of cyclic ^{3}H-AMP in the assay mixture was 3 μM, and the exact composition of the reaction mixture has been given by Mills and Smith (1970).

not account for the fact that the shape of the curves is similar even at very low cyclase stimulation by small amounts of PGE_1 (Fig. 3a). Figure 5 shows potentiation of the stimulation of incorporation of radioactivity into cyclic AMP by RA233 and by papaverine. These experiments show that inhibitors of PDE cause very little stimulation of cyclic AMP formation in resting platelets

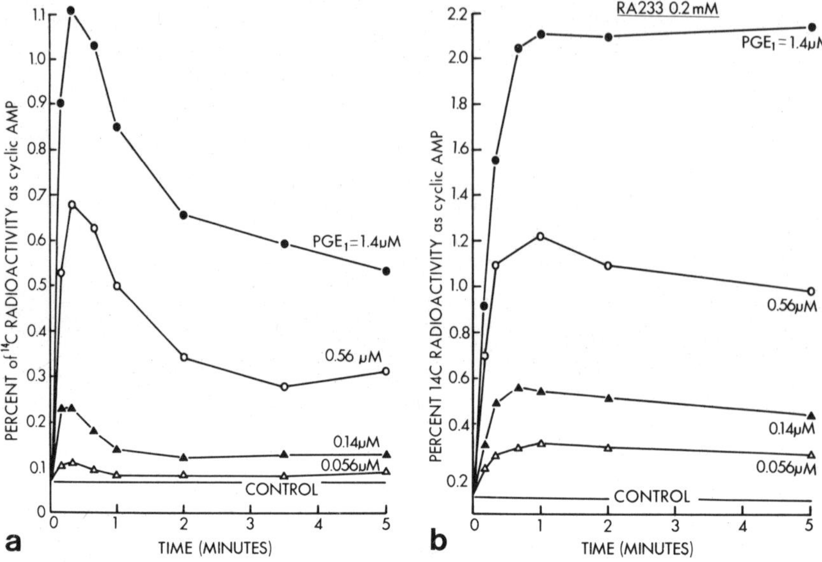

Figure 3. Radioactivity of cyclic AMP in platelets measured at successive times after the addition of PGE_1 to human platelet-rich citrate plasma prelabeled by incubation with ^{14}C-adenine. (a) PGE_1 alone. (b) PGE_1 added 30 sec after the phosphodiesterase inhibitor RA233, 0.2 m*M*. Final concentrations of PGE_1 were 0.056 μM (△——△), 0.14 μM (▲——▲), 0.56 μM (○——○), and 1.4 μM (●——●).

compared with their effect in the presence of PGE_1. This implies that the resting activity of the platelet adenylate cyclase is extremely low.

EFFECTS OF ADP AND ADRENALINE ON THE CYCLASE SYSTEM

In platelets that have been exposed to PGE_1 and in which the cyclic AMP content is consequently higher than the basal level, addition of adrenaline causes a fall in cyclic AMP (Robison *et al.*, 1969). Adrenaline also causes a reduction in the radioactivity of cyclic AMP in ^{14}C-adenine-labeled platelets previously exposed to PGE_1 (Moskowitz *et al.*, 1971; Marquis *et al.*, 1970; Haslam and Taylor 1971b) and a similar response occurs with ADP (Mills and Smith, 1972). Figure 6 shows that this reduction occurs very rapidly, and that it also occurs, although at a slower rate, in the presence of an inhibitor of PDE. The concentrations of ADP and

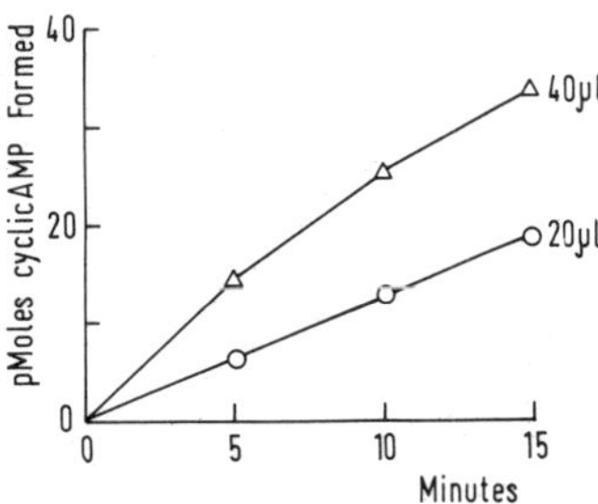

Figure 4. Adenylate cyclase activity of platelet homogenates. Platelets from plasma containing EDTA as anticoagulant were resuspended in 0.13 *M* NaCl containing 0.015 *M* Tris-HCl, pH 7.4, and homogenized briefly with a Polytron ultrasonic homogenizer. Intact cells were removed by centrifugation (5 min at 500 × *g*) and the supernatant used directly. Incubation mixtures (0.10 ml) contained 50 µl of reaction mixture, 10 µl of PGE_1 (10 µ*M*), and 20 or 40 µl of the homogenate. The reaction mixture contained ATP (1 m*M*), ^{14}C-ATP (5 µCi/ml), phosphoenolpyruvate (5 m*M*), pyruvate kinase (0.25 mg/ml), bovine serum albumin (0.4 mg/ml), cyclic AMP (0.2 m*M*), $MgCl_2$ (20 m*M*), and Tris-HCl (pH 7.4; 8 m*M*). Reactions were terminated by the addition of 10 µl of 0.8 *M* $HClO_4$ containing 0.05 µCi/ml cyclic ^{3}H-AMP. Cyclic ^{14}C-AMP was assayed by the method of Krishna *et al.* (1968).

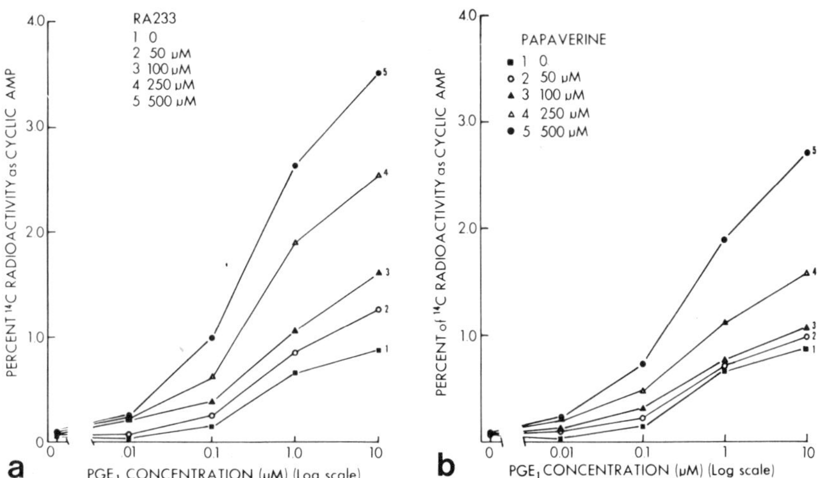

Figure 5. Radioactivity of cyclic AMP in samples of platelet-rich acid citrate dextrose plasma preincubated with ^{14}C-adenine and exposed to different concentrations of PGE_1 and (a) RA233 or (b) papaverine. The samples (1.0 ml) of platelet-rich plasma were incubated at 37°C with RA233 or papaverine for 2 min before, and for a further 3 min after, the addition of PGE_1.

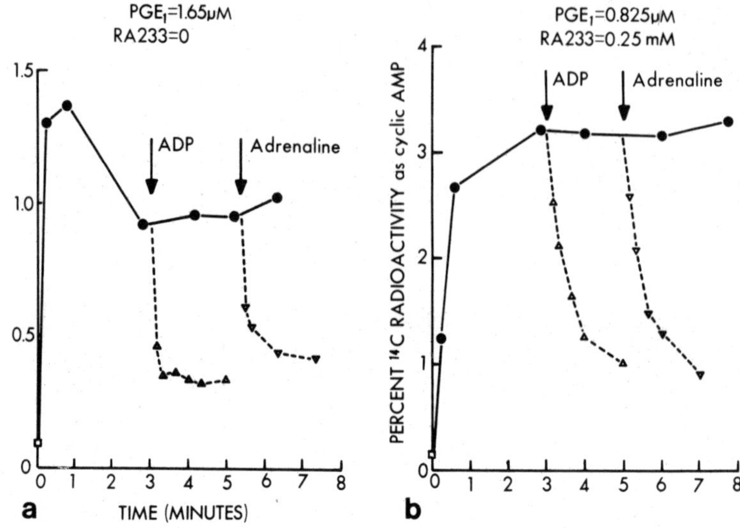

Figure 6. Effect of ADP and of adrenaline on the radioactivity of cyclic AMP in platelets in citrated plasma incubated with (b) a mixture of PGE_1 (0.825 *μM*) and RA233 (0.2 m*M*) and (a) PGE_1 (1.65 *μM*) alone. For each experiment, 18 ml of platelet-rich plasma, prelabeled with ^{14}C-adenine, were incubated at 37°C with PGE_1 or PGE_1 plus RA233. Samples of 1.0 ml were withdrawn at intervals for measurement of cyclic AMP radioactivity (●——●). At the points indicated by the arrows, samples were withdrawn and added to tubes containing either ADP (△– – –△) or adrenaline (– – –) to give a final concentration of 5 *μM*. The incubations were terminated by the addition of perchloric acid containing cyclic AMP and cyclic ^{3}H-AMP for recovery standard. (Reproduced from Mills and Smith (1972) with permission of the publishers.)

adrenaline that produce this effect correspond to the concentrations that provoke platelet aggregation when PGE_1 is absent (Fig. 7). This, together with evidence that ADP and adrenaline can lower the basal cyclic AMP levels in unstimulated platelets (Salzman and Neri, 1969), suggests that these agents may cause aggregation as a result of their effects on cyclic AMP levels, as has been cogently argued by Salzman (1971). However, Haslam and Taylor (1971a) have given strong reasons for believing that this is not necessarily so. Using three aggregating agents, ADP, adrenaline, and vasopressin, these authors have shown an inverse relationship between the ability to cause aggregation and the ability to inhibit the PGE_1-stimulated formation of cyclic AMP. In their system

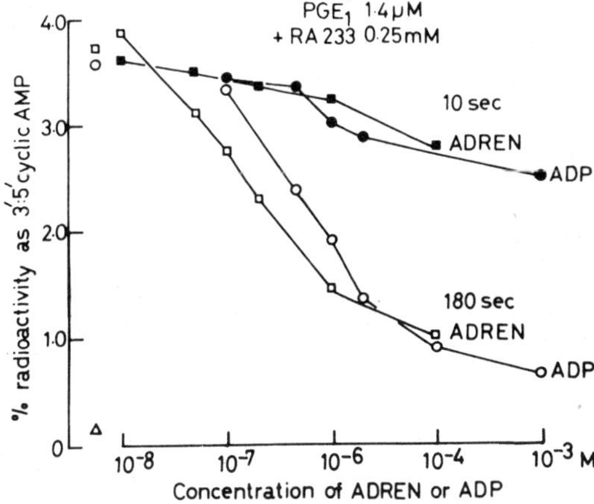

Figure 7. Effect of different concentrations of ADP and adrenaline on cyclic AMP radioactivity in platelets preincubated with ^{14}C-adenine and exposed to a combination of PGE_1 (1.4 *μM*) and compound RA233 (0.25 m*M*). The results are plotted as percentage of the total ^{14}C radioactivity in the platelets recovered as cyclic AMP, either 10 sec (closed symbols) or 180 sec (open symbols) after the addition of ADP (●, ○) or adrenaline (ADREN) (■, □). Controls without ADP or adrenaline (○, □) and without PGE_1 or RA233 (△) are shown at the left of the figure.

vasopressin is the most powerful aggregating agent, and the least active inhibitor of cyclic AMP formation, whereas adrenaline is most active in antagonizing the effect of PGE_1 and the weakest aggregating agent. That any one of these agents, and adrenaline is the most likely, may cause aggregation by inhibiting adenylate cyclase, is plausible; that all three do so seems highly unlikely. Adrenaline inhibits adenylate cyclase in broken cell preparations from both platelets (Zieve and Greenough, 1969) and other cells (Robison *et al.*, 1971). So far attempts to show a similar action of ADP have not been successful. Moreover, although the inhibition by ADP of PGE_1-stimulated cyclic AMP formation is blocked by the sulfhydryl reagent N-ethylmaleimide (NEM), the inhibition caused by adrenaline is not (Mills and Smith, 1972). The effects of NEM will be considered in detail below.

In thrombasthenia, platelets do not aggregate in response to ADP (Hardisty *et al.*, 1964), although they change shape in a normal way (Fig. 8) with both ADP and 5-hydroxytryptamine (5HT). Thrombasthenic platelets also respond in a qualitatively

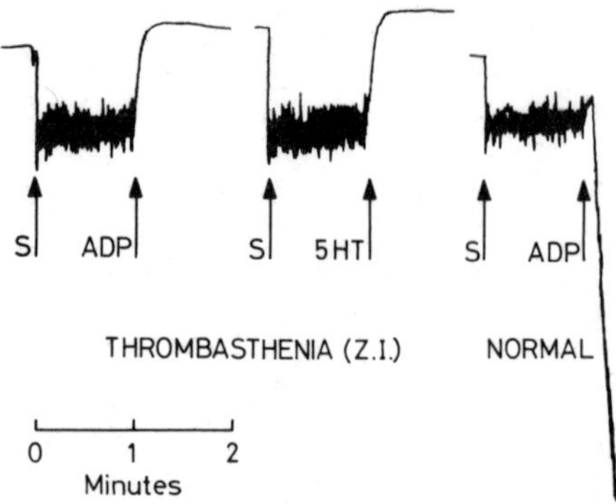

Figure 8. Aggregometer records made of thrombasthenic platelets on addition of ADP and 5HT, and of normal platelets with ADP. The stirring motor was started at the arrow marked S causing an immediate reduction in the transmitted light and the appearance of oscillations characteristic of discoid platelets. Traces were made with the apparatus and conditions described by Mills and Roberts (1967), with the sensitivity increased to emphasize the initial reactions. ADP and 5HT were added in 10 μl of saline solution to give final concentrations of 10 μM.

normal manner to stimulation of adenylate cyclase by PGE_1 (Fig. 9), and the subsequent addition of ADP causes a similar fall in the steady state level of cyclic AMP radioactivity to that observed with normal platelets. From this it appears that thrombasthenic platelets, at least those of the two unrelated patients so far examined, are normal with respect to those aspects of the adenylate cyclase system that we have been able to measure.

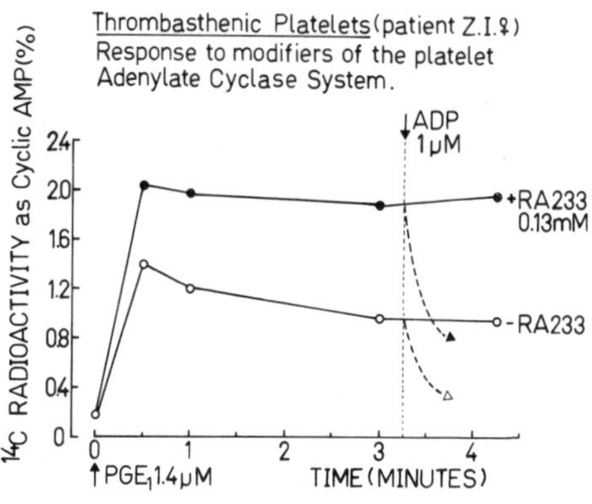

Figure 9. Radioactivity of cyclic AMP in thrombasthenic platelets after exposure to PGE_1 (1.4 μM, open symbols) or PGE_1 plus RA233 (0.13 mM, closed symbols). At the time indicated by the vertical dashed line, subsamples were added to ADP (final concentration, 1 μM) and cyclic AMP radioactivity determined 30 sec later (△, ▲).

EFFECTS OF OTHER AGGREGATING AGENTS

A number of reports, summarized by Salzman (1971), have shown that aggregating agents including thrombin, collagen, and 5HT may inhibit adenylate cyclase or lower cyclic AMP levels in platelets. In particular, the experiments of Brodie *et al.* (1972) have shown that exposure of intact platelets to low concentrations of thrombin followed by homogenization leads to a reduction of basal and PGE_1-stimulated adenylate cyclase activity in the platelet fragments. Addition of thrombin to the homogenate inhibits the cyclase only at excessively high concentrations. Brodie *et al.* (1972) suggest that thrombin may act primarily by destroying the adenylate cyclase of intact platelets, causing aggregation by lower-

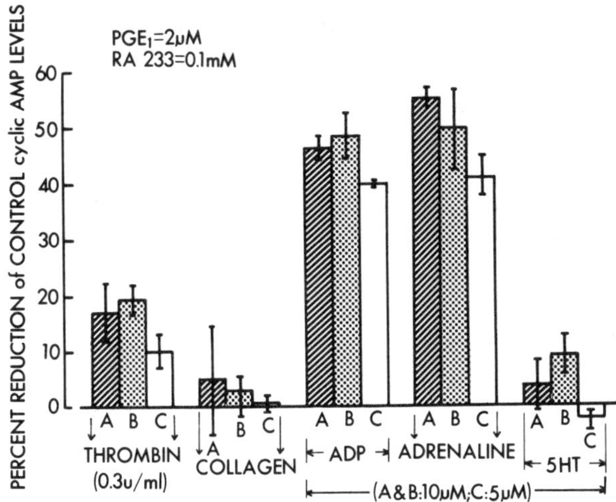

Figure 10. Effect of different aggregating agents on the radioactivity of cyclic AMP in platelets. Human platelets in acid citrate dextrose plasma were preincubated with ^{14}C-adenine and then exposed to a combination of PGE_1 (2 μM) and RA233 (0.1 mM). Results are expressed as the mean reduction in cyclic AMP radioactivity after exposure to the various aggregating agents. Three experiments are shown. In experiments A and B, using the same sample of labeled platelet-rich plasma, the incubations were terminated 30 and 60 sec after the addition of the aggregating agent, respectively. In experiment C, using a different sample of platelets, the time was 30 sec. In A and B the results are given as the means of two determinations with the individual results shown by the vertical bars. In C, the means and ranges of triplicate determinations are given.

ing intracellular cyclic AMP levels. Our experiments with PGE_1-stimulated platelets (Fig. 10) show that, when used at concentrations that produce marked aggregation of normal citrated platelet-rich plasma, neither collagen nor 5HT caused any appreciable lowering of cyclic AMP radioactivity, and the effect of thrombin was small in comparison with that observed under the same conditions with ADP or adrenaline. However, numerous objections can be raised to this experiment. The effect of thrombin observed by Brodie *et al.* (1972) is inhibited by PGE_1; also, the small effect of thrombin added after PGE_1 could be the result of the action of released ADP, although PGE_1 at the concentrations used is a powerful inhibitor of release (Kinlough-Rathbone *et al.*, 1970).

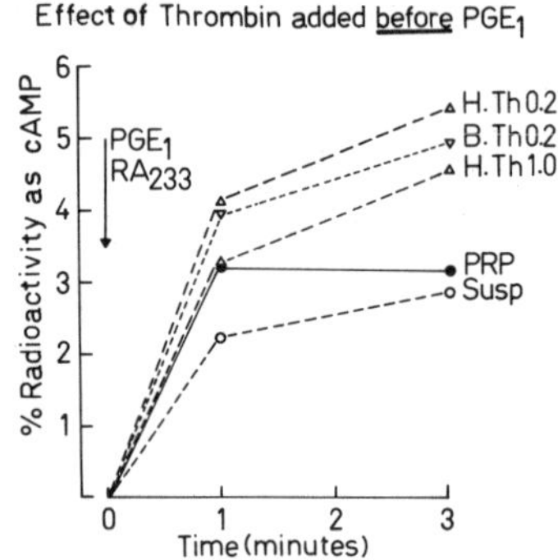

Figure 11. Effect of preincubation of platelets with thrombin on their response to PGE_1. Citrated human platelet-rich plasma (PRP) was labeled with ^{14}C-adenine for 60 min at 37°C. The plasma was then cooled in melting ice for 5 min, and EDTA (0.1 *M*, pH 7.2) was added to a final concentration of 10 m*M*. The platelets were separated by centrifugation at 4°C in plastic 10-ml tubes at 3500 × *g* for 10 min and resuspended in 0.13 *M* NaCl containing 0.015 *M* Tris-HCl, pH 7.4, and glucose (10 m*M*). Aliquots of this suspension (Susp) were incubated with different concentrations of thrombin (bovine (B.Th.), Parke-Davis Thrombin Tropical or human (H. Th.), United States Standard Thrombin (Human) from the Division of Biological Standards, National Institutes of Health) for 6 min at 37°C. EDTA was then added to final concentration of 5 m*M* and the suspensions cooled and centrifuged at 4°C for 10 min at 2000 × *g*. The platelets were resuspended in fresh saline-Tris-glucose medium, prewarmed to 37°C and incubated with a combination of PGE_1 (5 μ*M*) and RA233 (0.4 m*M*). A sample of the original platelet-rich plasma, preserved on ice during the preparation of the suspensions served as a control (●——●). Platelets pretreated with human (△– – –△) and bovine (▽– – –▽) thrombin are compared with platelets processed identically, but without exposure to thrombin (○– – –○).

Also, thrombin causes the synthesis of prostaglandin E_2 (PGE_2) by platelets (Smith and Willis, 1970) and PGE_2 may antagonize the effects of PGE_1 on the adenylate cyclase (Shio *et al.*, 1972). To resolve this confused situation, we have treated adenine-labeled platelets with thrombin, washed and resuspended them (thereby removing both released ADP and any PGE_2 that might be formed), and then exposed them to PGE_1. The increased incorporation of radioactivity into cyclic AMP in the resuspended platelets that occurred after the addition of PGE_1 was not prevented by previous exposure to either bovine or human thrombin (Fig. 11). Rather, the thrombin-treated platelets responded more vigorously to adenylate cyclase stimulation by PGE_1 than either the control resuspended platelets or the original platelet-rich plasma, despite the fact that thrombin treatment caused a depletion of the platelet ATP content owing to the formation of hypoxanthine that occurs concomitantly with the release reaction (Ireland, 1967; Holmsen *et al.*, 1972). An increase in the cyclic AMP content of platelets exposed to thrombin has been reported by Droller and Wolfe (1972). These results indicate that platelet adenylate cyclase is not destroyed by thrombin, although possibly thrombin renders the enzyme more susceptible to inactivation during homogenization.

EFFECTS OF N-ETHYLMALEIMIDE (NEM)

An attractive explanation for the effects of adrenaline and ADP on the adenylate cyclase system is that these two aggregating agents induce an energy-consuming reaction connected with the reorganization of the platelet membrane that leads to the exposure of normally concealed "adhesive sites." This process might be ex-

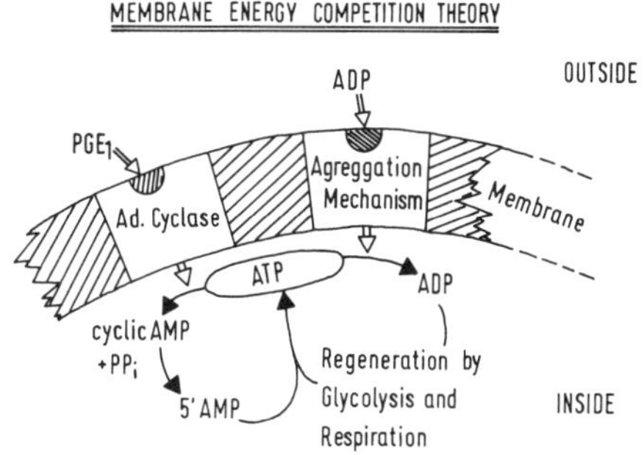

Figure 12. A model of the theory of membrane energy competition between the adenylate cyclase (Ad. Cyclase) and the aggregation mechanism used to explain the effects of ADP on the PGE_1-stimulated cyclase.

pected to consume ATP, the substrate for the adenylate cyclase reaction, and consequently to inhibit the cyclase by deprivation of substrate. Similarly, activation of the cyclase might reduce the availability of ATP to support aggregation (Fig. 12). The effects of NEM were examined because NEM is an inhibitor of platelet aggregation (Robinson *et al.*, 1963) and because NEM also reacts with actomyosin contractile systems (Webb, 1966). The shape change induced by ADP strongly suggests that it acts on a contractile system in the platelets (White, 1968).

It was expected that NEM would prevent the activation by ADP of the contractile mechanism, and consequently prevent the depletion of ATP, thereby allowing the adenylate cyclase unhindered access to its substrate. Platelets were therefore incubated with different concentrations of NEM before being exposed to PGE_1 (Fig. 13). This produced the surprising result that NEM caused a dose-dependent increase in the response of platelets to PGE_1, up to a maximum at about 0.4 m*M* NEM. The PGE_1-stimulated accumulation of radioactive cyclic AMP is also enhanced by NEM in platelets suspended in buffered saline solutions (Fig. 14). In this case the maximum stimulation was found at about 10-fold lower concentrations of NEM, indicating that in platelet-rich plasma the platelets are to some extent protected from the actions of NEM, probably by combination of NEM with readily accessible

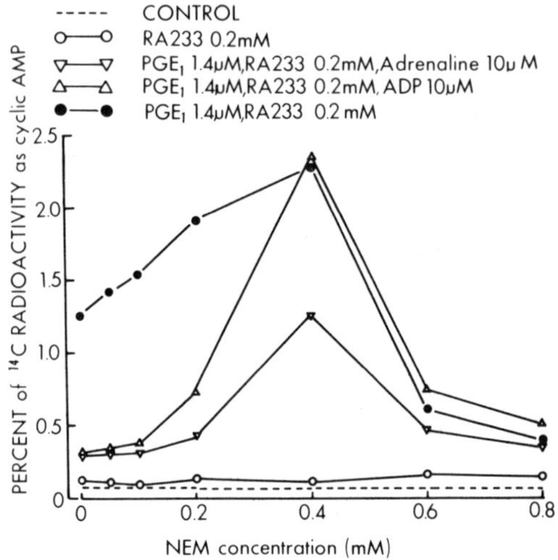

Figure 13. Effect of different concentrations of N-ethylmaleimide on the radioactivity of cyclic AMP in platelets prelabeled with ^{14}C-adenine. Platelet-rich plasma was incubated with NEM for 1 min before the addition of the other agents, and for a further 1 min thereafter. The other additions are indicated in the figure. (Reproduced from Mills and Smith (1972) with permission of the publishers.)

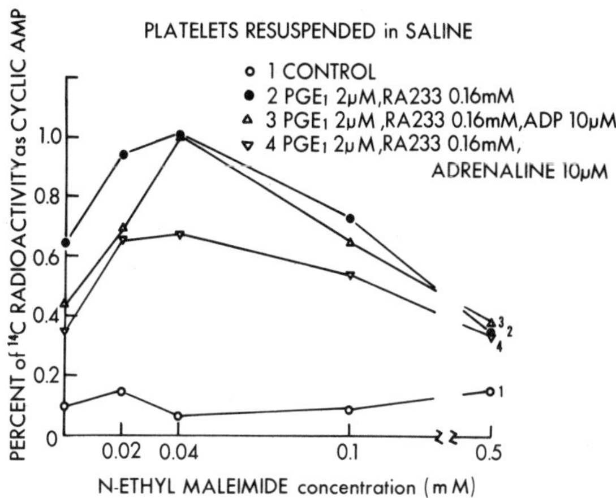

Figure 14. Radioactivity of cyclic AMP in resuspended platelets isolated from acid citrate dextrose platelet-rich plasma labeled with ^{14}C-adenine. The resuspension medium contained NaCl, 130 m*M*; KCl, 5 m*M*; $MgCl_2$, 2 m*M*; Tris-HCl, pH 7.4, 15 m*M*; and glucose, 55 m*M*. Platelet suspensions were incubated at 37°C with NEM for 4 min before the addition of the other agents and for a further 4 min thereafter.

sulfhydryl groups in plasma (Ellman, 1959). This observation agrees well with the finding that NEM inhibits the aggregation of washed platelets at considerably lower concentrations than are required in platelet-rich plasma.

NEM did not stimulate adenylate cyclase by itself, either in the presence or absence of the phosphodiesterase inhibitor RA233 (Fig. 13). The PGE_1-stimulated adenylate cyclase of platelet fragments is progressively inhibited by NEM (Fig. 15) in the concentration range that stimulated the response to PGE_1 of intact platelets resuspended in saline (Fig. 14). This suggests that the biphasic effect of increasing concentrations of NEM in Figs. 13 and 14 is due to a combination of stimulation at low concentrations and inhibition at high concentrations.

A further possible explanation for the enhancement of PGE_1-induced cyclic AMP formation by NEM is that NEM is an inhibitor of phosphodiesterase (PDE). A number of different experiments have convinced us that this is not the case. When the time course of cyclic AMP radioactivity in platelets stimulated by PGE_1 is followed (Fig. 16), the effect of NEM is seen to be quite different from that of the known PDE inhibitor, RA233. Whereas RA233

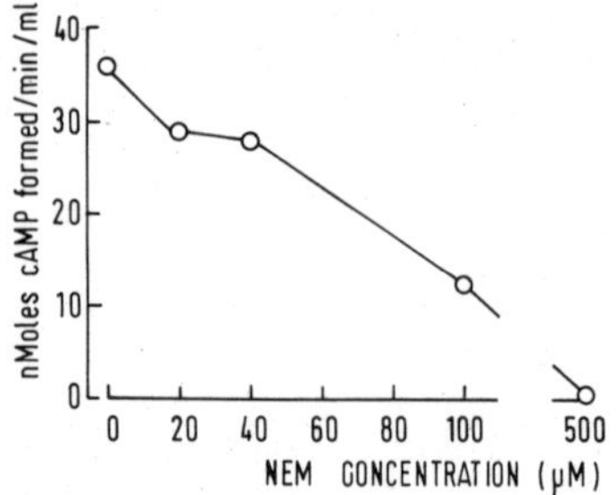

Figure 15. **Effect of NEM on the adenylate cyclase activity of platelet homogenates.** Platelets suspended in 0.13 *M* NaCl containing 0.015 *M* Tris-HCl, pH 7.4, were frozen and thawed three times by successive immersion in Dry Ice-methanol and water at 37°C. The preparation was centrifuged for 5 min at 500 × *g* to remove intact cells and then used directly. The incubation mixtures contained 50 μl of reaction mixture (see caption to Fig. 4); 30 μl of the platelet lysate, 10 μl of 10 μ*M* PGE_1, and 10 μl of water or NEM solution. The reaction was terminated after 5 or 10 min incubation at 37°C and the results are given as the means of the 5- and 10-min results which, when expressed as rates of cyclic AMP formation, were in close agreement.

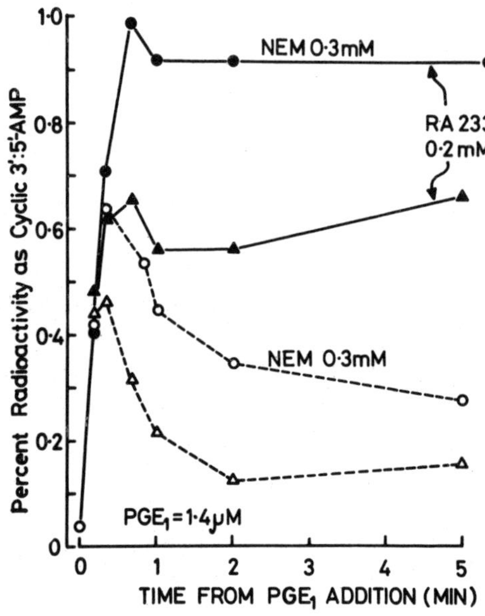

Figure 16. Effect of N-ethylmaleimide (NEM) on the stimulation of incorporation of radioactivity into platelet cyclic AMP by PGE_1 in the presence (closed symbols) and absence (open symbols) of RA233. Prelabeled platelets were incubated at 37° C for 1 min with 0.3 m*M* NEM (●——●), or without NEM (▲——▲, △— — —△) before the addition of PGE_1 (1.4 μ*M*) or PGE_1 plus RA233 (0.2 m*M*). The radioactivity of cyclic AMP was determined on successive 1.0-ml samples. (Reproduced from Mills and Smith (1972) with the permission of the publishers.)

causes a marked increase in the steady state level of cyclic AMP radioactivity as compared with a small increase in the initial peak, NEM enhances both phases of the response curve to a similar extent. Also, the effect of NEM critically depends on whether it is added to the platelets before or after they have been stimulated by PGE_1. Adding RA233 during the steady state attained after exposure of platelets to PGE_1 increases the radioactivity of cyclic AMP in a manner that would be expected if this steady state represents a rapid turnover of cyclic AMP in the cell (Mills and Smith, 1972). In contrast, addition of NEM at this point causes a reduction in cyclic AMP radioactivity (Fig. 17). This implies both that NEM is not acting as a PDE inhibitor and that after platelets have been exposed to PGE_1 a change takes place that results in a reduction of the stimulatory activity of NEM, so that its inhibitory action, normally only seen at high concentrations, becomes dominant. Finally, Table 1 shows that NEM, at the concentrations that enhance PGE_1-stimulated adenylate cyclase activity in platelet-rich plasma have very little effect on PDE activity of platelet lysates.

As expected on the basis of the substrate-competition theory (Fig. 12), NEM blocked the effect of ADP on the PGE_1-stimulated cyclase (Fig. 13). In platelet-rich plasma, the effect was greatest at the same concentration (0.4 m*M* NEM) that caused the maximum enhancement of the effect of PGE_1. This coincidence has led us to

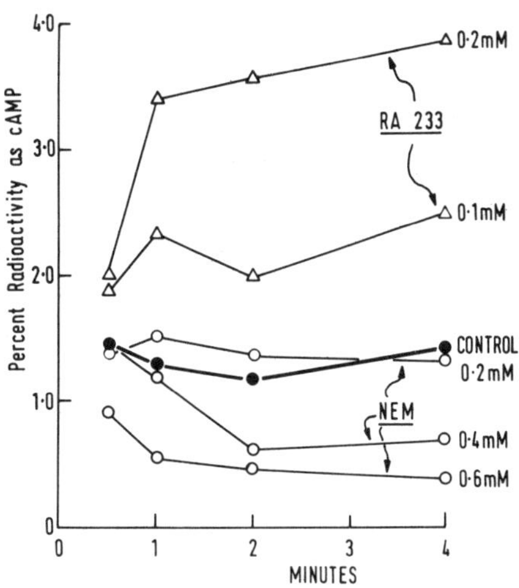

Figure 17. Effect of RA233 (△) or NEM (○) on the radioactivity of cyclic AMP in platelets exposed to PGE_1 (2 μM) added 3 min previously. The radioactivity of cyclic AMP in control platelets, exposed to PGE_1 but with no further additions, is shown (●) over the same period to be relatively constant.

Table 1. Effect of NEM on phosphodiesterase activity of ammonium sulfate-fractionated platelet lysates

NEM concentration (μM)	Cyclic ^{3}H-AMP hydrolyzed (pmoles/min/mg protein)	
	A	B
0	308	608
1	324	616
10	308	617
33	320	577
100	284	616
330	296	586
1000	270	553

Phosphodiesterase was prepared from human platelets by washing the platelets, resuspending them in 0.13 *M* NaCl containing 0.015 *M* Tris-HCl, pH 7.4, and sonicating them three times for 10 sec. The sonicate was centrifuged at 500 × *g* for 5 min to remove intact cells, and the enzyme was precipitated by the addition of ammonium sulfate. Fraction A was precipitated by 35 per cent saturation in ammonium sulfate, and fraction B between 35 and 60 per cent saturation. The activities of fractions A and B were 0.47 and 1.34 mμ/mg protein when tested in an assay system containing 3 μM cyclic ^{3}H-AMP (100 Ci/mole), 20 m*M* $MgCl_2$, 25 m*M* Tris-HCl, pH 7.3, and up to 0.6 mg/ml enzyme protein. Incubations (0.1 ml) were done for 5 min at 37°C and stopped by dilution with 2 ml of water, followed by 0.2 ml of 10 per cent barium hydroxide. Unreacted cyclic ^{3}H-AMP remaining in the supernatant after two precipitations with barium and zinc (Krishna *et al.*, 1968) was determined by liquid scintillation counting.

suspect that the two phenomena may be intimately connected. However, in contrast to the stimulation by NEM of PGE_1-activated cyclase activity, which requires that NEM addition should precede exposure to PGE_1, the ability of NEM to block the effect of ADP occurs when NEM is added after or before PGE_1 (Fig. 18).

The actions of NEM can be attributed justifiably to its ability to react with thiol groups. No extensive preincubation is required with platelets before the effects are apparent, and the reaction conditions are mild with respect to pH and temperature. NEM reacts with numerous other chemical groups, but usually under more vigorous conditions (Webb, 1966). The effects of NEM are prevented by the prior addition of a slight molar excess of cysteine, although cysteine added after NEM has no effect (Fig. 19).

NEM does not block the inhibition of cyclic AMP formation caused by adrenaline under the same conditions in which the effect of ADP is abolished (Figs. 13 and 14). It appears from this

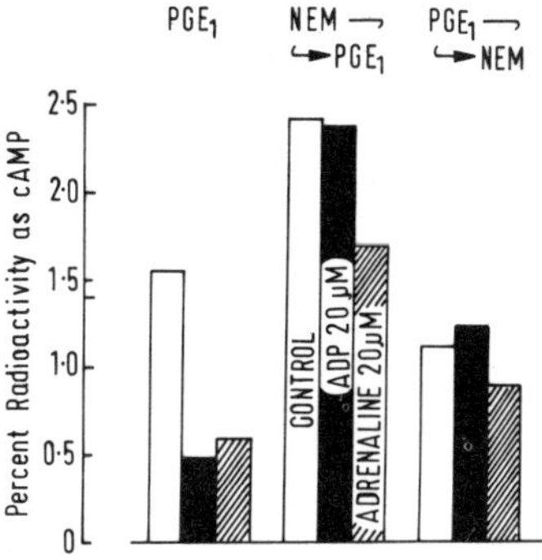

Figure 18. **Effect of the order of addition of PGE_1 (2 μM) and NEM (0.4 mM) on the increase in platelet cyclic AMP radioactivity brought about by PGE_1 (open bars), PGE_1 plus ADP (20 μM; solid bars), or PGE_1 plus adrenaline (20 μM; hatched bars). In the columns at the left, no NEM was added. In the center columns NEM was added 30 sec before PGE_1 and in the right-hand columns NEM was added 3 min after PGE_1. ADP or adrenaline, when included, was added 3.5 min after PGE_1 and the reaction was stopped 4.5 min after addition of PGE_1. In all incubation mixtures, RA233 (0.2 mM) was added together with PGE_1.**

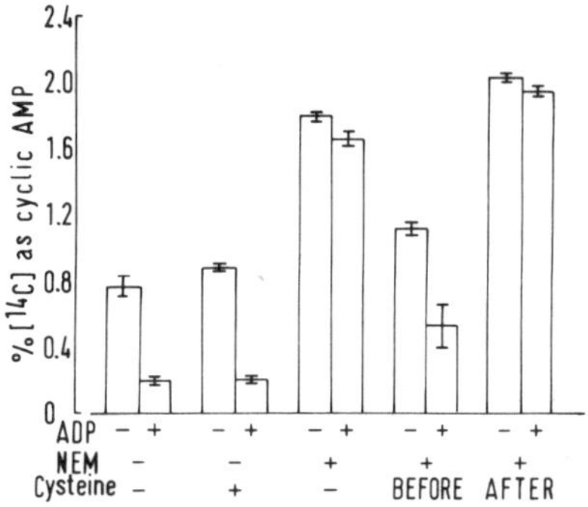

Figure 19. **Effect of cysteine added before or after NEM on the interaction of platelets with PGE_1 and ADP. Platelets prelabeled by incubation with ^{14}C-adenine were incubated for between 2 and 3 min with PGE_1 (2 μM) and RA233 (0.2 mM). During this period, aliquots of platelet-rich plasma (1.0 ml) were added to tubes containing ADP (20 μl; final concentration, 20 μM) or saline, and incubated for a further 1.0 min, before stopping the reaction with perchloric acid. NEM (0.4 mM), when included, was added 1.0 min before PGE_1. Cysteine-HCl at pH 7 (0.5 mM), when included, was added 1.5 min before PGE_1, except for the right-hand columns, which describe the result of adding cysteine 0.5 min after the addition of NEM.**

fact that ADP and adrenaline produce their inhibitory effects on the cyclase by fundamentally different mechanisms. As the adenylate cyclase of platelet fragments is inhibited by adrenaline (Zieve and Greenough, 1969), but no such effect occurs with ADP, it is reasonable to suspect that the action of adrenaline occurs through a direct effect of this hormone on an inhibitory adrenergic receptor in the platelet membrane, and the ADP acts indirectly through a complex intracellular mechanism, possibly through competition for ATP. It seems likely that this mechanism involves an unidentified sulfhydryl mediator that is inactivated by NEM. This explanation is offered as an alternative to the substrate competition mechanism outlined above for the following reasons. The initial reaction of platelets to ADP, the change in shape from discs to irregular spheres (MacMillan and Oliver, 1965), is associated with a shift in the energy balance of the metabolically active adenine nucleotides in the cells (Mills, 1973). This is measured as a reduction in the energy charge of the adenylate pool, defined as the ratio of the high energy phosphate (2ATP + ADP) to twice the total size of the pool 2(ATP + ADP + AMP) that is governed by the equilibrium conditions of the adenylate kinase reaction. The effect of ADP on the energy charge can be attributed reasonably to the activation of an energy-consuming process connected with the shape change. At concentrations of NEM that abolish the effect of ADP on the PGE_1-stimulated adenylate cyclase, we should expect that the effect of ADP on the energy charge would also be prevented, if ADP acts by reducing the amount of ATP available to the cyclase. In fact, NEM causes only a small, variable reduction of the effect of ADP on the energy charge. These results, which will be presented elsewhere, make it unlikely that the substrate competition theory alone will be adequate to explain the effects of ADP on the cyclase system.

ACKNOWLEDGMENTS

This work was supported in part by the National Heart and Lung Institute, Grant HL 14217. I am indebted to Mrs. Carol Lipson for excellent technical assistance. Prostaglandin E_1 was a generous gift from Dr. J. E. Pike of the Upjohn Co., Kalamazoo, Mich., and RA233 (2,6-bis-(diethanolamino)-4-piperidinopyrimido-[5,4d]-pyrimidine) were kindly provided by Dr. J. W. Bell of Boehringer Ingelheim Ltd., Isleworth, Middlesex. I thank Prof. R. M. Hardisty for permission to publish my investigations of one of his thrombasthenic patients.

REFERENCES

Ardlie, N. G., Glew, G., Schultz, B. G., and Schwartz, C. J. 1967. Inhibition and reversal of platelet aggregation by methyl xanthines. Thromb. Diath. Haemorrh. 18: 670.

Ball, G., Brereton, G. G., Fulwood, M., Ireland, D. M., and Yates, P. 1970. Effect of prostaglandin E_1 alone and in combination with theophylline or aspirin on collagen induced platelet aggregation and on platelet nucleotides including adenosine 3′:5′ cyclic monophosphate. Biochem. J. 102: 709.

Ball, G., Fulwood, M., Ireland, D. M., and Yates, P. 1969. Effect of some inhibitors of platelet aggregation on platelet nucleotides. Biochem. J. 114: 669.

Born, G. V. R. 1962. Aggregation of blood platelets by adenosine diphosphate and its reversal. Nature 194: 927.

Brodie, G. N., Baenziger, N. L., Chase, L. R., and Majerus, P. W. 1972. The effects of thrombin on adenyl cyclase activity and a membrane protein from human platelets. J. Clin. Invest. 51: 81.

Butcher, R. W. 1970. Prostaglandins and cyclic AMP, pp. 173–183. *In* P. Greengard and E. Costa (eds.) Role of cyclic AMP in cell function. Raven Press, New York.

Droller, M. J., and Wolfe, S. M. 1972. Uncertain role of cAMP in platelet function. New Engl. J. Med. 286: 948.

Ellman, G. L. 1959. Tissue sulfhydryl groups. Arch. Biochem. Biophys. 82: 70.

Hardisty, R. M., Dormandy, K., and Hutton, R. A. 1964. Thrombasthenia: Studies on three cases. Brit. J. Haematol. 10: 371.

Harwood, J. P., Moskowitz, J., and Krishna, G. 1972. Dynamic interactions of prostaglandin and norepinephrine in the formation of adenosine 3′:5′-monophosphate in human and rabbit platelets. Biochim. Biophys. Acta 261: 444.

Haslam, R. J., and Taylor, A. 1971a. Role of cyclic 3′:5′-adenosine monophosphate in platelet aggregation, pp. 85–93. *In* J. P. Caen (ed.) Platelet aggregation. Masson et Cie, Paris.

Haslam, R. J., and Taylor, A. 1971b. Effects of catecholamines on the formation of adenosine 3′:5′ cyclic monophosphate in human blood platelets. Biochem. J. 125: 377.

Holmsen, H., Day, H. J., and Setkowsky, C. A. 1972. Secretory mechanisms. Behaviour of adenine nucleotides during the platelet release reaction induced by adenosine diphosphate and adrenaline. Biochem. J. 129: 67.

Ireland, D. M. 1967. Effect of thrombin on the radioactive nucleotides of human washed platelets. Biochem. J. 105: 857.

Kinlough-Rathbone, R. L., Packham, M. A., and Mustard, J. F. 1970. The effect of prostaglandin E_1 on platelet function *in vitro* and *in vivo.* Brit. J. Haematol. 19: 559.

Kloeze, J. 1967. Influence of prostaglandins on platelet adhesiveness and platelet aggregation, pp. 241–252. *In* S. Bergstrom and B. Samuelsson (eds.) Proceedings of 2nd Nobel Symposium. Interscience, New York.

Krishna, G., Weiss, B., and Brodie, B. B. 1968. A simple, sensitive method for the assay of adenyl cyclase. J. Pharmacol. Exp. Ther. 163: 379.

MacMillan, D. C., and Oliver, M. F. 1965. The initial changes in platelet morphology following the addition of adenosine diphosphate. J. Atheroscler. Res. 5: 440.

Marquis, N. R., Becker, J. A., and Vigdahl, R. L. 1970. Platelet aggregation. III. An epinephrine induced decrease in cyclic AMP synthesis. Biochem. Biophys. Res. Commun. 39: 783.

Mills, D. C. B. 1973. Nature New Biol. 243: 220.

Mills, D. C. B., and Roberts, G. C. K. 1967. Effects of adrenaline on human blood platelets. J. Physiol. (London) 193: 443.

Mills, D. C. B., and Smith, J. B. 1971. The influence on platelet aggregation of drugs that effect the accumulation of adenosine 3′:5′ cyclic monophosphate in platelets. Biochem. J. 121: 185.

Mills, D. C. B., and Smith, J. B. 1972. The control of platelet responsiveness by agents that influence cyclic AMP metabolism. Ann. N.Y. Acad. Sci. 201: 391.

Moskowitz, J., Harwood, J. P., Reid, W. D., and Krishna, G. 1971. The interaction of norepinephrine and prostaglandin E_1 on the adenyl cyclase of human and rabbit blood platelets. Biochim. Biophys. Acta 230: 279.

Poch, G., Juan, H., and Kukovetz, W. R. 1969. Influence of cardio- and vasoactive substances on phosphodiesterase activity. Naunyn-Schmiedebergs Arch. Pharmakol. Exp. Pathol. 264: 293.

Robinson, C. W., Jr., Mason, R. G., and Wagner, R. H. 1963. Effect of sulfhydryl inhibitors on platelet agglutinability. Proc. Soc. Exp. Biol. Med. 113: 857.

Robison, G. A., Arnold, A., and Hartmann, R. C. 1969. Divergent effects of epinephrine and prostaglandin E_1 on the level of cyclic AMP in human blood platelets. Pharm. Res. Commun. 1: 325.

Robison, G. A., Butcher, R. W., and Sutherland, E. W. 1971. Cyclic AMP. Academic Press, New York.

Salzman, E. W. 1971. Cyclic AMP and platelet function. New Engl. J. Med. 286: 358.

Salzman, E. W., and Neri, L. L. 1969. Cyclic 3′:5′ adenosine monophosphate in human blood platelets. Nature 224: 609.

Sattin, A., and Rall, T. W. 1970. The effect of adenosine and adenine nucleotides on the cyclic adenosine 3′:5′ phosphate content of guinea pig cerebral cortex slices. Mol. Pharmacol. 6: 13.

Shio, H., Ramwell, P. W., and Jessup, S. J. 1972. Prostaglandin E_2: Effects on aggregation, shape change and cyclic AMP of rat platelets. Prostaglandins 1: 29.

Smith, J. B., and Mills, D. C. B. 1970. Inhibition of adenosine 3′:5′ cyclic monophosphate phosphodiesterase. Biochem. J. 120: 20.

Smith, J. B., and Willis, A. L. 1970. Formation and release of prostaglandins by platelets in response to thrombin. Brit. J. Pharmacol. 40: 545.

Webb, J. L. 1966. Enzyme and metabolic inhibitors, Vol. 3. Academic Press, New York.

White, J. G. 1968. Fine structural alterations induced in platelets by adenosine diphosphate. Blood 31: 604.

Zieve, P. D., and Greenough, W. B., III. 1969. Adenyl cyclase in human platelets: activity and responsiveness. Biochem. Biophys. Res. Commun. 35: 462.

The Storage of Serotonin in Human Platelets

P. K. Schick and B. P. Yu

The effects of methylene blue and phospholipase C on the storage of serotonin in human platelets were investigated. Methylene blue (2×10^{-4} M) induces a linear rate of release of 48 per cent of platelet serotonin during 15 min. Methylene blue selectively releases serotonin and does not release storage pool ADP, cytoplasmic potassium, or metabolic pool ADP. Following the incubation of platelets with methylene blue, "holes" can be seen after 5 min in virtually all α-granules in otherwise morphologically normal platelets. Serotonin organelles (dense bodies) remain undisturbed even after 30-min incubation with methylene blue. This study indicates that methylene blue alters the affinity between serotonin and platelet storage organelles. Methylene blue may induce the release of serotonin stored in α-granules but not from dense bodies.

Phospholipase C does not usually cause the clumping of platelets, but occasionally clumping occurs following the addition of the enzyme. Phospholipase C, 0.4 units/ml, causes the hydrolysis of 32 per cent of platelet phospholipids and the release of 18 per cent of serotonin in unclumped platelets during 10 min. In clumped platelets phospholipase C, 0.4 units/ml, causes the destruction of 65 per cent of membrane phospholipids and releases only 23 per cent of serotonin during 10 min. This indicates that phospholipase C does not attack serotonin storage organelles despite massive destruction of granule membranes, and that the enzyme releases small amounts of serotonin stored in the plasma membrane.

The platelet has only recently been recognized to be a highly complex cell with numerous metabolic activities. There are intricate mechanisms present in blood platelets for the transport and storage of serotonin. This biogenic amine is not present in significant amounts in other blood cells or in human plasma (Paasonen, 1965). Aggregating agents such as thrombin or collagen can release both platelet serotonin and ADP (Holmsen *et al.*, 1969). The role of platelet serotonin and its release is not clear but conceivably may be important for platelet physiological activities (Baumgartner, 1969).

Drugs such as reserpine and chlorpromazine can induce the release of serotonin from platelets as well as from the neuron. The platelet has been used as an easily obtained model system for the investigation of serotonin transport and storage (Paasonen, 1965).

Methylene blue and phospholipase C have recently been shown to release platelet serotonin (Schick and Yu, 1972, 1973). In this paper the effects of methylene blue and phospholipase C on the storage of serotonin in platelets will be considered.

MATERIALS AND METHODS

Methylene Blue and Phospholipase C

Methylene blue was obtained from Applied Science. Phospholipase C from *Clostridium welchii* was obtained from Sigma (St. Louis, Missouri). The enzyme was purified and tested for neuraminidase and proteolytic activity by methods described by Macchia and Pastan (1967). Phospholipase activity was determined and expressed in units as described by Rodbell (1966).

Preparation of Platelet Suspensions

Platelet-rich plasma (PRP) was prepared as previously described (Schick *et al.*, 1972), except that the freshly drawn blood had been anticoagulated with 3.2 per cent trisodium citrate (9 parts blood to 1 part citrate). The effect of methylene blue on serotonin release was investigated by using PRP that had been buffered with Trismaleate (75 m*M*) at pH 7.8. For the phospholipase C studies, platelets were resuspended in artificial medium buffered at pH 7.4 as described by Haslam (1964), except that it contained glucose (0.005 *M*) and $CaCl_2$ (0.1 m*M*). Cell counts were performed as previously described (Schick *et al.*, 1972). Platelet counts varied between 450,000 and 650,000/mm^3 in PRP and between 250,000 and 500,000/mm^3 in modified Haslam medium. Erythrocyte and leukocyte contamination was not significant. Only siliconized glassware was used.

Platelet Serotonin Release

Serotonin release was determined by using platelets that were preloaded with ^{14}C-serotonin by methods previously described (Schick *et al.*, 1972). The percentage of serotonin released was calculated by measuring the radioactivity in aliquots of filtrates and PRP using the following formula:

$$\% \text{ Serotonin released} = \frac{\text{CPM (test filtrate)} - \text{CPM (control filtrate)}}{\text{CPM (PRP)} - \text{CPM (control filtrate)}} \times 100.$$

Phospholipase C-Induced Hydrolysis

Estimates of the degree of phospholipase C-induced destruction of platelet membranes and serotonin release were performed concomitantly. Platelets were preloaded with ^{14}C-serotonin prior to their resuspension in modified Haslam medium. Phospholipase C dissolved in 0.1 ml of diluent was added to 1.9 ml of platelets resuspended in artificial medium to achieve the desired final concentration. The reaction mixtures were shaken gently in a Dubnoff metabolic shaker at 37°C. At the end of the incubation period the reaction mixtures were chilled in an ice bath and filtered. Phospholipids were extracted from platelets that had been collected on GF/A filters, and the lipid phosphorus in the extracts was determined as previously described (Schick *et al.*, 1972). The percentage of hydrolysis of platelet phospholipids was calculated from the ratio of lipid phosphorus present in enzyme-treated platelet to that in control experiments. The filtrates were assayed for the percentage of serotonin released as described above. The presence of platelet clumping was checked visually as well as under phase-contrast microscopy in the course of the incubations.

Release of Metabolic Pool ADP

Platelet metabolic pool ADP was labeled by incubating PRP with ^{14}C-adenine (New England Nuclear, NEC-005, specific activity 5.5 mCi/m*M*), 0.9 nmoles/ml PRP, for 60 min at 37°C. The percentage of leakage of ^{14}C-ADP was measured by the calculation described above under serotonin release.

Release of Storage Pool ADP

Perchloric acid extracts, 2 *N*, of filtrates of the reaction mixtures were neutralized with 3 *M* K_2CO_3 and then assayed for nonradioactive ADP by the method described by Holmsen *et al.* (1972).

Release of Platelet Potassium

Potassium present in filtrates of reaction mixtures was measured by atomic absorption spectrometry. For potassium studies platelets were resuspended in Haslam medium (Haslam, 1964) enriched with glucose (0.005 *M*).

Electronmicroscopy

Platelets were prepared for electronmicroscopy by the method described by White (1968). The specimens were examined with a Phillips EM 300 electronmicroscope.

RESULTS

Table 1 shows that the rate of methylene blue-induced serotonin release is linear, and that methylene blue (2×10^{-4} *M*) releases 48.5 per cent of platelet serotonin during 15 min. Table 2 demonstrates that concentrations of methylene blue that release more than 50 per cent of platelet serotonin do not release significant amounts of storage pool ADP, metabolic pool ADP, or cytoplasmic potassium.

The influence of methylene blue on the platelet's ultrastructure is shown in Fig. 1a. Methylene blue in concentrations that release substantial amounts of platelet serotonin also induced the development of "holes" in α-granules in virtually every platelet after

Table 1. Rate of methylene blue-induced serotonin release

Time (min)	Per cent serotonin released by methylene blue ($2 \times 10^{-4} M$)
2.5	8.5 ± 1.1
5	15.5 ± 2.0
10	34.0 ± 2.5
15	48.5 ± 2.8

Values are expressed as means ± SD of four experiments.

5-min incubations. Platelets incubated with the dye seem to be otherwise morphologically normal, and dense bodies are undisturbed even after 30-min periods, as shown in Fig. 1a. Figure 1b is a photomicrograph of a representative platelet from a 30-min control experiment.

Phospholipase C did not usually cause the clumping of platelets, but in occasional experiments the addition of the enzyme was followed by platelet clumping.

Table 3 shows the relationship between the concentration of phospholipase C and the percentage of phospholipid hydrolysis. The effects of phospholipase C on unclumped and clumped platelets are demonstrated. Platelets that had not clumped seemed to be resistant, and the phospholipase C concentration of 0.4 units/ml only induced the hydrolysis of 32.7 per cent of platelet phospho-

Table 2. Release of platelet constituents other than serotonin

Inducing agent	^{14}C-ADP (metabolic pool) (%)	ADP (storage pool) (5×10^8 cells) (nmoles)	Potassium (5×10^8 cells) (μmoles)
MB ($2 \times 10^{-4} M$)	53 ± 4.8	0.33 ± 0.31	0.09 ± 0.03
Freeze-thaw	75 ± 5.0		0.40 ± 0.04
Thrombin (10 units)		5.16 ± 0.50	
Control	0*	0	0.19 ± 0.19†

Values are expressed as means ± SD of four experiments.

* Controls were adjusted to zero.

† Potassium present in control filtrates represented carry-over from plasma.

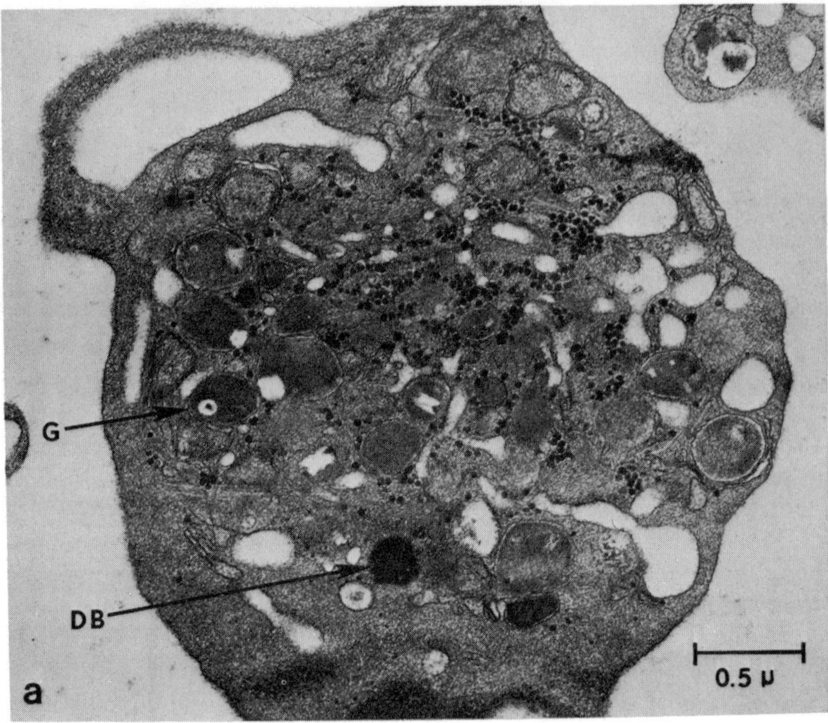

Figure 1a. Photomicrograph of the ultrastructural features of a methylene blue-treated platelet. A representative cell is shown from an experiment in which platelet-rich plasma was incubated with methylene blue (2×10^{-4} *M*) for 30 min. More than 50 per cent of platelet serotonin was released. DB, dense body; G, granule. × 11,200.

lipids during 10 min. Clumped platelets were considerably more susceptible, and maximal destruction of 65.1 per cent of platelet phospholipids occurred at enzyme concentrations of 0.2 units/ml during 10 min.

Table 3 also demonstrates that the relationship between the percentage of serotonin released and the concentration of phospholipase C is not linear. Very little serotonin is released by low concentrations of the enzyme, and high concentrations only release 18.2 per cent during 10 min. The magnitude of serotonin released was proportional to the degree of phospholipid destruction in unclumped platelets. The massive destruction of platelet phospholipids that occurred in clumped platelets did not result in

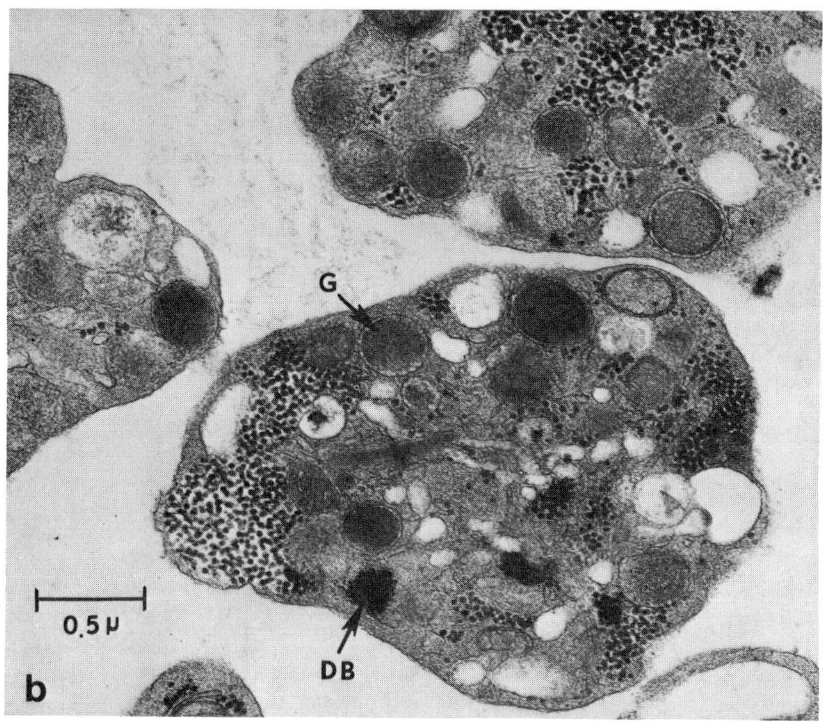

Figure 1b. Photomicrograph of the ultrastructural features of representative platelets from a 30-min control experiment. DB, dense body; G, granule. × 11,200.

the release of significant amounts of additional serotonin during 10 min. In contrast, Table 4 shows that the relationship of the rate of platelet serotonin released to the concentration of methylene blue is linear at low concentrations of the dye. Maximal serotonin release occurs at concentrations of 2×10^{-4} M methylene blue which releases 30.5 per cent of serotonin during 10 min. Platelets seem to be resistant to the induction of serotonin release by phospholipase C but not to the action of methylene blue.

DISCUSSION

A number of agents are known to release platelet serotonin, but most likely only a few mechanisms exist for the release of this amine. Methylene blue and phospholipase C are newly discovered

Table 3. Effect of phospholipase C on human platelets

Phospholipase C (concentration, units/ml)	Per cent phospholipid hydrolysis during 10 min	Per cent serotonin released during 10 min
	In unclumped platelets	
0.1	1.5 ± 1.3	0.7 ± 0.5
0.2	3.0 ± 2.0	4.7 ± 1.2
0.3	9.5 ± 3.2	9.5 ± 2.8
0.4	32.7 ± 5.8	18.2 ± 5.2
	In clumped platelets	
0.1	31.7 ± 3.7	0.8 ± 0.6
0.2	65.1 ± 5.8	7.3 ± 3.0
0.3	63.0 ± 6.1	10.1 ± 3.1
0.4	65.4 ± 7.2	23.2 ± 5.0

Values are expressed as means ± SD of four experiments.

Table 4. Release of serotonin in relation to concentration of methylene blue

Methylene blue (*M*)	Per cent serotonin released during 10 min
0.5×10^{-4}	11.5 ± 1.1
1×10^{-4}	20.0 ± 1.9
2×10^{-4}	30.5 ± 2.8
3×10^{-4}	31.5 ± 2.7
4×10^{-4}	31.3 ± 2.9

Values are expressed as means ± SD of four experiments.

releasers of platelet serotonin (Schick and Yu, 1972, 1973), and appear to act at different serotonin storage sites.

Serotonin is thought to be stored in several platelet compartments, primarily in dense bodies and possibly also in the plasma membrane (Baumgartner and Born, 1969). The rapidity of methylene blue-induced serotonin release suggests that the dye either selectively alters the affinity between serotonin and its storage organelles or causes leakage of serotonin by damaging the platelet. Reserpine and metabolic inhibitors such as iodoacetate cause a considerably slower rate of serotonin release, about 30 per cent during 1 hr (Buckingham and Maynert, 1964). Reserpine is thought to block the uptake of serotonin into dense bodies, and metabolic inhibitors interfere with the active transport of the amine (Pletscher *et al.*, 1967).

This study clearly shows that methylene blue specifically releases serotonin, but does not cause the leakage of cytoplasmic potassium or metabolic pool ADP. Chlorpromazine and *p*-chloromercuribenzoic acid are thought to increase platelet permeability for potassium and amino acids as well as serotonin (Buckingham, 1964). Methylene blue, unlike thrombin or collagen (Holmsen *et al.*, 1969), does not trigger the release reaction, since the dye does not release storage pool ADP. Therefore, methylene blue does not seem to damage the platelet plasma membrane, and the rapid release is probably due to the dye's action on a major serotonin storage site, most likely in platelet organelles.

White (unpublished data) has demonstrated the effects of methylene blue on platelets. Following the incubation of platelets with methylene blue, "holes" could be seen in α-granules in otherwise morphologically normal platelets. He has interpreted these changes as representing the removal of a portion of the nucleoid of α-granules. Serotonin storage organelles (dense bodies) were undisturbed. We have observed the same phenomenon after 5-min incubations. If the dye released serotonin that had been stored in these "holes," then this study indicates that methylene blue induces the releases of serotonin from an organelle storage site which is separate from dense bodies. Currently, serotonin is thought to be stored primarily in specialized platelet organelles known as dense bodies (Tranzer *et al.*, 1966). Not excluded is the possibility that the methylene blue-induced "holes" may be due to an effect of the dye not related to its ability to release serotonin.

In order to interpret the significance of phospholipase C-induced release of platelet serotonin, we must consider the effect of the enzyme on platelets. Phospholipase C can hydrolyze membrane phosphatidylcholine and sphingomyelin, which represent about 60 per cent of platelet phospholipids (Schick *et al.*, 1972). Therefore, about 60 per cent of platelet phospholipids can potentially serve as substrate for phospholipase C.

In intact platelets high concentrations of phospholipase C only hydrolyzed 32 per cent of platelet phospholipids, possibly because the enzyme did not penetrate the plasma membrane and only destroyed phospholipids on the platelet surface. Occasionally, unexplained clumping of platelets occurred following the addition of phospholipase C. Low concentrations of the enzyme caused the hydrolysis of 65 per cent of platelet phospholipids in clumped platelets, indicating that massive destruction of both plasma and organelle membranes had occurred.

The marked difference in the degree of membrane destruction in clumped and unclumped platelets provided an opportunity to investigate the role of platelet membranes in serotonin storage. Phospholipase C probably releases small amounts of serotonin stored in the platelet's plasma membrane. This is suggested by the observation that in unclumped platelets the amount of serotonin release is proportional to the degree of "plasma membrane" destruction. Our assumption that in unclumped platelets phospholipase C only attacks the plasma membrane is discussed above. The absence of significant release of additional serotonin when phospholipase C had induced massive destruction of both plasma and granule membranes in clumped platelets indicates that the storage of serotonin in granules is not dependent on the integrity of granule membranes.

Methylene blue appears to release selectively serotonin stored in platelet organelles. Most likely granule storage sites are not attacked by phospholipase C, and the enzyme may only release serotonin that is stored in the plasma membrane. The further use of these agents should help clarify the mechanisms for the storage of serotonin in human platelets.

ACKNOWLEDGMENTS

This investigation was supported by grants from The Pennsylvania Heart Association and The Medical College of Pennsylvania. The authors would like to acknowledge the assistance of Drs. Walter Rubin and Wesley Stile in the electronmicroscopic studies, and that of Dr. Joel Steinberg in the purification of phospholipase C. The released nonradioactive ADP was kindly measured by Dr. David Mills.

REFERENCES

Baumgartner, H. R. 1969. 5-Hydroxytryptamine uptake and release in relation to aggregation of rabbit platelets. J. Physiol. (London) 201: 409.

Baumgartner, H. R., and Born, G. V. R. 1969. The relation between the 5-hydroxytryptamine content and aggregation of rabbit platelets. J. Physiol. (London) 201: 397.

Buckingham, S., and Maynert, E. W. 1964. The release of 5-hydroxytryptamine, potassium, and amino acids from platelets. J. Pharm. Exp. Therap. 143: 332.

Haslam, R. J. 1964. Role of adenosine diphosphate in aggregation of human blood-platelets by thrombin and by fatty acids. Nature 202: 765.

Holmsen, H., Day, H. J., and Stormorken, H. 1969. The blood platelet release reaction. Scand. J. Haematol. Suppl. 8: 1.

Holmsen, H., Storm, E., and Day, H. J. 1972. Determination of ATP and ADP in blood platelets: A modification of the firefly luciferase assay for plasma. Anal. Biochem. 46: 489.

Macchia, U., and Pastan, I. 1967. Action of phospholipase C on the thyroid. J. Biol. Chem. 242: 1864.

Paasonen, M. K. 1965. Release of 5-hydroxytryptamine from blood platelets. J. Pharm. Pharmacol. 17: 681.

Pletscher, A., Burkard, W. P., Tranzer, J. P., and Gey K. F. 1967. Two sites of 5-hydroxytryptamine uptake in blood platelets. Life Sci. 6:273.

Rodbell, M. 1966. Metabolism of isolated fat cells. J. Biol. Chem. 241: 130.

Tranzer, J. P., DaPrado, M., and Pletscher, A. 1966. Ultrastructural localization of 5-hydroxytryptamine in blood platelets. Nature 212: 1574.

Schick, P. K., Spaet, T. H., and Jaffé, E. R. 1972. The effects of phenazinemethosulfate and methylene blue on human platelet phospholipid synthesis. Proc. Soc. Exp. Med. Biol. 141: 114.

Schick, P. K., and Yu, B. P. 1972. Serotonin release in human platelets. Clin. Res. 20: 499 (abstr.).

Schick, P. K., and Yu, B. P. 1973. Methylene blue-induced serotonin release in human platelets. J. Lab. Clin. Med. In press.

White, J. G. 1968. Fine structural alterations induced in platelets by adenosine diphosphate. Blood 31: 604.

Prostaglandins: Are They Intracellular Messengers?

J. B. Smith, M. J. Silver, C. Ingerman, and J. J. Kocsis

The concept that endogenous prostaglandins function as intracellular messengers of hormonal response is discussed with reference to: (*a*) the interactions between exogenous prostaglandins and endogenous cyclic AMP in various tissues; (*b*) the associations between endogenous prostaglandins and endogenous cyclic AMP; (*c*) the actions of exogenous prostaglandins on platelet function and platelet cyclic AMP; (*d*) evidence which links the synthesis of endogenous prostaglandins to platelet function. Several possible mechanisms of action of endogenous platelet prostaglandins are outlined.

The concept that endogenous prostaglandins (PG) may function as intracellular regulators of the hormonal response has developed from investigations with a variety of cell types (Shio *et al.*, 1971). There is now considerable information about the actions of exogenous prostaglandins on platelets and platelet enzymes, and also some recent findings about prostaglandins that are intrinsic to platelets. Therefore, it seems worthwhile to consider whether endogenous prostaglandins could play a role in regulating platelet response.

EXOGENOUS PROSTAGLANDINS AND CYCLIC AMP

Prostaglandins are related to "prostanoic acid," a 20-carbon carboxylic acid containing a cyclopentane ring (Fig. 1). Prostaglandins E_1 and E_2 contain a keto group at position 9, an hydroxyl group at position 11, a double bond at position 13, and a second hydroxyl group at position 15. Prostaglandin (PG) E_2 differs from prostaglandin E_1 by the presence of an additional double bond at position 5. Prostaglandins E_1 or E_2, or both, have been reported to activate adenylate cyclase, increase cyclic AMP, and mimic the effect of the stimulating hormone in the anterior pituitary, corpus luteum, and thyroid (Ramwell and Shaw, 1970). Moreover, prostaglandins E_1 or E_2 have an amazing diversity of biological effects (Weeks, 1972), and promote the formation of cyclic AMP in bone, diaphragm, heart, leukocytes, lung, lymphocytes, ovary, placenta, red cells, and spleen (Hinman, 1972). However, in adipose tissue prostaglandins E_1 and E_2 antagonize the hormonally induced increases in cyclic AMP and inhibit lipolysis. In fat cells prostaglandin E_1 inhibits epinephrine-induced in-

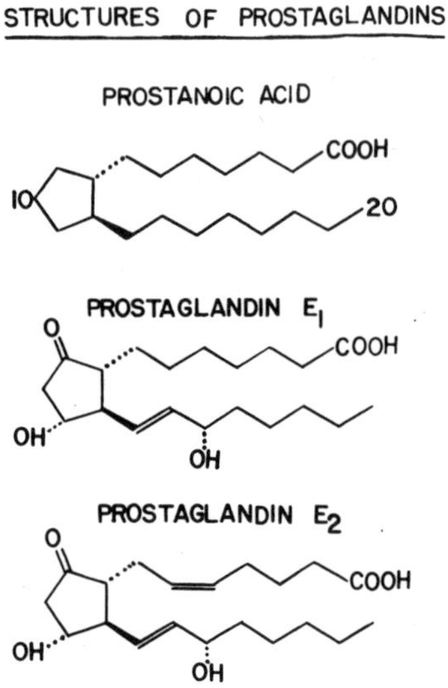

Figure 1. Prostanoic acid is a hypothetical structure with 20 carbon atoms and a cyclopentane ring. It is the carbon skeleton of most of the naturally occurring prostaglandins, such as prostaglandin E_1 and prostaglandin E_2.

creases in cyclic AMP at a concentration of 4×10^{-11} *M* (Butcher and Baird, 1968), and in red cells prostaglandin E_2 activates adenylate cyclase at a concentration as low as 10^{-13} *M* (Allen and Rasmussen, 1971).

Where investigated, other naturally occurring prostaglandins such as the PGA, PGB, or PGF compounds have been found to be less active than the PGE compounds in modifying the levels of cyclic AMP.

ENDOGENOUS PROSTAGLANDINS AND CYCLIC AMP

Prostaglandins were discovered in human semen, where they are present in high concentration (Bergström, 1967). It is noteworthy that the concentration of cyclic AMP in human semen is also very high (10^{-5} *M*) (Broadus *et al.*, 1971). Indeed, there are some intriguing associations in mammals between the formation of prostaglandins and the formation of cyclic AMP. First, it is becoming apparent that the production of prostaglandins is almost as ubiquitous as that of cyclic AMP with respect to both tissues and species. Second, the biosynthesis of prostaglandins is believed to be intimately linked to changes in the cell membrane, as is the synthesis of cyclic AMP (Robison and Sutherland, 1971). For prostaglandin biosynthesis it is supposed that, in response to

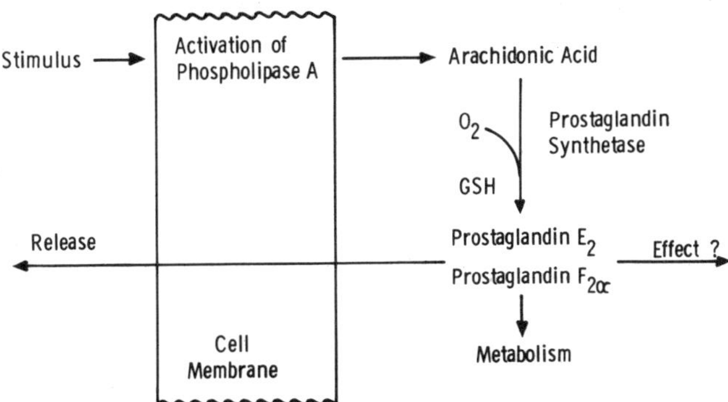

Figure 2. Conceptual scheme for the endogenous biosynthesis of prostaglandins. Formation of prostaglandins depends initially on the release of free unsaturated fatty acids from ester linkage with membrane phospholipid. Released arachidonic acid is converted to prostaglandins E_2 and F_{2a} whereas released 8,11,14-eicosatrienoic acid would be converted to prostaglandins E_1 and F_{1a}.

various types of stimulation, a phospholipase A is activated and liberates unsaturated fatty acids from the membrane phospholipids (Fig. 2). Certain of these fatty acids, such as arachidonic acid, are then converted into prostaglandins by a microsomal enzyme system, prostaglandin synthetase. This reaction involves the incorporation of molecular oxygen and is stimulated by glutathione (Samuelsson, 1969). The third association between prostaglandins and cyclic AMP is that stimulation of the synthesis of either results in their being released from the cell or degraded intracellularly. These associations, and the ability of E-type prostaglandins to modify cyclic AMP levels when used in very low concentrations, have led some investigators to propose that endogenous prostaglandins may be intermediary between hormonal stimulation and changes in cyclic AMP (Shio *et al.*, 1971).

Study of the role of endogenous prostaglandins or endogenous cyclic AMP has been hampered because of the small amounts of them which are formed upon hormonal stimulation and the even lower levels of these compounds which occur in unstimulated cells. However, techniques are now available for the measurement of prostaglandins by radioimmunoassay (Hinman, 1972) and of cyclic AMP by radioimmunoassay or protein binding (Chasin, 1972). These methods are specific, sensitive, and accurate enough to answer many of the questions that earlier studies have raised. For example, Shaw and Ramwell (1968) have reported that adipose tissue releases prostaglandin E_1 on hormonal stimulation, whereas Christ and Nugteren (1970) believe that this tissue releases principally prostaglandin E_2. The observation of Salzman and Neri (1969) that ADP or epinephrine lowers the basal levels of cyclic AMP in platelets awaits confirmation. Studies of prostaglandin formation by human platelets using biological assay led to the conclusion that they synthesize prostaglandins E_2 and $F_{2\alpha}$ from endogenous fatty acids (Smith and Willis, 1970). That $PGF_{2\alpha}$ is formed during platelet aggregation has now been demonstrated by radioimmunoassay (Silver *et al.*, this symposium).

EXOGENOUS PROSTAGLANDINS AND PLATELETS

The initial observation that prostaglandin E_1 inhibits the aggregation of platelets (Kloeze, 1967) has been confirmed by many investigators. Apart from some closely related synthetic analogues, such as ω-homo-PGE_1 (Kloeze, 1969) and 2-*trans*-PGE (Van

Dorp, 1971), it is the most potent inhibitor of aggregation yet described and produces a marked effect at a concentration of 5×10^{-8} *M*. Platelets differ from most other tissues in that there appears to be a qualitative difference between the effect of prostaglandin E_1 and that of prostaglandin E_2. With platelets from various species other than humans, prostaglandin E_2 in low concentrations (5×10^{-8} to 1×10^{-6} *M*) stimulates aggregation (Kloeze, 1967). The divergent effects of prostaglandins E_1 and E_2 on the collagen-induced aggregation of human platelets are shown in Fig. 3. The addition of prostaglandin E_1 before collagen inhibits aggregation and this effect is reduced by previous addition of prostaglandin E_2. However, the effects of prostaglandin E_2 on the aggregation of human platelets are not straightforward as will be

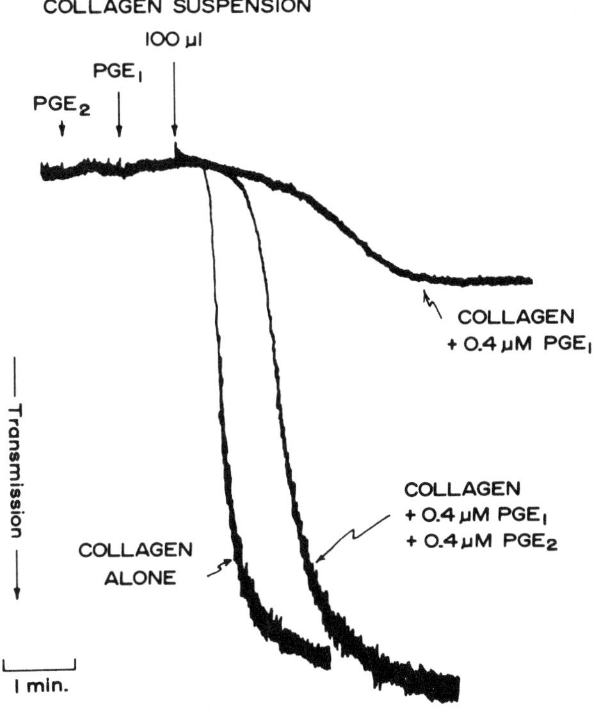

Figure 3. Effects of prostaglandin E_1 alone and in combination with prostaglandin E_2 on the aggregation of human platelets induced by collagen. Three tracings are superimposed and increasing light transmission indicates increasing platelet aggregation.

considered later. Prostaglandin E_1 or, to a much lesser extent, prostaglandin E_2 activates platelet adenylate cyclase (Wolfe and Shulman, 1969, Marquis *et al.*, 1969). By contrast, whereas prostaglandin E_1 dramatically increases the level of cyclic AMP in platelets (Cole *et al.*, 1971), prostaglandin E_2 reduces prostaglandin E_1-induced cyclic AMP accumulation (Shio *et al.*, 1972). Salzman (1972) has found that PGE_2 by itself reduced cyclic AMP in platelets. Prostaglandins of the A-, B-, or F-types are less effective than the E-types as modifiers of platelet aggregation or of the platelet adenylate cyclase system.

ENDOGENOUS PROSTAGLANDINS AND PLATELETS

Our belief that endogenous prostaglandins play a regulatory role in platelet function rests on three findings. First, prostaglandins E_2 and $F_{2\alpha}$ are formed by human platelets in response to agents which release endogenous ADP and induce aggregation. Second, the drugs aspirin and indomethacin, which inhibit the release of endogenous ADP and aggregation, inhibit platelet prostaglandin biosynthesis. These findings are dealt with in the following paper. The third finding is that arachidonic acid, the precursor of prostaglandins E_2 and $F_{2\alpha}$, induces the release of labeled serotonin from platelets (Leonardi *et al.*, 1972). It also induces irreversible platelet aggregation, presumably because of the release of endogenous ADP (Fig. 4). Other fatty acids, such as linolenic acid, do not elicit these effects. In platelet-rich plasma, aggregation is brought about by arachidonic acid in concentrations of 0.1 m*M* or greater and prostaglandin E_2 formation can be demonstrated concomitant with aggregation (unpublished observations). All-*cis* 8,11,14-eicosatrienoic acid causes platelets to form prostaglandin E_1 but does not cause aggregation. However, there is one paradoxical finding. Even though exogenous prostaglandin E_2 does enhance the second wave of ADP-induced aggregation of human platelets, it does not induce aggregation (Shio and Ramwell, 1972). Taken together, these four findings are indicative, but certainly not conclusive, that endogenous platelet prostaglandins play some role in aggregation.

If endogenous prostaglandins do play some role in platelet function, how could they be working? The evidence that aggregation is mediated by a diminution of endogenous cyclic AMP and that inhibition of aggregation is mediated by an increase of cyclic

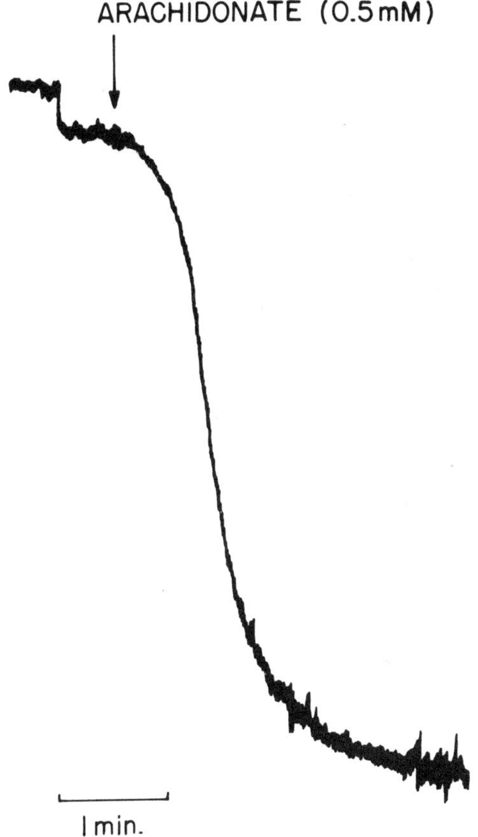

Figure 4. Aggregation induced by 0.5 m*M* arachidonic acid in human citrated platelet-rich plasma.

AMP has been reviewed elsewhere (Salzman and Levine, 1971). The observation that exogenous prostaglandin E_2 decreases endogenous cyclic AMP (Salzman, 1972) is of great interest and suggests that this is the mechanism of action of endogenous prostaglandins, but the observation requires confirmation. Several other possible mechanisms of action of endogenous platelet prostaglandins seem equally plausible at the present time. Abdulla and McFarlane (1971) have reported that prostaglandin E_2 significantly increases ADP in platelet homogenates by activation of adenylate kinase. Alternatively, Goldberg (1972) suggests that there are mechanisms by which cyclic GMP opposes effects mediated by cyclic AMP linked hormones or effectors. He calls this the "Yin–Yang" theory after the Oriental concept of the balance of opposing forces and has evidence which links release of cyclic GMP to the stimulation of uterine muscle by F-type prostaglandins. Perhaps prostaglandin $F_{2\alpha}$, formed during platelet aggregation, acts to increase cyclic GMP in platelets and so modify aggregation. Finally, it has been shown that prostaglandins can influence calcium movement (Ramwell and Shaw, 1970) and, since calcium plays a central role in platelet function, this could underlie a regulatory role of platelet prostaglandins.

ACKNOWLEDGMENT

This work was supported in part by Grants HL-6374 and HL-14890 from the National Institutes of Health.

REFERENCES

Abdulla, Y. H., and McFarlane, E. 1971. Control of adenylate kinase by prostaglandins E_2 and E_3. Biochem. Pharmacol. 20: 1726.

Allen, J. E., and Rasmussen, H. 1971. Prostaglandin- and isoproterenol-induced changes in the RBC membrane. Clin. Res. 19: 559.

Bergström, S. 1967. Prostaglandins: Members of a new hormonal system. Science 157: 382.

Broadus, A. E., Hardman, J. G., Kaminsky, N. I., Ball, J. H., Sutherland, E. W., and Liddle, G. W. 1971. Extracellular cyclic nucleotides. Ann. N.Y. Acad. Sci. 185: 50.

Butcher, R. W., and Baird, C. E. 1968. Effects of prostaglandins on adenosine 3′,5′-monophosphate levels in fat and other tissues. J. Biol. Chem. 243: 1713.

Chasin, M. (ed.), 1972. Methods in cyclic nucleotide research. p. 315. Marcel Dekker, Inc., New York.

Christ, E. J., and Nugteren, D. H. 1970. The biosynthesis and possible function of prostaglandins in adipose tissue. Biochim. Biophys. Acta 218: 296.

Cole, B., Robison, A., and Hartmann, R. C. 1971. Studies on the role of cyclic AMP in platelet function. Ann. N.Y. Acad. Sci. 185: 477.

Goldberg, N. D. 1972. Possible biological role(s) of cyclic 3′,5′-guanosine monophosphate (cyclic GMP). 5th International Congress on Pharmacology, San Francisco, July 23 (abstr.) (also quoted in Chem. Eng. News, October 16).

Hinman, J. W. 1972. Prostaglandins. Annu. Rev. Biochem. 41: 161.

Kloeze, J. 1967. Influence of prostaglandins on platelet adhesiveness and platelet aggregation, pp. 241–252. *In* S. Bergström and B. Samuelsson (eds.) Prostaglandins (Proceedings of the Second Nobel Symposium). Interscience Publishers, London.

Kloeze, J. 1969. Relationship between chemical structure and platelet aggregation activity of prostaglandins. Biochim. Biophys. Acta 187: 285.

Leonardi, R. G., Alexander, B., and White, F. 1972. Statement in oral presentation of paper at meeting of Federation of American Societies of Experimental Biology, Atlantic City, N. J.

Marquis, N. R., Vigdahl, R. L., and Tavormina, P. A. 1969. Platelet aggregation. I. Regulation by cyclic AMP and prostaglandin E_1. Biochem. Biophys. Res. Commun. 36: 965.

Ramwell, P. W., and Shaw, J. E. 1970. Biological significance of the prostaglandins. Recent Progr. Hormone Res. 26: 139.

Robison, G. A., and Sutherland, E. W. 1971. Cyclic AMP and the function of eukaryotic cells: an introduction. Ann. N.Y. Acad. Sci. 185: 5.

Salzman, E. W. 1972. Discussion, pp. 90–92. *In* P. W. Ramwell and B. B. Pharriss (eds.) Prostaglandins in cellular biology and the inflammatory process. Plenum Press, New York.

Salzman, E. W., and Levine, L. 1971. Cyclic 3′,5′-adenosine monophosphate in human blood platelets. II. Effect of N^6-2′-0-dibutyryl cyclic 3′,5′-adenosine monophosphate on platelet function. J. Clin. Invest. 50: 131.

Salzman, E. W., and Neri, L. L. 1969. Cyclic 3′,5′-adenosine monophosphate in human blood platelets. Nature 224: 609.

Samuelsson, B. 1969. Biosynthesis and metabolism of prostaglandins. Progr. Biochem. Pharmacol. 5: 109.

Shaw, J. E., and Ramwell, P. W. 1968. Release of prostaglandins from rat epididymal fat pad on nervous and hormonal stimulation. J. Biol. Chem. 243: 1498.

Shio, H., and Ramwell, P. W. 1972. Effect of prostaglandin E_2 and aspirin on the secondary aggregation of human platelets. Nature New Biol. 236: 45.

Shio, H., Ramwell, P. W., and Jessop, S. J. 1972. Prostaglandin E_2: Effects on aggregation, shape change and cyclic AMP of rat platelets. Prostaglandins 1: 29.

Shio, H., Shaw, J., and Ramwell, P. 1971. Relation of cyclic AMP to the release and actions of prostaglandins. Ann. N.Y. Acad. Sci. 185: 327.

Smith, J. B., and Willis, A. L. 1970. Formation and release of prostaglandins by platelets in response to thrombin. Brit. J. Pharmacol. 40: 545P.

Van Dorp, D. 1971. Recent developments in the biosynthesis and the analyses of prostaglandins. Ann. N.Y. Acad. Sci. 180: 181.

Weeks, J. R. 1972. Prostaglandins. Annu. Rev. Pharmacol. 12: 317.

Wolfe, S. M., and Shulman, N. R. 1969. Adenyl cyclase activity in human platelets. Biochem. Biophys. Res. Commun. 35: 265.

Persistent Inhibition by Aspirin of Collagen-induced Platelet Prostaglandin Formation

M. J. Silver, J. Hernandovich, C. Ingerman, J. J. Kocsis, and J. B. Smith

Platelets form prostaglandins E_2 and $F_{2\alpha}$ in blood during clotting and in stirred platelet-rich plasma in response to thrombin, collagen, epinephrine, or ADP. Evidence that there is an association between the hemostatic processes of platelet aggregation and blood clotting and the formation of platelet prostaglandins is summarized. This is supported by new data showing that, in humans, ingested aspirin inhibits both prostaglandin synthesis in response to collagen and platelet aggregation for several days, while these inhibitory effects are short-lived after ingestion of indomethacin. The combined data suggest that platelet prostaglandin synthesis may play a role in hemostasis.

Prostaglandins may influence a variety of important biological activities and intracellular biochemical events, as discussed in the preceding paper in this symposium.

Workers in the field of hemostasis and thrombosis became interested in the prostaglandins after the finding by Kloeze (1967) that exogenous prostaglandin (PG) E_1 was a very potent inhibitor

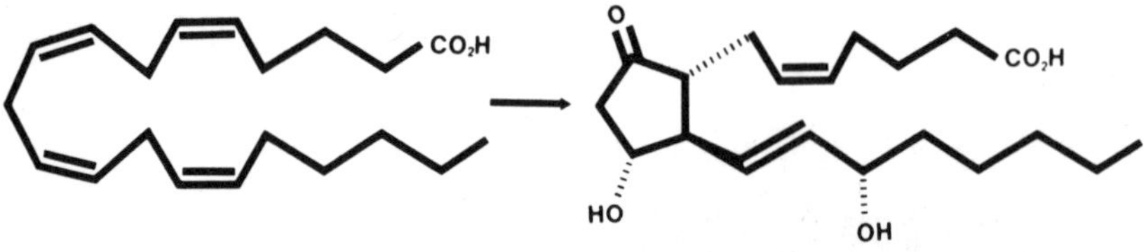

5, 8, 11, 14 — Eicosatetraenoic Acid PGE$_2$

Figure 1. Structure of arachidonic acid and prostaglandin E_2.

of platelet aggregation. More recently, Smith and Willis (1970, 1971) found that washed human platelets could in fact synthesize prostaglandins in response to thrombin, and that this synthesis could be inhibited by the nonsteroidal anti-inflammatory agents aspirin and indomethacin. Since the antihemostatic effects of aspirin are well established, it seems reasonable to hypothesize that there may be a relationship between hemostasis and the synthesis of prostaglandins by platelets. Therefore, we decided to see whether a parallelism existed between the duration of the effects of ingested aspirin on platelet aggregation and on prostaglandin production in response to collagen.

The two prostaglandins which are known to be produced by platelets in platelet-rich plasma (Silver *et al.*, 1972) and by washed platelets (Smith and Willis, 1970) are PGE_2 and $PGF_{2\alpha}$. The structure of PGE_2 along with its precursor, arachidonic acid or 5,8,11,14-eicosatetraenoic acid, is shown in Fig. 1.

METHODS

The preparation of platelet-rich plasma (PRP), the extraction and partial purification of prostaglandins from plasma, the biological assay of prostaglandin E_2, and radioimmunoassay of prostaglandin $F_{2\alpha}$ have all been described elsewhere (Silver *et al.*, 1972).

RESULTS AND DISCUSSION

Formation of Prostaglandins by Platelets during Blood Clotting and during Platelet Aggregation

Previous findings have shown that prostaglandins E_2 and $F_{2\alpha}$ are formed by platelets in blood during clotting (Silver *et al.*, 1972), in PRP in response to thrombin (Silver *et al.*, 1972), and in PRP during aggregation by well known aggregating agents (Smith *et al.*, 1972). Figure 2 shows the amounts of prostaglandins E_2 and F_{2a} found in serum from normal donors who had not ingested any drugs for a week prior to the study. Also indicated is the fact that considerable amounts of both prostaglandins are formed if platelet-rich plasma is treated with thrombin (1 unit/ml). These prostaglandins were not detected in citrated whole blood, in untreated platelet-rich plasma, or in platelet-poor plasma or platelet-poor plasma treated with thrombin. Thus, newly formed PGE_2 and PGF_{2a} found in PRP after treatment with thrombin must come from the platelets and must represent net synthesis.

Figure 3 shows the amounts of PGE_2 synthesized by human platelets in platelet-rich plasma in response to the aggregating agents collagen, epinephrine, and adenosine diphosphate (ADP). It

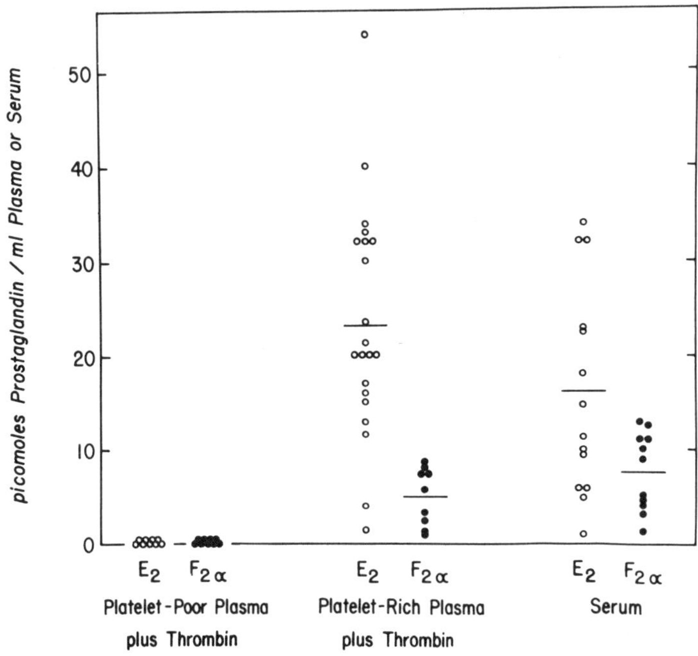

Figure 2. Concentration of prostaglandins E_2 (bioassay) and F_{2a} (radioimmunoassay) found in platelet-poor plasma treated with thrombin, platelet-rich plasma treated with thrombin, and serum prepared from whole blood allowed to clot at 37°C. In each column individual dots represent different blood donors. Horizontal lines indicate the means. (Reproduced from Silver *et al.*, 1972.)

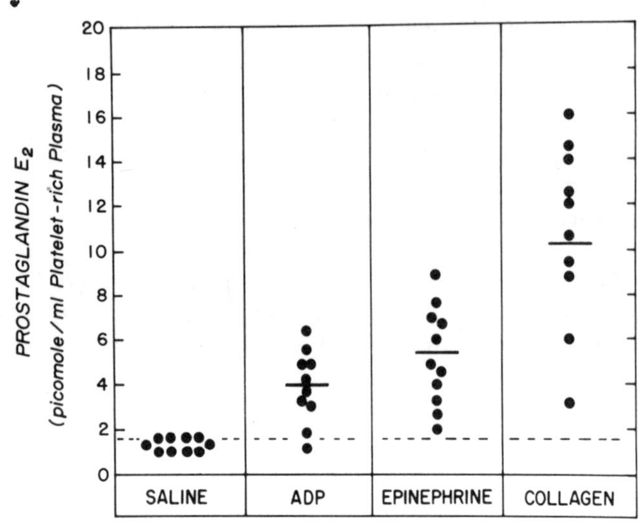

Figure 3. Concentrations of prostaglandin E_2 (bioassay) found in platelet-rich plasma after aggregation in response to several aggregating agents.

can be seen that considerable amounts of PGE_2 were formed in response to collagen, less with 40 μM epinephrine, and the least amount with 40 μM ADP.

Studies on the time course of prostaglandin synthesis indicated that prostaglandins were formed as aggregation began in response to collagen or as the second wave of aggregation appeared in response to epinephrine.

The close association between blood clotting and platelet aggregation on the one hand and the synthesis of platelet prostaglandins on the other strongly suggests that platelet prostaglandin synthesis may play a role in hemostasis and thrombosis. The evidence for this is summarized in Table 1. The first point in this table has been discussed above. Evidence for the second point comes from the work of Kloeze (1967), who showed that prostaglandin E_2 enhances aggregation of rat platelets, and from the work of Shio and Ramwell (1972), who showed that the second wave of aggregation of human platelets could be enhanced by exogenous prostaglandin E_2. Items 3 and 4 indicate that arachidonic acid, which is the precursor of prostaglandins E_2 and F_{2a}, can cause both platelet aggregation and the simultaneous formation of prostaglandins E_2 and F_{2a} when added to stirred platelet-rich plasma. These are new

Table 1. Evidence suggesting that platelet prostaglandins participate in hemostasis

1. PGE_2 and $PGF_{2\alpha}$ are formed by platelets during aggregation and clotting.
2. Exogenous PGE_2 enhances platelet aggregation.
3. Arachidonic acid causes platelet aggregation.
4. Arachidonic acid causes the formation of PGE_2 and $PGF_{2\alpha}$ during platelet aggregation.
5. Aspirin and indomethacin inhibit PG synthesis and platelet aggregation and cause prolonged bleeding time or increased loss of blood in humans.

data from our laboratory. The evidence for this will be published elsewhere. Finally it is known that aspirin and indomethacin inhibit both prostaglandin synthesis and platelet aggregation and cause prolonged bleeding times (Weiss *et al.*, 1968) or excessive loss of blood from bleeding time cuts (de Gaetano *et al.*, 1971).

Parallelism in Duration of Inhibition of Ability of Human Platelets to Synthesize Prostaglandins and Duration of Antihemostatic Effects after Ingestion of Aspirin or Indomethacin

The antihemostatic effects of aspirin and indomethacin have been the subject of many investigations (Mustard and Packham, 1970). These nonsteroidal anti-inflammatory agents inhibit collagen-induced platelet aggregation and the second wave of aggregation induced by ADP or epinephrine (O'Brien, 1968).

When aspirin or indomethacin is taken orally by humans, prostaglandin synthesis is inhibited in samples of washed platelets obtained 1 hr after ingestion of either drug (Smith and Willis, 1971). It is now recognized that aspirin and indomethacin will inhibit the synthesis of prostaglandins in a wide variety of tissues, including lung (Vane, 1971), spleen (Ferreira *et al.*, 1971), and seminal vesicles (Smith and Lands, 1971). Indeed, they have recently been shown to suppress prostaglandin output in humans (Hamberg, 1972).

Aspirin will also inhibit platelet aggregation in humans for several days, while the effects of indomethacin last less than 24 hr

(O'Brien, 1970). However, we did not know how long the inhibitory effects of these drugs on platelet prostaglandin synthesis lasted. Therefore, we considered it important to study both the inhibition of platelet aggregation and prostaglandin synthesis over a period of days after ingestion of these drugs. If the inhibitory effects of each of these drugs on platelet prostaglandin formation were to last as long as inhibition of platelet aggregation, this would be strong supporting evidence for the proposed relationship between hemostasis and prostaglandin synthesis. In these studies we followed platelet prostaglandin production in the platelet-rich plasma of four healthy donors before and at intervals after the ingestion of aspirin (13 mg/kg) or indomethacin (1.3 mg/kg). Portions of each sample of PRP were employed for aggregation studies and for estimating prostaglandin production after being stirred for 3 min at 37°C with or without collagen. Table 2 shows the amounts of prostaglandin (measured as PGE_2) produced in response to collagen in PRP samples taken before (0 hr) and at intervals after ingesting the drugs. It can be seen that, before taking the drugs, prostaglandins were detected in the PRP samples from all four donors. In control runs of stirred PRP without collagen, PGE_2 was not detected. One hour after the ingestion of aspirin or indomethacin, prostaglandins were not detected in the PRP samples in response to collagen. When aspirin was ingested prostaglandin synthesis was blocked for between 48 and 96 hr. On the other hand, when indomethacin was ingested, inhibition lasted less than 24 hr in three donors and less than 48 hr in the other donor. In each case, the platelet-rich plasma samples, taken before ingestion of either drug, produced a second wave of aggregation in response to epinephrine. One hour after ingestion of either drug the second wave of aggregation was abolished. In the case of aspirin, this effect persisted for 3–5 days. However, after indomethacin this effect on aggregation lasted less than 24 hr. In the studies where collagen was used as the aggregating agent the persistence of inhibition of aggregation was similar to that shown here for epinephrine.

The fact that the inhibitory effects of these drugs on platelet aggregation persist as long as their effects on prostaglandin production indicates that there is, indeed, a close relationship between platelet prostaglandin formation and hemostasis. Our present work is directed toward determining the exact nature of this relationship.

Table 2. Duration of inhibition of collagen-induced prostaglandin synthesis by platelets in platelet-rich plasma

		Prostaglandin E_2 (pmoles/ml PRP) at hours after ingestion of drug							
Subject	Treatment	0	1	6	24	48	72	96	120
B.S.	Aspirin	10.0*	<1	<1	<1	<1	2.5*	—	—
	Indomethacin	7.6*	<1	<1	4.0*	10.0*	—	—	—
D.A.	Aspirin	5.2*	<1	<1	<1	<1	1.5	2.1*	—
	Indomethacin	2.0*	<1	<1	<1*	3.0*	—	—	—
L.L.	Aspirin	2.4*	<1	<1	<1	<1	<1	2.0*	8.3*
	Indomethacin	1.5*	<1	<1	2.4*	1.3*	—	—	—
J.F.	Aspirin	2.6*	<1	<1	<1	<1	<1	<1	3.2*
	Indomethacin	4.0*	<1	<1	2.3*	3.7*	—	—	—

* Two waves of aggregation were recorded in PRP in response to epinephrine.

— Measurement not made.

ACKNOWLEDGMENTS

This work was supported in part by Grants HL-14890 and HL-6374 from the National Institutes of Health. The authors wish to thank Mr. Sergei Harkaway for excellent assistance with the biological assay and the ONO Pharmaceutical Co Ltd., Osaka, Japan, for the pure prostaglandin E_2 used in this work.

REFERENCES

Ferreira, S. H., Moncada, S., and Vane, J. R. 1971. Indomethacin and aspirin abolish prostaglandin release from spleen. Nature 231: 237.

De Gaetano, G., Donati, M. B., and Vermylen, J. 1971. Some effects of indomethacin on platelet function, blood coagulation and fibrinolysis. Int. Z. Klin. Pharmakol. Ther. Toxikol. 5: 196.

Hamberg, M. 1972. Inhibition of prostaglandin synthesis in man. Biochem. Biophys. Res. Commun. 49: 720.

Kloeze, J. 1967. Influence of prostaglandins on platelet adhesiveness and platelet aggregation, pp. 243–252. *In* S. Bergström and B. Samuelsson (eds.) Second Nobel Symposium: Prostaglandins. Almquist and Wiksell, Stockholm.

Mustard, J. F., and Packham, M. A. 1970. Factors influencing platelet function: adhesion, release and aggregation. Pharmacol. Rev. 22: 97.

O'Brien, J. R. 1968. Effects of salicylates on human platelets. Lancet 1: 779.

O'Brien, J. R. 1970. A comparison of an effect of different anti-inflammatory drugs on human platelets. J. Clin. Pathol. 23: 522.

Shio, H., and Ramwell, P. W. 1972. Effect of prostaglandin E_2 and aspirin on the secondary aggregation of human platelets. Nature 236: 45.

Silver, M. J., Smith, J. B., Ingerman, C., and Kocsis, J. J. 1972. Human blood prostaglandins: Formation during clotting. Prostaglandins 1: 429.

Smith, J. B., Silver, M. J., Ingerman, C., and Kocsis, J. J. 1972. Prostaglandin production during platelet aggregation, p. 246. Abstract, Third Congress of International Society on Thrombosis and Haemostasis, Washington, D. C.

Smith, J. B., and Willis, A. L. 1970. Formation and release of prostaglandins in response to thrombin. Brit. J. Pharmacol. 40: 545P. (abstr.)

Smith, J. B., and Willis, A. L. 1971. Aspirin selectively inhibits prostaglandin production in human platelets. Nature 231: 235.

Smith, W. L., and Lands, W. E. M. 1971. Stimulation and blockade of prostaglandin biosynthesis. J. Biol. Chem. 246: 6700.

Vane, J. R. 1971. Inhibition of prostaglandin synthesis as a mechanism of action for aspirin-like drugs. Nature 231: 232.

Weiss, H. J., Aledort, L. M., and Kochwa, S. 1968. The effect of salicylates on the hemostatic properties of platelets in man. J. Clin. Invest. 47: 2169.

Fibrin Retraction Induced by Platelets and Fibroblasts

S. Niewiarowski

Human and rabbit platelets, undifferentiated mouse L cells, and human skin fibroblasts retracted fibrin formed from fibrinogen by thrombin, but the retraction was inhibited when Reptilase (*Bothrops atrox* thrombin-like enzyme) was substituted for thrombin. The type of fibrin was not relevant since preincubation of rabbit platelets with thrombin followed by the incubation of this enzyme with hirudin resulted in the retraction of Reptilase-fibrin. Preincubation of rabbit platelets with collagen and preincubation of human platelets with ADP, epinephrine, or collagen also resulted in the retraction of fibrin. Prostaglandin E_1 and dibutyryl cyclic AMP inhibited platelet- or fibroblast-induced fibrin retraction in a system with thrombin.

It has been suggested that both platelet and fibroblast membranes may have sites which are susceptible to thrombin. A possible biological significance of fibrin retraction has been briefly discussed.

The phenomenon of the retraction of blood clot has been well known since the nineteenth century. Early investigators observed the absence of clot retraction in platelet diseases and suggested an involvement of platelets in this process. Duke (1912) suggested that the absence of clot retraction *in vitro* in cases of thrombocytopenia might be due to the fact that platelets were not present to anchor together the filaments of fibrin. Budtz-Olsen (1951) provided definite proof that clot retraction is due to a special function of platelets in which fibrin only plays a passive role. Bloom (1955) and Sokal (1960) accumulated further evidence indicating that fibrin plays a passive role in clot retraction and is simply carried along by actively contracting elements of platelet origin.[1]

Ability of platelets to retract fibrin depends on the generation of energy in the process of oxidative phosphorylation and anaerobic glycolysis within the cell (Bettex-Galland and Lüscher, 1965; Mürer, 1969). Bettex-Galland and Lüscher (1961) isolated platelet contractile protein (thrombosthenin, platelet actomyosin). It is now generally accepted that this protein plays a major role in fibrin retraction. Nachman *et al.* (1967) demonstrated that the specific antibody against thrombosthenin inhibits fibrin retraction. According to these authors thrombosthenin is located in the platelet membranes. This would imply a possibility of direct interaction between fibrin and thrombosthenin. However, Lüscher *et al.* (1972) consider that thrombosthenin might not be present on the outer surface of completely intact platelets but it might become available on the cell surface after profound alteration of the membrane structure, as invariably occurs in the course of irreversible "viscous metamorphosis" and comparable manifestations of platelet activity.

Morse *et al.* (1967) demonstrated that clot retraction does not occur in a system composed of washed platelets and fibrin if Reptilase is used as a clotting enzyme instead of thrombin. We have confirmed this observation. The adherence of platelets to polymerizing Reptilase-fibrin leads to the establishment of links between platelet membranes and fibrin (Niewiarowski *et al.*, 1972a). However, this does not result in fibrin retraction unless thrombin is present in the system (Niewiarowski *et al.*, 1972b). We have reported previously that undifferentiated mouse fibroblasts

[1]The term "fibrin retraction" rather than "clot retraction" is used throughout this paper. Retraction means an act of retracting, the ability to retract, and the state of being retracted (Webster's Seventh New Collegiate Dictionary, 1970). The last meaning only is applicable to fibrin retraction.

and human skin fibroblasts cause fibrin retraction (Niewiarowski *et al.*, 1972c, 1973b).

The purpose of this communication is to compare certain characteristics of fibrin retraction brought about by platelets and the fibroblasts. An experimental system is described to study the effect of various agents which may stimulate or inhibit the ability of cells to retract fibrin.

MATERIAL AND METHODS

Preparation of Platelets

Suspension of washed platelets of rabbit was prepared by the method of Ardlie *et al.* (1970). The final platelet count was 10^8/ml. Human platelet-rich plasma (PRP) was prepared from the citrate blood.

Undifferentiated Mouse L Cells

These cells were kindly supplied by Dr. L. Prevec (Department of Biology, McMaster University, Hamilton, Ontario). They were kept in a constant exponential growth phase by daily 2-fold dilution with Joklik-modified Eagle's minimal essential medium. After two washings they were resuspended in Tyrode albumin solution, containing 2×10^{-3} *M* calcium and 10^{-3} *M* magnesium. The cell count was adjusted to 1.05×10^7/ml.

Human Skin Fibroblasts

Cells from a fetus and from a normal adult male were kindly supplied by Dr. S. Goldstein (Department of Medicine, McMaster University, Hamilton, Ontario). They were developed and maintained by standard techniques (Goldstein *et al.*, 1969). Early passage cells had undergone 20–40 mean cell generations. Fibroblasts were harvested from monolayers by a 5–10 min exposure to 0.125 per cent trypsin. They were then washed extensively in growth medium and resuspended in Tyrode albumin solution. The final cell count was 2×10^6/ml.

Reagents

Human fibrinogen (Kabi grade L, Stockholm, Sweden), thrombin (Parke Davis, Detroit, Mich.), *Bothrops atrox* thrombin-like enzyme (Reptilase®, gift by Pentapharm, Basel, Switzerland) suspension of collagen (Sigma) was made as described by Evans *et al.* (1968). Prostaglandin E_1 (PGE_1, gift by Upjohn Co.) was dissolved as described previously (Niewiarowski *et al.*, 1972a). Epinephrine (Sigma), serotonin (Sigma), vasopressin (Sigma), ADP (Sigma), and N^6-2′-O-dibutyryl cyclic AMP (Sigma) were dissolved in 0.9 per cent NaCl.

Measurements of Fibrin Retraction

Fibrin retraction was measured usually in a system composed of 0.8 ml of cell suspension, 0.1 ml of 0.25 per cent fibrinogen, 0.1 ml of thrombin (20 units/ml) or 0.1 ml of 3 per cent Reptilase. In some experiments 0.8 ml of PRP was used instead of 0.8 ml of platelet suspension and 0.1 ml of fibrinogen. Samples were incubated in a water bath at 37° C and the volume of fluid separated from the clot was measured at various time intervals by means of a 1-ml syringe. Special care was taken to keep the needle tip at least 1–3 mm from the clot to avoid mechanical syneresis of fibrin. Retraction was usually done simultaneously in three test tubes and the mean value of three measurements was calculated.

RESULTS

Retraction of Clots Formed from Human Platelet-rich Plasma (PRP)

Clots formed upon addition of thrombin to PRP retracted readily but there was no retraction when Reptilase was used instead of thrombin (Table 1). Preincubation of PRP with epinephrine, collagen, or ADP altered platelets so that they retracted Reptilase fibrin.

Retraction of Clots Formed from Washed Rabbit Platelets and Fibrinogen

Figure 1 shows platelet-rich clots after a 60-min observation period. The retraction was complete in the tube which contained intact platelets and thrombin. There was virtually no retraction if

Table 1. Retraction of clots formed from human platelet-rich plasma (PRP)*

Reagent incubated with PRP for 3 min (final concentration)	Clotting enzyme†	Fibrin clot volume (% of initial) (incubation time in min.)		
		10	30	60
NaCl, 0.9%	Thrombin	41	15	14
NaCl, 0.9%	Reptilase	100	100	96
Epinephrine, 0.1 mg/ml	Reptilase	30	28	13
Collagen	Reptilase	81	60	40
ADP, 5×10^{-5} *M*	Reptilase	73	33	

* Mean values from three experiments.

† 0.1 ml of thrombin, 20 units/ml, or 0.1 ml of 3% reptilase.

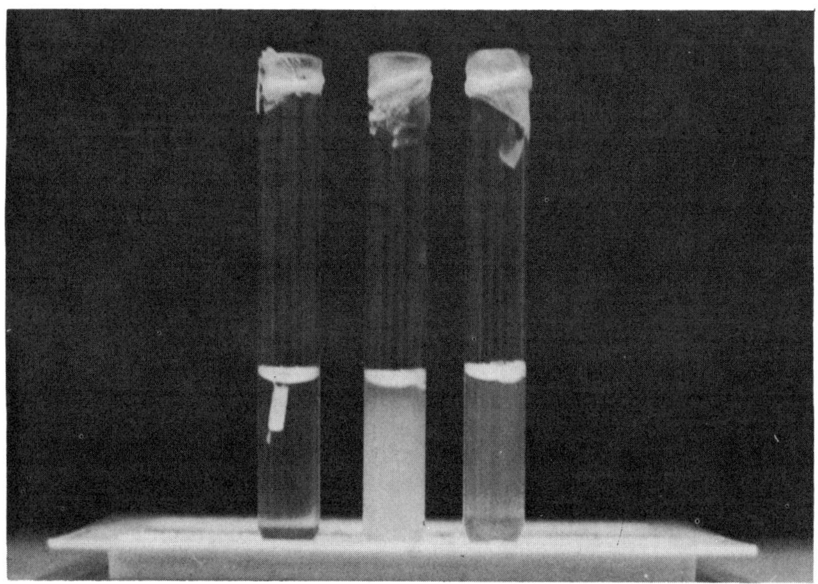

Figure 1. Fibrin retraction induced by rabbit platelets. Tubes from left to right contain: (*a*) 0.8 ml of intact platelet suspension, 0.1 ml of fibrinogen, 0.1 ml of thrombin; (*b*) 0.8 ml of intact platelet suspension, 0.1 ml of fibrinogen, 0.1 ml of Reptilase; (*c*) 0.8 ml of sonicated platelet suspension, 0.1 ml of fibrinogen, 0.1 ml of thrombin. Platelet count, 5×10^8 ml; observation period, 60 min; 37° C.

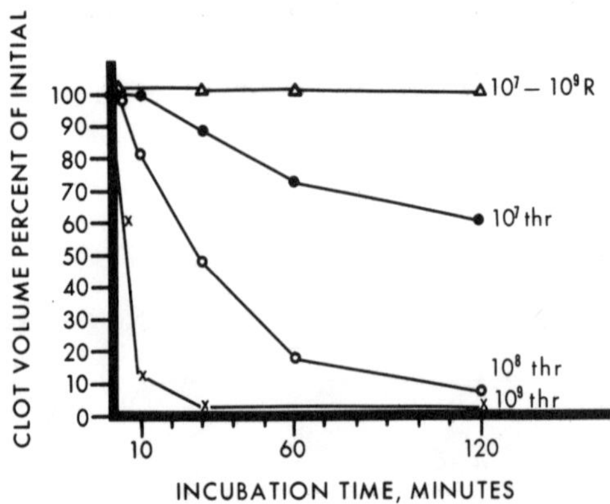

Figure 2. Effect of platelet count on the fibrin retraction in a system with thrombin (thr) and Reptilase (R).

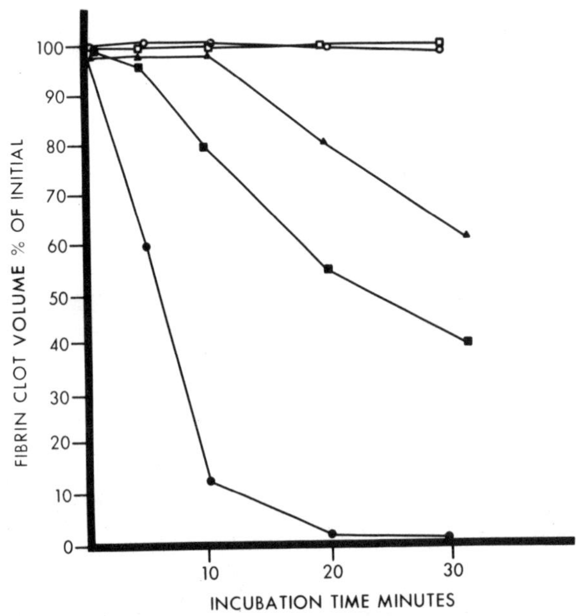

Figure 3. Effect of pretreatment of rabbit platelets with various reagents on the fibrin retraction. Each tube contains 0.8 ml of platelet suspension (5×10^8/ml). Following reagents were added to platelets. ●——●, 0.1 ml of 0.9 per cent NaCl, 0.1 ml of fibrinogen and 0.1 ml of thrombin (20 units/ml). □——□, 0.1 ml of 0.9 per cent NaCl, 0.1 ml of fibrinogen, and 0.2 ml of 3 per cent Reptilase. ○——○, 0.1 ml of thrombin (1 unit) and, after complete platelet aggregation (in aggregometer cuvettes with stirring for 90 sec), 0.1 ml of fibrinogen and 0.1 ml of 3 per cent Reptilase. ■——■, 0.1 ml of thrombin (2 units). After 20-sec incubation without stirring (no visible aggregation occurred) thrombin was neutralized by 0.1 ml of hirudin (10 units). Then 0.1 ml of fibrinogen and 0.1 ml of 3 per cent Reptilase were added. ▲——▲, 0.1 ml of collagen and, after 90-sec incubation (in aggregometer with stirring), 0.1 ml of fibrinogen and 0.1 ml of 3 per cent Reptilase.

Reptilase was substituted for thrombin or if platelets were homogenized by sonification. The rate of fibrin retraction in a system with thrombin depended on the concentration of platelets (Fig. 2). By contrast, there was no retraction at all if Reptilase was substituted for thrombin even at 10^9/ml concentration of platelets. The preincubation of platelets with thrombin (without stirring) followed by the inhibition of this enzyme by hirudin altered the platelets so that they were able to retract Reptilase-fibrin (Fig. 3). On the other hand, platelets aggregated with thrombin before addition of fibrinogen lost their ability to retract fibrin. Collagen incubated with platelets for 90 sec stimulated these cells to retract Reptilase-fibrin. However, the effect of collagen was much less pronounced than that of thrombin. Fibrin retraction induced by rabbit platelets in a system with thrombin was inhibited by PGE_1 and by dibutyryl cyclic AMP (Fig. 4).

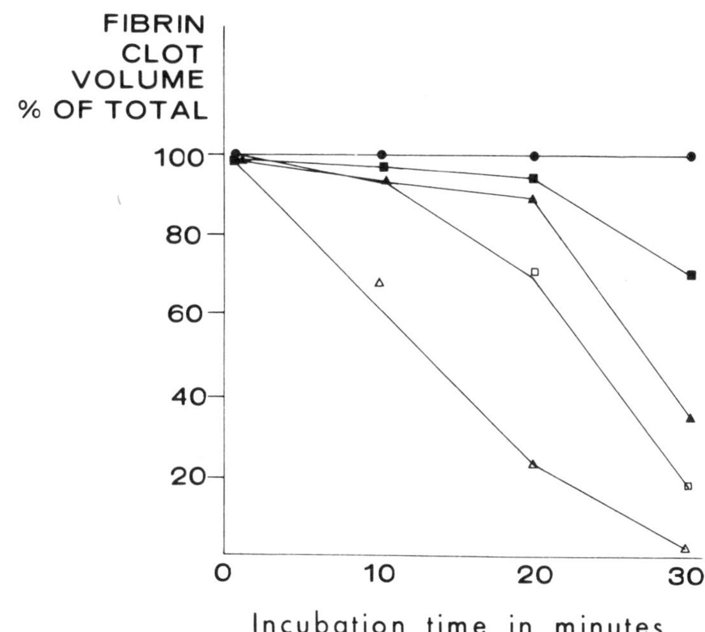

Figure 4. Inhibition of platelet-induced fibrin retraction by PGE_1 and dibutyryl cyclic AMP. Each tube contains 0.8 ml of rabbit platelets (10^8/ml), 0.1 ml of PGE_1 (or cyclic AMP or saline), 0.1 ml of fibrinogen, and 0.1 ml of thrombin (20 units/ml). △—△, control; □—□, cyclic AMP, 5×10^{-4} *M*; ▲—▲, PGE_1, 10^{-6}; ■—■, PGE_1, 10^{-5}; ●—●, PGE_1, 3×10^{-4} *M*.

Retraction of Clots Formed from Fibroblasts and Fibrinogen

Mouse L cells retracted the clots formed from fibrinogen by thrombin (Fig. 5, first tube from the left). There was very little retraction when Reptilase was substituted for thrombin (second tube) and no retraction with sonicated fibroblasts and thrombin (third tube). Mouse L cells, human fetal fibroblasts, and fibroblasts from a young man caused fibrin retraction to a similar extent in a system with thrombin (Table 2). In all experiments significantly less retraction occurred in a system with Reptilase.

Fibrin retraction induced by human fibroblasts was inhibited by PGE_1 and by dibutyryl cyclic AMP (Table 3). On the other hand, this process was not influenced by epinephrine, serotonin, or vasopressin (Table 4).

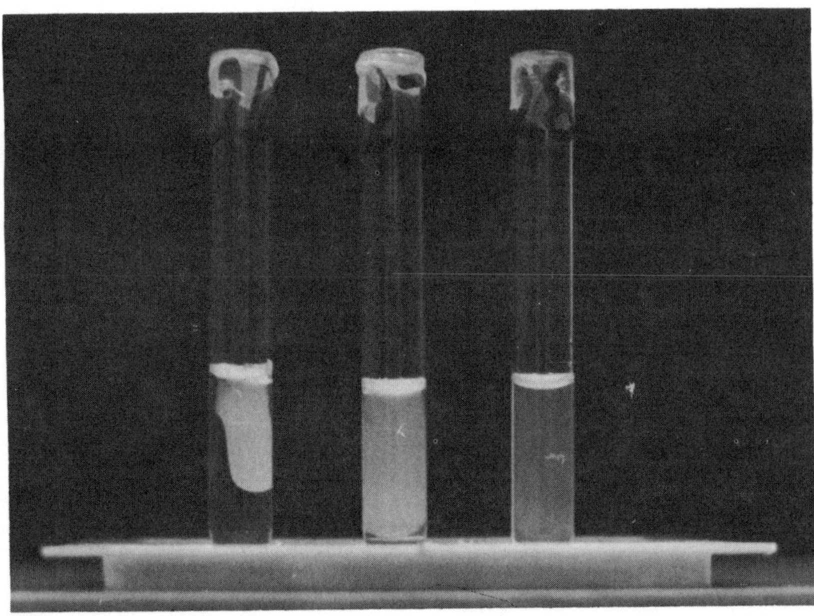

Figure 5. Fibrin retraction induced by undifferentiated mouse L cells. The tubes from left to right contain: (*a*) 0.8 ml of cell suspension, 0.1 ml of fibrinogen, 0.1 ml of thrombin; (*b*) 0.8 ml of cell suspension, 0.1 ml of fibrinogen, 0.1 ml of Reptilase; (*c*) 0.8 ml of sonicated fibroblast suspension, 0.1 ml of fibrinogen, 0.1 ml of thrombin. Cell count, 10^7/ml; observation period, 120 min; 37° C.

Table 2. Retraction of thrombin-fibrin and of Reptilase-fibrin by the fibroblasts

Species of cells	No. of observations	Fibrin clot volume (% inhibition)	
		Thrombin-fibrin	Reptilase-fibrin
Mouse L cells (10^7)	7	31.6 ± 23.8	78.4 ± 20.6
Human fetal fibroblasts (2×10^6)	4	37.3 ± 20.6	93.8 ± 9.5
Fibroblasts of young man (2×10^6)	7	42.1 ± 23.9	92.7 ± 9.3

Mean values and standard deviations after 120-min incubation.

Table 3. Effect of PGE_1 (10^{-5} *M*) and dibutyryl cyclic AMP (10^{-3} *M*) on the fibrin retraction brought about by the fibroblasts in the system with thrombin.

Species of cells	No. of observations	Fibrin clot volume (% initial)		
		Control	PGE_1	Cyclic AMP
Human fetal fibroblasts	5	45.6 ± 14.0	81.7 ± 10.6	
Fibroblasts of young man	8	44.1 ± 19.7	94.5 ± 8.2	84.4 ± 5.9

Mean values and standard deviations after 120-min incubation.

Table 4. Fibrin retraction induced by human fibroblasts in the presence of epinephrine, serotonin, or vasopressin

	Clot volume (% initial volume)	
Reagent (final concentration)	Thrombin-fibrin	Reptilase-fibrin
Control	47.5	100
Epinephrine, 0.1 mg/ml	50.1	100
Serotonin, 0.1 mg/ml	46.8	100
Vasopressin, 0.1 mg/ml	52.3	100

Mean values from three experiments after 120-min incubation.

DISCUSSION

Our experiments demonstrated the similarity of the processes of fibrin clot retraction brought about by platelets and by fibroblasts. Fibrin retraction can occur only in the presence of intact cells. The ability of cells to retract fibrin probably depends on contractile proteins which have been isolated from platelets (Bettex-Galland and Lüscher, 1961) and fibroblasts (Hoffmann-Berling, 1956). These proteins are also implied in other cellular functions such as aggregation (Booyse and Rafelson, 1969; Jones *et al.*, 1970), release reaction of secretion (Grette, 1962), and in cell movement (Hoffmann-Berling, 1959).

The intracellular level of cyclic AMP seems to influence the ability of cells to retract fibrin. Mürer (1971) demonstrated that dibutyryl cyclic AMP and PGE_1 inhibit fibrin retraction in the system with platelets. We confirmed this observation and found that the same is also true with fibroblasts. It is well known that PGE_1 activates adenyl cyclase in platelets (Robison *et al.*, 1969; Wolfe and Shulman 1969; Zieve and Greenbough, 1969) and in fibroblasts (Manganiello *et al.*, 1972), and this leads to the formation of intracellular cyclic AMP.

Both platelets and fibroblasts retract fibrin formed by thrombin. There is very little retraction of Reptilase-fibrin with fibroblasts and no retraction of Reptilase-fibrin with human or rabbit platelets. Morse *et al.* (1967) originally observed that Reptilase did not cause retraction of clots formed from washed platelets and fibrinogen, but it did cause retraction of clots formed from PRP.

This was probably due to contamination of Reptilase with factor X converting enzyme which caused thrombin formation in plasma. There are two possible explanations for the difference in the retraction of fibrin formed by Reptilase or thrombin. (*a*) The type of fibrin formed may be responsible for the difference. It has been established that during fibrin formation, thrombin splits off fibrinopeptides A and B from fibrinogen while Reptilase splits off fibrinopeptide A only (Blomback, 1958). (*b*) The ability of cells to retract fibrin may depend on their stimulation by thrombin but not on the type of fibrin. The experimental data support the second possibility. Washed rabbit platelets preincubated with thrombin cause retraction of Reptilase-fibrin (Niewiarowski *et al.*, 1972b). In addition, agents other than thrombin could stimulate platelets to retract Reptilase-fibrin. As demonstrated by de Gaetano *et al.* (1972) and by ourselves, epinephrine, ADP, and collagen stimulated human platelets to retract Reptilase-fibrin. The presence of collagen in rabbit platelet suspension resulted in the retraction of Reptilase-fibrin. Another snake venom enzyme, ancrod (Arvin), clots fibrinogen but it does not cause platelet release reaction and fibrin clot retraction (Brown *et al.*, 1972). However, Bounameaux (1970) observed that ancrod-fibrin formed from human PRP preincubated with collagen retracted.

Recently de Gaetano *et al.* (1972) tried to link clot retraction to the platelet aggregation and adhesion reaction. We consider that these phenomena may reflect different functions of platelets. Platelets project pseudopodes and adhere readily to polymerizing Reptilase-fibrin (Niewiarowski *et al.*, 1972a, b); however, this is not followed by the fibrin retraction unless a stimulating agent is present in the system.

Since thrombin seems to be essential in the fibroblast-induced fibrin retraction as well as in the platelet-induced fibrin retraction, it is possible that there are sites on the fibroblast membrane which are susceptible to the thrombin action.

Fibrin retraction differs from the contraction of smooth muscles and from that of granulation tissue. The latter processes are triggered by such hormones as epinephrine, serotonin, and vasopressin (Majno *et al.*, 1971). In our hands these substances did not stimulate fibrin retraction induced by human fibroblasts. Recently Majno and associates (1972) reached a similar conclusion studying platelet-induced fibrin retraction by means of the kymographic technique.

The biological significance of fibrin retraction is not fully understood. Budtz-Olsen (1951) suggested that clot retraction is a redundant phylogenetic relic of no inportance in higher animal life. However, this point of view is not generally accepted. It is possible that the reduction of the size of the hemostatic plug may contribute to secondary bleeding. Bettex-Galland and Lüscher (1965) suggested that clot retraction may facilitate canalization of the thrombi and that the orientation of the fibrin fibers under the influence of retraction may favor wound regeneration. We have recently demonstrated that factor XIII inhibits platelet-induced fibrin retraction. The increased resistance of cross-linked fibrin to the retraction brought about by platelets and fibroblasts may represent one of the mechanisms by which factor XIII exerts its function in hemostasis and in tissue repair processes (Niewiarowski *et al.*, 1973a).

It is possible that the observed phenomenon of fibrin retraction induced by fibroblasts and by other cells may reflect a mechanism whose significance is far beyond thrombosis and hemostasis. These cells may pull together the fibers of collagen and of other extracellular material in a way similar to the way they pull fibrin strands. If so, the studied properties of cells may have significance in maintaining the coherence of tissues.

ACKNOWLEDGMENTS

The author is indebted to Miss E. Freeman, Miss M. Markiewicz, and Mr. A. Senyi for invaluable technical assistance. The work has been supported by an Ontario Health (RD-3) grant and by grants from the National Institutes of Health (HL-15226-01), Hoechst Pharmaceutical Co., and by an institutional grant of the American Cancer Society to Temple University Medical School (IN-88).

REFERENCES

Ardlie, N. G., Packham, M. A., and Mustard, J. F. 1970. Adenosine diphosphate induced platelet aggregation in suspensions of washed platelets. Brit. J. Haematol. 10: 7.

Bettex-Galland, M., and Lüscher, E. F. 1961. Thrombosthenin. A contractile protein from thrombocytes. Its extraction from human blood platelets and some of its properties. Biochim. Biophys. Acta 49: 520.

Bettex-Galland, M., and Lüscher, E. F. 1965. Thrombosthenin, the contractile protein from blood platelets and its relation to other contractile proteins. Advan. Protein Chem. 20: 1.

Blomback, B. 1958. Studies on the action of thrombic enzymes on bovine fibrinogen as measured by N-terminal analysis. Ark. Kemi 12: 321.

Bloom, G. 1955. The morphology of human blood platelets and the coagulation of human blood *in vitro*. Histochemie 42: 365.

Booyse, F. M., and Rafelson, M. E., Jr. Studies on human platelets. III. A contractile protein model for platelet aggregation. Blood 33: 100.

Bounameaux, Y. 1970. Exploration fonctionnelle des plaquettes. Description d'un test original, p. 374. *In* Proceedings of VIth International Congress Clinical Chemistry, Geneve/Evian, S. Karger, Basel.

Brown, C. H., Bell, W. R., Shreiner, D. P., and Jackson, D. P. 1972. Effects of arvin on blood platelets. *In vitro* and *in vivo* studies. J. Lab. Clin. Med. 79: 758.

Budtz-Olsen, O. E. 1951. Clot retraction, p. 149. Blackwell Scientific Publications, Oxford.

De Gaetano, G., Bottecchia, D., and Vermylen, J. 1973. Retraction of reptilase-clots in the presence of agents inducing or inhibiting the platelet adhesion-aggregation reaction. Thromb. Res. 2:71.

Duke, W. W. 1912. The pathogenesis of purpura hemorrhagica with especial reference to the part played by blood platelets. Arch. Intern. Med. 10: 445.

Evans, G., Packham, M. A., Nishizawa, E. E., Mustard, J. F., and Murphy, E. E. 1968. The effect of acetylsalicylic acid on platelet function. T. Exper. Med. 128: 877.

Goldstein, S., Littlefield, J. W., and Soeldner, J. S. 1969. Diabetes mellitus and aging: diminished plating efficiency of cultured human fibroblasts. Proc. Nat. Acad. Sci. U.S.A. 64: 155.

Grette, K. 1962. Studies on the mechanism of thrombin-catalyzed hemostatic reactions in blood platelets. Acta Physiol. Scand. 56 (suppl. 195): 1.

Hoffmann-Berling, H. 1956. Das kontraktile Eiweiss undifferenzierter Zellen. Biochim. Biophys. Acta 19: 453.

Hoffmann-Berling, H. 1959. The role of cell structures in cell movements, pp. 45–62. *In* D. Rudnick (ed.) Cell, Organism and Milieu, Ronald Press, New York.

Jones, B. M., Kemp, R. B., and Groschel-Stewart, U. 1970. Inhibition of cell aggregation by antibodies directed against actomyosin. Nature 226: 261.

Lüscher, E. F., Probst, E., and Bettex-Galland, M. 1972. Thrombosthenin: Structure and function. Ann. N.Y. Acad. Sci. 201: 122.

Majno, G., Gabbiani, G., Kirschel, B. J., Ryan, G. B., and Statkov, P. R. 1971. Contraction of granulation tissue *in vitro:* similarity to smooth muscle. Science 173: 548.

Majno, G., Bouvier, C. A., Gabbiani, G., Ryan, G. B., and Statkov, P. 1972. Kymographic recording of clot retraction: effects of papaverine, theophylline and cytochalasin B. Thromb. Diath. Haemorrh. 28: 49.

Manganiello, V., Breslow, J., and Vaughan, M. 1972. An effect of dexamethasone on the cyclic AMP content of human fibroblasts stimulated by catecholamines and prostaglandin E_1. J. Clin. Invest. 51: 60a.

Morse, E. E., Jackson, D. P., and Conley, C. L. 1967. Effects of reptilase and thrombin on human blood platelets and observations on the molecular mechanism of clot retraction. J. Lab. Clin. Med. 70: 106.

Mürer, E. H. 1969. Clot retraction and energy metabolism of platelets. Biochim. Biophys. Acta 172: 266.

Mürer, E. H. 1971. Compounds known to affect the cyclic adenosine monophosphate level in blood platelets: effect on thrombin-induced clot retraction and platelet release. Biochim. Biophys. Acta 237: 310.

Nachman, R. L., Marcus, A. J., and Safier, L. B. 1967. Platelet thrombosthenin: subcellular localization and function. J, Clin. Invest. 46: 1380.

Niewiarowski, S., Regoeczi, E., Stewart, G. J., Senyi, A. F., and Mustard, J. F. 1972a. Platelet interaction with polymerizing fibrin. J. Clin. Invest. 51: 685.

Niewiarowski, S., Regoeczi, E., and Mustard, J. F. 1972b. Platelet interaction with fibrinogen and fibrin. Ann. N.Y. Acad. Sci. 201: 72.

Niewiarowski, S., Regoeczi, E., and Mustard, J. F. 1972c. Adhesion of fibroblasts to polymerizing fibrin and retraction of fibrin induced by fibroblasts. Proc. Soc. Exp. Biol. Med. 140: 199.

Niewiarowski, S., Markiewicz, M., and Nath, N. 1973a. Inhibition of the platelet dependent fibrin retraction by the fibrin stabilizing factor (FSF, Factor XIII). J. Lab. Clin. Med. 81: 641.

Niewiarowski, S., and Goldstein, S. 1973b. Interaction of cultured human fibroblasts with fibrin and its modification by aging and drugs. J. Lab. Clin. Med. in press.

Robison, G. A., Arnold, A., and Hartmann, R. C. 1969. Divergent effects of epinephrine and prostaglandin E_1 on the level of cyclic AMP in human blood platelets. Pharm. Res. Commun. 1: 325.

Sokal, G. 1960. Plaquettes sanguines et structure du caillot. Etude morphologique et thromboelastographique, p. 234. Editions Arscia S. A., Brussels.

Webster's Seventh New Collegiate Dictionary. 1970. p. 734. T. Allen and Son Ltd., Toronto. Based on Webster's Third International Dictionary.

Wolfe, S. M., and Shulman, N. R. 1969. Adenyl cyclase activity in human platelets. Biochem. Biophys. Res. Commun. 35: 265.

Zieve, P. D., and Greenbough, W. B., III. 1969. Adenyl cyclase in human platelets: activity and responsiveness. Biochem. Biophys. Res. Commun. 35: 462.

Research on the Mechanisms of the Intravascular Adhesion of Circulating Cells

G.V.R. Born

Evolution from single to multicellular organisms has depended on the development of intercellular adhesion mechanisms; if they did not exist we would still be piles of cells on the ground. Cell adhesions are, of course, tissue specific. Experimentally it has been shown, for example, that when suspensions of single cells from embryonic kidney and liver are mixed, the cells from each organ tend to aggregate separately to the exclusion of the cells from the other organ (Moscona, 1962, 1965). Another example of a very specific recognition mechanism between different adhering cells is that between circulating lymphocytes and the endothelial cells in the venules of lymph nodes (see below). So far, these adhesion phenomena have remained in the purely descriptive stage, and almost nothing is known about the biochemical mechanisms responsible for the specificity of the interactions. I will describe and discuss recent experimental researches designed to initiate understanding of these mechanisms.

ADHESION OF SMALL LYMPHOCYTES IN LYMPH NODE VENULES

The phenomena of lymphocyte recirculation (Gowans, 1957, 1958) became particularly intriguing after the discovery that the small lymphocytes leave the circulating blood by an unexpected route: not, as one might have expected, *between* the cells which line the insides of blood vessels but actually *through* an unusual type of endothelial cell which normally occurs only in the postcapillary venules of lymph nodes. By using the large popliteal lymph node in sheep, it has been shown that about one in 10 of the small lymphocytes in the blood perfusing the node migrates out of the venules in this way. This emigration must depend on a highly selective recognition mechanism between the endothelial cells and the small lymphocytes because all other types of circulating cells, including other types of motile leukocytes, are excluded. How the recognition mechanism works is still unknown. Pretreatment of small lymphocytes with certain enzymes, *e.g.*, neuraminidase or trypsin, greatly diminishes the rate of the emigration (Gessner and Ginsberg, 1964), presumably by removing some essential components from the cell surface. A similar diminution is brought about by exposing small lymphocytes to the large molecular mucopolysaccharide *heparin*, which apparently hinders recognition by becoming bound to the cell surface (Bradfield and Born, 1969).

The rate of emigration of lymphocytes from the blood into lymphoid tissues is, within limits, a linear function of the concentration of lymphocytes in the blood. It is not yet known whether this cellular emigration mechanism can become saturated with very high concentrations of lymphocytes, analogous to the maxima in the active transport of dissolved molecules such as glucose across cell membranes.

As Ford and Gowans (1969) pointed out, the recirculation of a large population of small lymphocytes between blood and lymphoid tissue is such an arresting phenomenon that to suggest that it had no functional significance would indicate an unusual distaste for teleology; and they proposed as the most likely function some sort of facilitation of the induction of immune responses. By now there is some experimental evidence in support of this proposition. However, there is an alternative or additional possibility which comes to mind when one thinks of small lymphocytes as the cellular carriers of *immunological memory*. Like other memories, this kind of memory can be very long-lasting; indeed, it is well known that it totally prevents the recurrence of some infectious diseases in a person's entire lifetime. Now a property of nerve cells, which presumably are the repositories of nonimmunological memories, is that they have no turnover and that most of the cells themselves as well as their DNA live as long as the individual to whom they belong. There is evidence that nerve cells depend for their longevity on the neuroglial cells with which they are intimately intermingled and connected in the central nervous system. This analogy suggests that the small lymphocytes, as the cellular carriers of long-lasting immunological memory, owe their longevity to some process of rejuvenation which recurs at frequent intervals as they enjoy the singularly intimate contact provided by passage *through* the endothelial cells during recirculation. This idea gains strength from the contrast between the long life of small lymphocytes *in vivo* and the extraordinary difficulty of keeping them alive, even for a few hours, under the optimal *in vitro* conditions so far devised. It may well be, of course, that the unique transcellular migration process subserves both immunological and nutritional or survival functions.

MECHANISM OF THE ADHESIVENESS BETWEEN BLOOD VESSEL WALLS AND CIRCULATING GRANULOCYTES

Next I should like to describe some work in progress in which Mrs. Anne Atherton and I are trying for the first time to quantitate an important phenomenon that has been known qualitatively for well over a hundred years. In the first half of the nineteenth century, descriptions were given of the tendency of the white cells of the blood to roll along the walls of blood vessels at a much slower velocity than that of the main bloodstream (Dutrochet, 1824; Wagner, 1833, 1839; Addison, 1843). Some of these cells were seen to come to rest, and their appearance was likened to "so many pebbles or marbles over which a stream runs without disturbing them" (Waller, 1848). This phenomenon was observed to be much more prominent in inflamed tissues in which the inner walls of veins become paved by an unbroken lining of leukocytes without the admixture of a single red blood cell, an arrangement spoken of as "pavementing of the leukocytes."

What follows then can best be described in the vivid words of Cohnheim in his Lectures on General Pathology, published in 1877:

But the eye of the observer hardly has time to catch all the details of the picture before it is arrested by a very unexpected occurrence. Usually it is a vein with the typical peripheral arrangement of the white corpuscles, but sometimes a capillary, that first displays the phenomenon. A pointed projection is seen on the external contour of the vessel wall; it pushes itself further outwards, increases in thickness, and the pointed projection is transformed into a colourless rounded hump; this grows longer and thicker, throws out fresh points, and gradually withdraws itself from the vessel wall, with which at last it is connected only by a long thin pedicle. Finally this also detaches itself, and now there lies outside the vessel a colourless, faintly glittering, contractile corpuscle with a few short processes and one long one, of the size of a white blood cell and having one or more nuclei; in a word, a colourless blood corpuscle.

This process by which the white blood cells pass through the walls of the vessels is known as the emigration of the leukocytes. It is confined to the veins, particularly the smaller ones, although some believe that it occurs also in capillaries. The process has been described time and again in many different preparations, particularly well in the rabbit ear chamber (Clark and Clark, 1935). When inflammation is the result of bacterial infection, the emigrated leukocytes engulf and digest the foreign microorganisms and, in the process, many or most are themselves killed; this mixture of dead and autolysing cells is what we call pus. Although the *function* of leukocyte emigration was established many years ago, its *mechanism* is still completely unknown. The reason for this ignorance is presumably that, unlike the movement of molecules across the wall of blood vessels, the corresponding movement of whole cells had not been considered amenable to quantitative investigation. The only previous attempt to estimate this movement *in vivo* depended on counting the cells in histological sections of skin 45 min after the intradermal injection of substances claimed to promote leukocyte emigration (Spector and Willoughby, 1964, 1968). Clearly, such a technique can give no information about the early changes in the vessel wall and/or in the circulating cells by which adhesion and emigration are initiated.

We have recently begun to explore a new technique with which it seems to be possible to make measurements on these earliest changes in living preparations, *viz.*, the hamster cheek pouch and the mouse mesentery (Atherton and Born, 1972, 1973). The outstanding characteristic of this technique is again its banal simplicity for which we feel almost apologetic. The principle is to observe a small venule, 30–100 μ in diameter, under the microscope at a magnification of up to 500 times and to count in successive time periods of 1 or 2 min those white cells which move sufficiently much slower than the main red stream of blood to be visible as individual cells rolling down one side of the vessel wall. In practice, a grid line in the eyepiece is made to appear crossing the chosen vessel at right angles and the individually visible leukocytes are counted as they cross the junction of the line with one side of the vessel. We are finding that the application of diverse agents said to induce directional movements of leukocytes *in vitro* (Sorkin, Borel, and Stecher, 1970) causes a temporary increase in the number of white cells that can be so counted. The conclusion that this effect must necessarily depend on an increase in the mutual adhesiveness between vessel wall and circulating cells is, of course, far from being established. But at least we can begin to investigate the phenomenon quantitatively. Among the assumptions the validity of which has to be assessed are that (*a*) the slow rolling movement indicates adhesiveness to the vessel wall; (*b*) the cells have to collide with the vessel wall in order to become visible; and (*c*) the numbers and other parameters, such as the distributions of velocity and path length of these visible cells, provide a measure of the adhesiveness between them and the vessel wall. We are devising techniques for measuring all these variables. An interesting result already obtained shows that although the visible cells move at somewhat different velocities, they are all very much (at least 10 times) slower than the mean flow velocity in the vessels. The flow velocity will, of course, be less along the vessel wall, but it is obviously still much faster than that of the visible leukocytes.

This particular investigation has been prompted as much as anything by curiosity about and the desire to understand the mechanism of an old and particularly intriguing observation. However, any progress on this may also throw light on other unanswered questions, two of which require urgent answers: (*a*) is it possible that leukocytes promote their own emigration by releasing enzymes which loosen the connections between endothelial cells? In contrast with small lymphocytes which, it should be remembered, emigrate out of blood vessels *through* certain cells, granulocytes are known to push their way out *between* the endothelial cells. (*b*) What is the mechanism whereby circulating malignant cells come to adhere to blood vessel walls to form metastases? Practically nothing is known about that medically important problem (Weiss, 1967).

APPLICABILITY OF *IN VITRO* OBSERVATIONS ON PLATELET AGGREGATION TO THEIR FUNCTION *IN VIVO*

Finally, some comments on the intravascular adhesion of platelets. There is a great deal of information about the sequence of reactions of platelets to aggregating agents *in vitro*. The reaction sequence is similar, at least qualitatively, for all common, naturally occurring agents with the exception of collagen. Collagen induces aggregation of platelets without a preceding change in their shape and after a lag period of several seconds; during this period the platelets release several substances, including adenosine diphosphate (ADP), which are responsible for the aggregation. Other naturally occurring agents, including adrenaline (Ahtee and Michal, 1972), first cause a morphological change in the platelets (Born, 1970). This initial reaction is very rapid; at 37°C it is over in 2–3 sec. This is followed by the mutual adhesion of the platelets, which may redisperse. Alternatively, the aggregated platelets become much more tightly packed together (Born and Hume, 1967); at the same time they release aggregating agents, including ADP and 5-hydroxytryptamine, from intracellular storage granules in a reaction similar to that induced by collagen. The biochemical mechanisms underlying these reactions are still unknown.

It is still uncertain whether the sequence of reactions observed *in vitro* takes place when circulating platelets adhere and aggregate *in vivo*, whether physiologically during hemostasis or pathologically during thrombosis. This contribution describes, first, recent experimental observations on the rapid morphological reaction of platelets *in vitro* which make it possible to find out whether this reaction also precedes platelet aggregation *in vivo*, and second, experimental evidence that the mechanism by which ADP causes platelets to aggregate *in vitro* can also make them adhere to vascular endothelium and aggregate *in vivo*.

Components of the Rapid Morphological Reaction

The change in shape of platelets stirred in citrated plasma at 37°C caused by the addition of ADP (Macmillan and Oliver, 1965) is associated with an increase in light scattering (Michal and Born, 1971). This optical effect provides a measure of the velocity and magnitude of the rapid reaction, which consists of more than one morphological component.

To find out what the optical effect means morphologically, samples of rabbit citrated platelet-rich plasma used for optical measurements were mixed rapidly with equal volumes of chilled 2.5 per cent glutaraldehyde in 0.1 *M* cacodylate buffer, pH 7.4, postfixed with buffered osmium tetroxide and processed for transmission electronmicroscopy. On the electronmicrographs, the perimeter of each sectioned bit of platelet was measured with a D-Mac pen follower. The measurements were collated by computer and the distribution of perimeter lengths was plotted against the percentage of total sections measured. About 500 sections were measured to establish each of the following results.

EDTA was always added first to prevent the platelets from aggregating when ADP was added later. After EDTA only for 15 sec, the platelet sections were mostly ellipsoid and there were also very small, mainly circular sections which accounted for about 38 per cent of the total. After ADP (1 μM) for 10 sec, the platelet sections were irregular and covered with small blebs; the ratio of small (> 2 μ) to larger (2–8 μ) sections had increased 3.0 times. After ADP for 2 min, the blebs mostly disappeared but the ratio increased further to 3.9. These observations indicate that the rapid reaction is made up of at least two morphological components, *viz.*, small blebs and long, thin projections. The spherical blebs disappear spontaneously within ½ min while the thin projections increase in number for at least 2–3 min.

It was established earlier (Born, 1970) that the rapid morphological reaction is associated with an increase of up to 60 per cent in volume of plasma trapped between platelets sedimented by centrifugation. This increase suggests that the long, thin projections prevent platelets from being packed together as closely as they can be normally and that these projections, therefore, are remarkably rigid. The morphological reaction is not associated with a change in mean platelet volume (Born, 1970). Clearly, however, the morphological changes must be associated with large changes in the surface membrane of the platelets; the nature of these changes and their functional implication are still unknown.

The Role of Thin Pseudopodia in the Adhesion of Other Cell Types

General considerations indicate that thin cellular extensions facilitate adhesion between cells (Bangham and Pethica, 1960). Calculations of repulsion barriers to adhesion between cells show that delicate protuberances on cell membranes are the most likely regions of initial contact (Pethica, 1961). A fairly small repulsive energy of about 1 erg/cm^2 in the potential energy barrier will be sufficient to prevent the close contact of two cells of, say, adhesion area 1 μm^2 (10^{-8} cm^2) being brought about by Brownian motion (Curtis, 1967). Under these conditions cells can, however, adhere to one another, at least temporarily, by fine projections on their surfaces of the kind that are referred to as microvilli or spikes (Bangham and Pethica, 1960). The tip of such projections may be treated as spheres with a radius of, for example, 0.1 μm. Such fine projections could receive sufficient Brownian (thermal) energy to overcome the small repulsion energy that they experience, whereas a larger spherical body would not. Because microvilli behave like small spheres, they can come into close contact, and from these initial points of contact the cells can be "zippered" together. Such a mechanism has been used to explain cell adhesion in general (Lesseps, 1963). When small lymphocytes or macrophages are stimulated with antigen they extend long, thin processes which can come together and form intercellular bridges (Clarke, Salzburg, and Willoughby, 1971). The mutual adhesion of single cells of the slime mould *Dictyostelium discoidium* is accompanied by the appearance of microvilli on the cell surfaces (Garrod and Born, 1971).

Relevance of *in Vitro* Observations to the Initiation of Platelet Adhesion *in Vivo*

The thin pseudopodia formed on platelets during the morphological reaction also have the right dimension for such an adhesion-promoting effect. The evidence so far reviewed suggests, therefore, that the rapid shape change of platelets subserves the function of initiating and facilitating their mutual aggregation, at least under experimental conditions *in vitro*. An important unanswered question is whether this applies also under the physiological or pathological conditions which cause adhesion and aggregation of platelets in the living organism. The answer is still unknown but is clearly of great importance, because it has been shown that the initial morphological reaction of platelets to the naturally occurring aggregating agents can be inhibited by different substances, including adenosine triphosphate, adenosine and some analogues, and prostaglandin E_1 together with phosphodiesterase inhibitors (Born, 1970; Born *et al.*, 1972); under these conditions, the subsequent aggregation and release reactions of platelets are also inhibited.

The problem is much more difficult to investigate experimentally *in vivo* than *in vitro*. The main reason for this is the rapidity of the morphological reaction, which makes it difficult to "catch it" when induced experimentally in living blood vessels. Much information has been accumulated about the behavior of platelets in vessels which have been injured in various ways, ranging from the macroscopic mechanical damage caused by a cut to the microscopic thermal damage caused by a laser beam. It is, however, difficult to control the amount of damage quantitatively as well as to quantitate its effects on the circulating platelets affected by the damage. Furthermore, behavior of platelets in the bloodstream is affected by changes in flow properties alone (Murphy *et al.*, 1962). Recently, the increasing use of artificial systems to replace functionally impaired organs, *e.g.*, dialyzers for kidneys or oxygenators for lungs, has shown that extracorporeal blood flow almost invariably becomes impeded by deposits and adhering aggregates of platelets (Richardson, 1972). It is, therefore, necessary to establish how the initiation and growth of these deposits depends quantitatively on the following variables: (*a*) the geometrical properties of the natural or artificial flow channel; (*b*) the rheological properties of the blood flow; (*c*) the nature, duration, and strength of any thrombogenic stimulus coming from the channel wall; (*d*) the concentration, distribution, and reactivity of the platelets in the bloodstream; and (*e*) the concentration of other factors in the blood known to influence platelet adhesion and aggregation, *i.e.*, calcium and proteins in the plasma and other circulating cells, particularly the erythrocytes.

Analysis of Adhesion and Aggregation in Uninjured Small Blood Vessels

To investigate the relevance of *in vitro* observations on aggregation to the formation of platelet deposits and thrombi *in vivo*, a method was introduced in which platelet thrombi or "white bodies" can be produced experimentally *in vivo* under conditions in which the variables can be measured or controlled (Begent and Born, 1970*a*). ADP is applied to the outside of small venules in the cheek pouch of the anesthetized hamster by iontophoresis through a micropipette. By using highly radioactive ADP, the rate at which it is released from the pipette tip can be determined (Begent and Born, 1970*b*). The iontophoretic currents needed for the release of thrombogenic quantities of ADP are three or more orders of magnitude smaller than the electrical currents that have been used to induce platelet thrombi by direct vascular injury (Sawyer, Suckling, and Wesolowski, 1960; French, Macfarlane, and Sanders, 1964; Berman, 1969).

We confirmed first (Begent and Born, 1970*a*) that the thrombogenic effect was specific to ADP and not possessed by closely related nucleotides such as guanosine diphosphate, which has similar chemical properties. We showed that the platelet thrombi grew exponentially and demonstrated a dependence of the growth rate constant on the mean blood velocity. The small venules in which this was demonstrated appeared to remain normal, both functionally and morphologically under the electronmicroscopy, except for some loss of electron density in the cytoplasm of the endothelial cells.

Role of the Endothelium

Those observations raised several questions. First, it had to be established whether the circulating platelets were induced to adhere and to aggregate by the applied ADP or via a secondary process induced by the ADP in the vessel wall, *e.g.*, in the endothelial cells.

The endothelial abnormality was seen with iontophoretic current of 300 nA. If it could be shown that platelet adhesion could be initiated with still smaller currents without any abnormality in the vessel wall demonstrable electronmicroscopically, it would be evidence for a direct effect of the applied ADP.

Furthermore, in moving from the pipette on the outside of the vessel into its lumen, ADP presumably would have to diffuse through the junction between the endothelial cells because, as a polyanion at physiological pH, ADP would be unable to pass through the endothelial cells themselves. If, therefore, it could be shown that the physiological production of gaps in the endothelial lining had the effect of accelerating the thrombogenic action of ADP, it would provide more evidence for a direct action of ADP. Histamine and serotonin cause contraction of the endothelial cells lining the venules in the cremaster muscle of the rat (Majno, Gilmore, and Leventhal, 1967; Majno, Shea, and Leventhal, 1969); histamine has a similar effect in venules of the hamster cheek pouch (Entrican, Simpson, and Stalker, 1971). The effect of this contraction is to separate the junctions between the endothelial cells so that gaps appear between them in which the basement membrane becomes exposed to the flowing blood. On the supposition that the appearance of these gaps should increase the rate of diffusion of externally applied ADP into the venules, we have examined the effect of histamine, which by itself has no effect on platelets, on the initiation of thrombogenesis by ADP applied iontophoretically to venules in the cheek pouch of anesthetized hamsters. We did not use serotonin because it has direct effects on platelets.

Effect of Histamine

The hamster cheek pouch was prepared for the microiontophoretic application of both ADP and histamine (Begent, Born, and Sharp, 1972). Histamine was applied with a positive potential through a second micropipette, the tip of which was micromanipulated to lie on the other side of the venule opposite the pipette filled with ADP. Histamine (10 m*M* in the pipette) was released by a current of 300 nA for 2 min before and during the application of ADP. To demonstrate this release, the pipette was placed against an arteriole which was seen to constrict when the current was passed, an effect shown earlier to be due to histamine (Duling, Berne, and Born, 1968).

The effects were quantitated by determining the time interval in seconds from the start of the iontophoretic current for ADP to the first visible platelet aggregate or white body adhering in the vessel opposite the micropipette tip. This was a clear endpoint and highly reproducible in that repeated applications of ADP at the same site caused no significant change in the time to first appearance of the white body.

Histamine applied alone had no effect on the venules or on the platelets circulating through them. When ADP alone was applied by currents of increasing strength, white bodies appeared after decreasing times. In seven experiments, histamine applied together with ADP caused a further decrease of up to 30 per cent in the time to the first appearance of white bodies at all iontophoretic currents for ADP. This accelerating effect of histamine was absent in cheek pouch preparations which appeared to be inflamed or had already been affected by the release of endogenous agents.

The accelerating effect of histamine was reversible. About 10 min after the iontophoretic current for histamine was switched off, the time to first appearance of the white bodies increased to that found before histamine was applied.

Conclusions

From these experiments, it can be concluded that the effectiveness of ADP applied outside the venule on platelets circulating inside the venule is increased in the presence of histamine which, by itself, has no effect on platelets. The most likely explanation for this is that histamine produces gaps between the endothelial cells, thus permitting the accelerated diffusion of ADP from outside the vessel. Another way to account for the observation would be that histamine enables platelets to collide with exposed basement membrane to which they tend to adhere (Tranzer and Baumgartner, 1967); whether this really matters under our experimental conditions is uncertain.

It seems, therefore, that the mechanism by which ADP mediates aggregation of platelets *in vitro* can also operate *in vivo* without anything else having to enter the sequence of events. What is not yet known is whether *all* of the effects of ADP demonstrable *in vitro*, *i.e.*, shape change, aggregation, and release, are necessary for the behavior of platelets *in vivo*. For example, there is evidence (Zuzel, 1971) that the release reaction is not necessary for the formation of aggregates *in vitro;* and the great rapidity of aggregation *in vivo* suggests that it may also progress far without requiring the release reaction.

REFERENCES

Addison, W. 1843. The actual process of nutrition in the living structure. J. Churchill, London.

Ahtee, L., and Michal, F. 1972. Brit. J. Pharmacol. 44: 363P.

Atherton, A., and Born, G. V. R. 1972. J. Physiol. 222: 447.

Atherton, A., and Born, G. V. R. 1973. J. Physiol. 233: 157.

Bangham, A. D., and Pethica, B. A. 1960. Proc. Roy. Soc. Edin. 28: 43.

Begent, N. A., and Born, G. V. R. 1970*a*. Nature 227: 926.

Begent, N. A., and Born, G. V. R. 1970*b*. Brit. J. Pharmacol. 40: 592P.

Begent, N. A., Born, G. V. R., and Sharp, D. E. 1972. J. Physiol. 223: 229.

Berman, H. L. 1969. P. 534 *In* S. Sherry, K. M. Brinkhouse, E. Genton, and J. M. Stengle (eds.) Thrombosis. Nat. Acad. Sci., Washington.

Born, G. V. R. 1970. J. Physiol. 209: 487.

Born, G. V. R., Foulks, J. G., Michal, F., and Sharp, D. E. 1972. J. Physiol. 225: 27.

Born, G. V. R., and Hume, M. 1967. Nature (London) 215: 1027.

Bradfield, J. W. B., and Born, G. V. R. 1969. Nature 222: 1183.

Clark, E. R., and Clark, E. C. 1935. Amer. J. Anat. 57: 385.

Clarke, J. A., Salsbury, A. J., and Willoughby, D. A. 1971. J. Pathol. 104: 115.

Curtis, A. S. G. 1967. Academic Press, London.

Duling, B. R., Berne, R. M., and Born, G. V. R. 1968. Microvasc. Res. 1: 158.

Dutrochet, M. H. 1824. Bailliere et Fils, Paris.

Entrican, J. H., Simpson, H. G., and Stalker, A. L. 1971. J. Pathol. Bacteriol. 104: iii.

Ford, W. L., and Gowans, J. L. 1969. Semin. Hematol. 6: 68.

French, J. E., Macfarlane, R. G., and Sanders, A. G. 1964. Brit. J. Exp. Pathol. 45: 467.

Garrod, D. R., and Born, G. V. R. 1971. J. Cell. Sci. 8: 751.

Gessner, B. M., and Ginsburg, V. 1964. Proc. Nat. Acad. Sci. U.S.A. 52: 750.

Lesseps, R. J. 1963. J. Exp. Zool. 153: 171.

Macmillan, D. C., and Oliver, M. R. 1965. J. Atheroscler. Res. 5: 440.

Majno, G., Gilmore, V., and Leventhal, M. 1967. Circ. Res. 21: 833.

Majno, G., Shea, S. M., and Leventhal, M. 1969. J. Cell Biol. 42: 647.

Michal, F., and Born, G. V. R. 1971. Nature 231: 220.

Moscona, A. A. 1962. Int. Rev. Exp. Pathol. 1: 371.

Moscona, A. A. 1965. Pp. 489–524. In E. N. Willmer (ed.) Cells and tissues in culture. Academic Press, New York.

Murphy, E. A., Rowsell, H. C., Downey, H. G., Robinson, G. A., and Mustard, J. F. 1962. Can. Med. Ass. 87: 259.

Pethica, B. A. 1961. Exp. Cell Res. (Suppl.) 8: 123.

Richardson, P. D. 1972. Bull. N. Y. Acad. Med. 48: 379.

Sawyer, P. N., Suckling, E. E., and Wesolowski, S. A. 1960. Amer. J. Physiol. 197: 1006.

Sorkin, E., Borel, J. F., and Stecher, V. 1970. Mononuclear phagocytes symposium, Blackwell, Oxford.

Spector, W. G., and Willoughby, D. A. 1964. J. Pathol. Bacteriol. 88: 557.

Spector, W. G., and Willoughby, D. A. 1968. The English Universities Press, London.

Tranzer, J. P., and Baumgartner, H. R. 1967. Nature 216: 1126.

Wagner, R. 1833. Leopold Voss, Leipzig.

Wagner, R. 1838. Leopold Voss, Leipzig.

Waller, A. 1846. Lond. Edinb. Dubl. Phil. Mag. 29: 271.

Weiss, L. 1967. Amer. J. Med. 43: 570.

Zuzel, M. 1971. *In* Abstracts of the Oslo Meeting of the International Society of Haemostasis and Thrombosis.

Platelet Kinetics

Allan J. Erslev

Available data on the rate of platelet production and destruction, on the clinical syndrome "periodic thrombocytopenia," and on the generation of thrombopoietin have been reviewed, and a feedback circuit which most harmoniously accounts for platelet homeostasis has been constructed. According to this circuit, the platelets control the release of a thrombopoietin which in turn controls the rate of stem cell differentiation to megakaryocytes. Data on a family with megathrombocytopenia suggest that the thrombopoietin release is determined not by platelet count, platelet function, or platelet mass, but rather by platelet surface.

The maintenance of an optimal number of cells in circulating blood demands the presence of feedback circuits responsible to the needs for blood cells and capable of adjusting their number appropriately (Erslev, 1971). The first such feedback circuit to be unraveled was the circuit governing the red blood cell count. This feat was facilitated by the fact that the normal red blood cell count is stable, the normal red cell life span is fixed, the rate of production of red cells can be assessed easily by reticulocyte counts, and a slight decrease in the number of red cells has metabolic consequences. These attributes led to the discovery of a fairly simple red cell feedback circuit linking the bone marrow to the kidney and being mediated in one direction by oxygen and in the opposite direction by erythropoietin (Fig. 1).

Because of the close developmental relationship between red cells and platelets, it has been assumed that a very similar feedback circuit would govern the platelet count. However, such a circuit has been difficult to establish because the normal platelet count fluctuates considerably, the life span and rate of production of platelets are difficult to measure, and the function of platelets is such that even a considerable decrease in platelet count would be unlikely to generate a measurable metabolic signal.

Recent studies appear to have removed some of these obstacles and cleared the way for the formulation of a reasonable platelet feedback circuit.

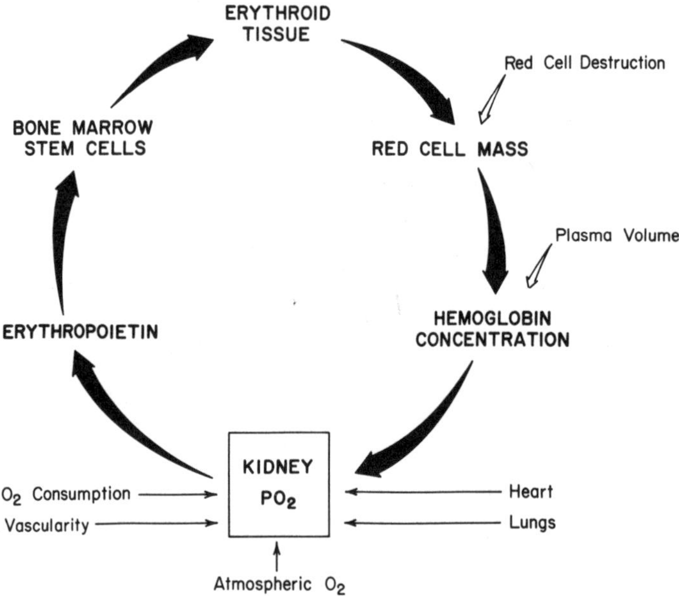

Figure 1. Proposed feedback circuit for the control of the red blood cell count (Erslev, 1971).

The first obstacle was the platelet count, which has a wide normal range (175,000–350,000/mm^3) and displays considerable daily fluctuations. Although the employment of improved counting apparatus such as the phase contrast microscope and the automatic particle counter has narrowed this spread, the actual number of circulating platelets undoubtedly varies widely. Recent observations by Aster (1966) indicate that one of the causes for this variability is the spleen. Under normal conditions, the platelets traverse the spleen relatively slowly and it is estimated that at any one time about 30 per cent of the total number of platelets are in transit through the maze of fenestrated splenic sinusoids. Since the size of these vascular channels is very responsive to epinephrine-like compounds, the platelet transit time and in turn the platelet count in blood depend to some extent on the highly variable concentration of vasoactive substances in the circulation. The importance of splenic sequestration of platelets is graphically demonstrated in Fig. 2, which depicts data from Gardner (1972) on the recovery of transfused platelets in patients without spleen,

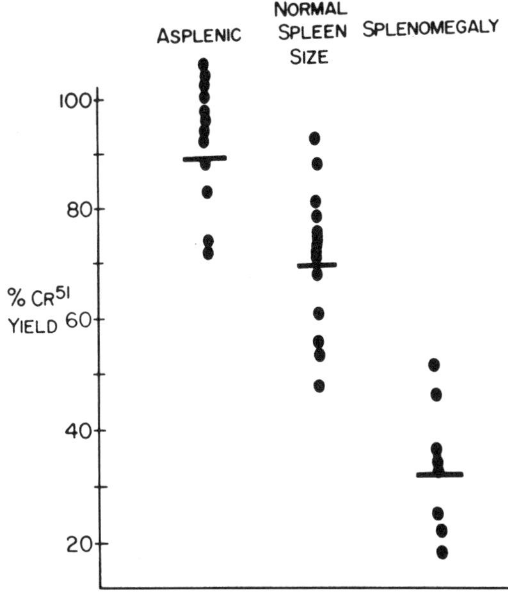

Figure 2. The recovery of transfused platelets in the circulating blood of asplenic patients, normal patients, and patients with congestive splenomegaly (Gardner, 1972).

with normal sized spleens, and with congestive splenomegaly. The unaccounted-for platelets in the patients with normal or large spleens are probably in slow transit through the spleen. Nevertheless, even in asplenic individuals the platelet counts do have a wide normal range, and it seems likely that the adjustment of the normal platelet mass is coarse without the fine discrimination observed in the regulation of the red blood cell count.

The second obstacle was the lack of reproducible techniques for measuring platelet life span and the rate of platelet production. Most estimates of platelet life span had provided data with such a wide confidence limit that they could be interpreted as either indicating an age-dependent fixed life span or a random destruction. Since it was assumed that platelets were destroyed at random during performance of their duties in defense and maintenance, it was difficult to imagine that the life span was age-dependent. However, recent studies of platelets labeled *in vitro* with radio-

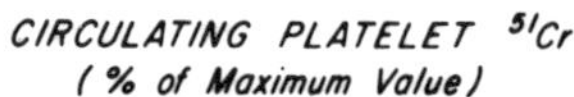

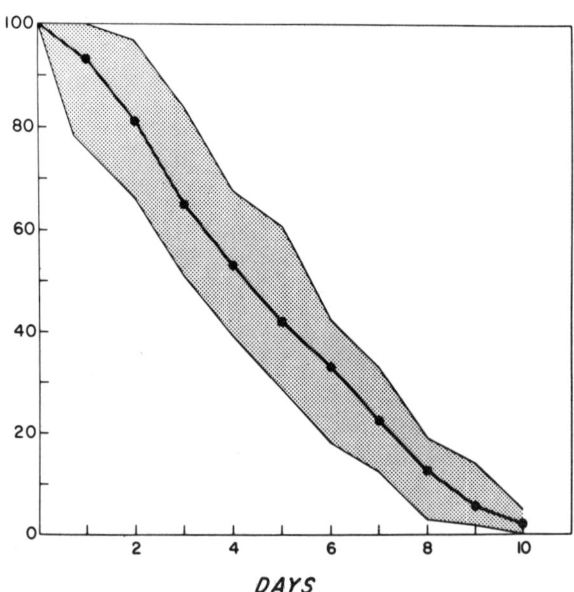

Figure 3. Survival of ^{51}Cr-labeled human platelets. Points represent average values expressed as percentage of initial recovery, and shaded area represents the range for 30 normal subjects (Aster, 1966).

chromium (Fig. 3) show unquestionably that most platelets live a fixed life span of about 8–10 days and that only very few are consumed at random in the daily surveillance for vascular leaks. This conclusion indicates that the platelet count, like the red cell count, must be controlled by cellular production rather than by cellular destruction.

Unfortunately, it is still quite difficult to determine the rate of platelet production. Young platelets are larger than old platelets, and careful sizing of platelets by Garg *et al.* (1972) has led to useful but not accurate estimations of the rate of platelet production. The enumeration and sizing of megakaryocytes in a bone marrow section by Harker and Finch (1969) has led to fairly accurate estimates of thrombopoiesis, but the technique is too cumbersome for routine use. Attempts to use an isotope label of megakaryocytic cytoplasm such as ^{75}selenium methionine have resulted in interesting data as to rate of utilization, but have not provided a measure of platelet production comparable with the measure provided for red cell production by the use of radioiron (Evatt and Levin, 1969). The best estimates of platelet turnover are obtained by measuring platelet count and platelet life span, but this method, unfortunately, demands steady state conditions.

Despite these shortcomings, the available techniques for platelet enumeration, platelet life span, and platelet production have been used successfully to demonstrate that a change in the platelet count or the platelet mass is followed by an appropriate change in platelet production. First, platelet survival studies have established that platelet production in idiopathic thrombocytopenic purpura is increased. This had been suspected before because of the increased number of bone marrow megakaryocytes, but their large size and unusual morphology had been wrongly interpreted as reflecting decreased rather than accelerated platelet production. A second piece of evidence, provided by Odell and co-workers (1962, 1967), has been that a rebound overshoot or rebound undershoot follows platelet depletion or platelet transfusion (Fig. 4). More recently, additional support has been derived from a reinterpretation of the pathogenesis of periodic thrombocytopenia by Morley *et al.* (1970). In some splenectomized patients with borderline thrombopoietic function, the platelet count oscillates regularly with a period of about 28 days (Fig. 5). Such a pattern was previously thought to be caused by cyclic hormonal changes. However, it now appears more likely that it is caused by the

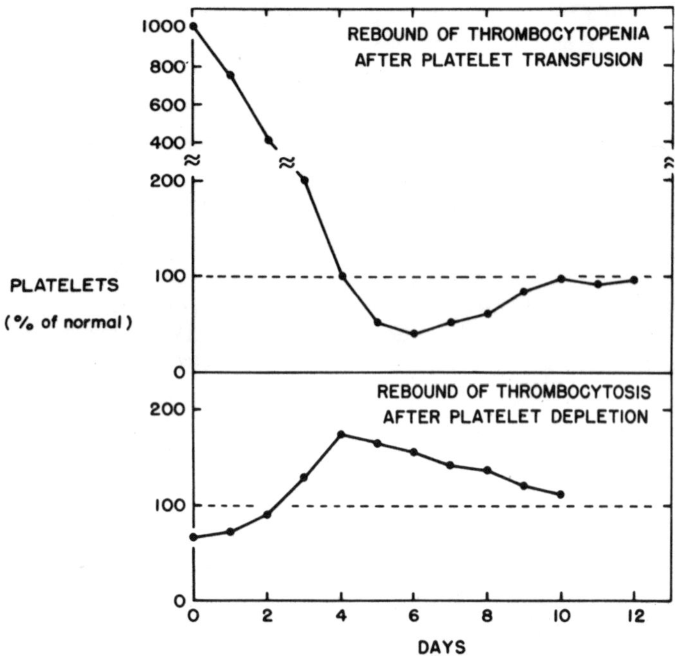

Figure 4. Rebound thrombocytopenia after platelet transfusion and rebound thrombocytosis after platelet depletion in normal rats (adapted from Odell *et al.* (1967) and Odell *et al.* (1962).

presence of a feedback circuit with low discrimination. If this is true, the period should be twice as long as the time it takes from the initiation of a signal for increased platelet production until the platelet has finished its life span. Since it takes about 4 days for a megakaryoblast to mature into a platelet-producing megakaryocyte and about 10 days for a platelet to finish its life span in the circulation, the observed oscillating period seems to fit reasonably well with the predicted value.

These considerations also indicate that the stimulus leading to a change in platelet production acts on the megakaryoblasts or more likely on the stem cells committed to the megakaryocytic line (Fig. 6). Studies by Harker and Finch (1969) indicate that the stimulus also acts on the maturing megakaryocyte causing additional endomitotic divisions and thereby increasing the platelet-producing cytoplasmic volume. The identity of the stimulus has as yet not been established, but evidence provided by Evatt and

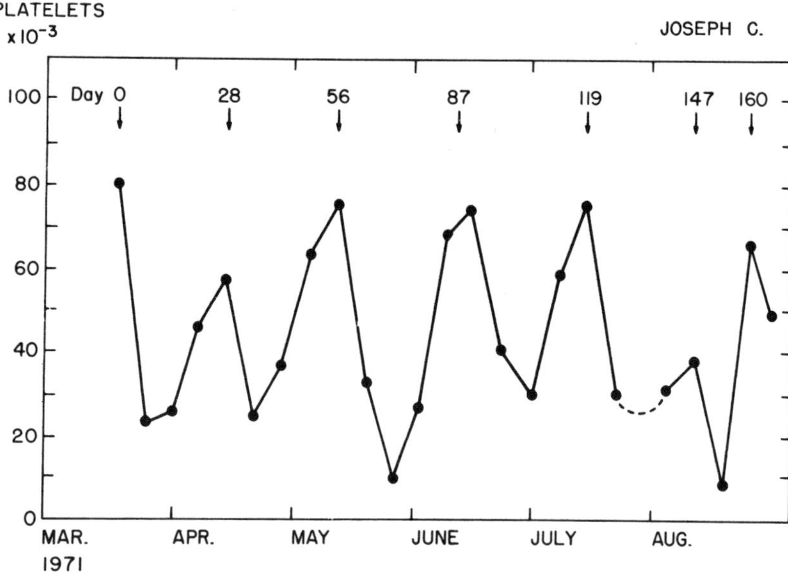

Figure 5. Oscillating pattern of the platelet count of a splenectomized male with chronic thrombocytopenia.

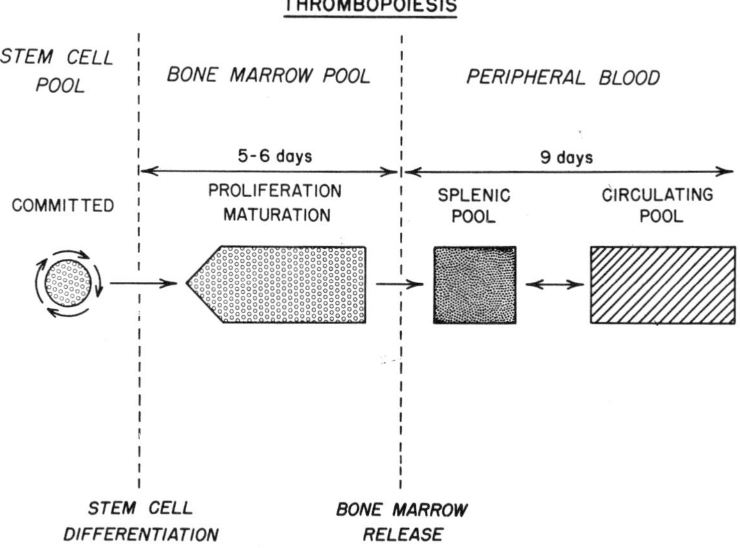

Figure 6. Thrombopoietic model outlining the path from stem cell differentiation to the eventual demise of platelets in the circulation.

Levin (1969) and Harker and Finch (1969) suggests that it is a humoral factor akin to erythropoietin. It has been named thrombopoietin and has been demonstrated in the plasma from severely thrombocytopenic animals. Several assay methods have been used, but the most promising has been developed by Schreiner and Levin (1970) and is based on the injection of a test plasma into animals in which endogenous platelet production has been suppressed by platelet transfusions. The effect of the injected plasma can be measured by the utilization of a compound such as ^{75}selenium methionine which labels megakaryocytic cytoplasma (Fig. 7). Although this technique is similar to the technique which has been used so successfully in the study of erythropoietin, the logistic problem of maintaining a preparatory thrombocytosis is so much greater than maintaining an erythrocytosis that so far little information has been obtained about the nature of thrombopoietin.

The mechanism by which a decrease in the platelet count generates thrombopoietin is unknown. Since the platelets serve as our first line of defense against blood loss, the most likely explanation would be that impaired hemostasis causes the release of a

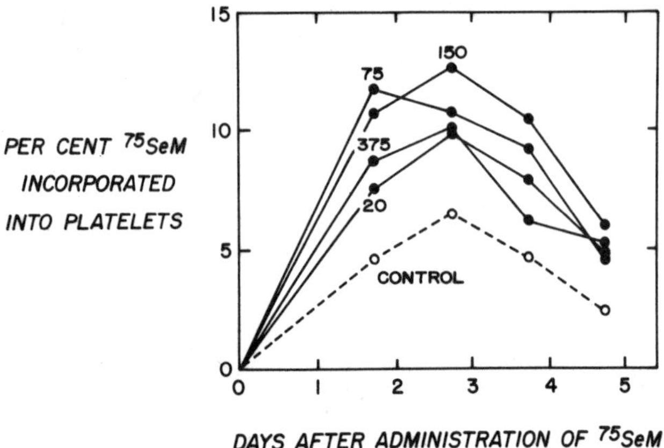

Figure 7. Effects of plasma upon incorporation of ^{75}selenium methionine (^{75}SeM) into the platelets of rabbits previously transfused with platelet concentrates. The plasma, in volume from 20–150 ml, was administered in three divided doses and ^{75}selenium methionine was given 6 hr after the last infusion (solid lines). The dashed line is the mean ^{75}selenium methionine utilization in six platelet-transfused control rabbits (Schreiner and Levin, 1970).

thrombopoietin. However, as shown by the age-dependent life span of platelets, most platelets do not get involved in hemostatic activities. Furthermore, clinical observations show normal hemostatic function until the platelet count is reduced to between 50,000 and 20,000/mm^3, far below the level at which a compensatory increase in platelet production is initiated. Finally, patients with congestive splenomegaly in whom up to 80 per cent of the total platelet mass is in the spleen show no compensatory increase in platelet production despite low circulating platelet count and impaired hemostatic function. These observations suggest that it is the platelet mass rather than the platelet count which triggers the release of thrombopoietin. However, it is very difficult to envision a sensor which could perceive the total mass of platelets in the spleen and in the circulation. It seems possible that it is the surface area, rather than the number or mass, which is involved in sensing and adjusting the concentration of a thrombopoietin in the circulation. The platelet surface is known to act as a sponge and absorb a variety of plasma factors. Actually, de Gabriele and Penington (1967) have shown that thrombopoietic activity of a plasma sample can be removed by preincubation with platelets. Another suggestive piece of evidence can be derived from measurements of the platelet number, platelet mass, and platelet surface in members of a family with hereditary megathrombocytopenia (Table 1). The

Table 1. Platelet parameters

	Mean count (mm^3)	Mean diameter (μ)	Mean surface (μ^2/mm^3)	Mean volume (μ^3/mm^3)
Normals (7)	294,000	2.1	3,986,000	1,592,000
Thrombocytopenia with megathrombocytes			% of normal	
J.C.	36,000	5.9	107	325
B.C.	105,000	3.8	127	253
S.M.	142,000	3.0	125	206
V.M.	68,000	3.5	92	191
L.W.	62,000	3.6	75	150
F.W. Sr.	135,000	3.4	144	280

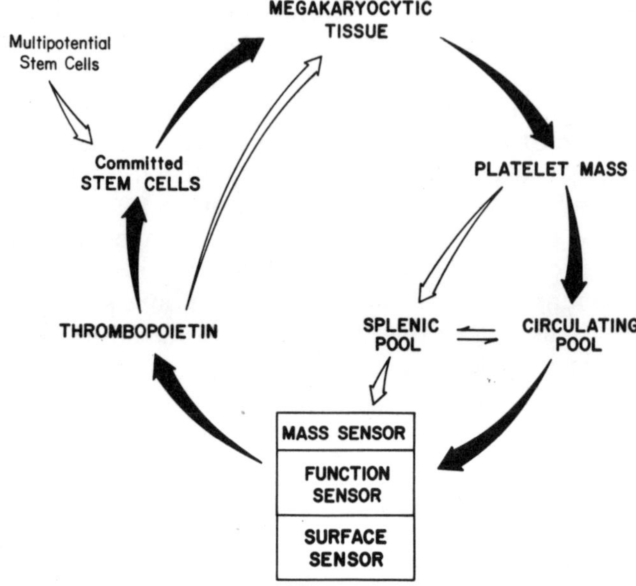

Figure 8. Proposed feedback circuit for the control of the platelet count.

capacity to produce platelets appears to be intact in this family, and the maintenance of a steady state thrombocytopenic level seems to be under active control. The only platelet parameter which was found to have an approximately normal value was the total surface area, suggesting that this parameter is involved in the feedback control of platelet production.

In conclusion, it can be stated that it seems most likely that platelet production is controlled by a feedback circuit in which a humoral factor, thrombopoietin, controls the proliferative activity of stem cells committed to megakaryocytes and of megakaryocytes themselves (Fig. 8). Some evidence has been presented suggesting that the concentration of thrombopoietin is regulated by the platelet surface rather than the platelet count or the platelet mass.

ACKNOWLEDGMENT

This work was supported in part by United States Public Health Service Grants H 6374 and H 4612.

REFERENCES

Aster, R. H. 1966. Pooling of platelets in the spleen: Role in the pathogenesis of "hypersplenic" thrombocytopenia. J. Clin. Invest. 45: 645.

De Gabriele, G., and Penington, D. S. 1967. Regulation of platelet production: "Thrombopoietin." Brit. J. Haematol. 13: 210.

Erslev, A. J. 1971. Feedback circuits in the control of stem cell differentiation. Amer. J. Pathol. 65: 629.

Evatt, B. L., and Levin, J. 1969. Measurement of thrombopoiesis in rabbits using ^{75}selenomethionine. J. Clin. Invest. 48: 1615.

Gardner, F. H. 1972. Platelet kinetics and lifespan. Clin. Haematol. 1: 307.

Garg, S. K., Lackner, H., and Karpatkin, S. 1972. The increased percentage of megathrombocytes in various clinical disorders. Ann. Intern. Med. 77: 361.

Harker, L. A., and Finch, C. A. 1969. Thrombokinetics in man. J. Clin. Invest. 48: 963.

Morley, A., King-Smith, E. A., and Stohlman, F., Jr. 1970. The oscillatory nature of hemopoiesis, pp. 3–14. *In* F. Stohlman, Jr. (ed.) Hemopoietic cellular proliferation. Grune and Stratton, New York.

Odell, T. T., Jr., Jackson, C. W., and Reiter, R. S. 1967. Depression of the megakaryocyte–platelet system in rats by transfusion of platelets. Acta Haematol. 38: 34.

Odell, T. T., Jr., MacDonald, T. P., and Asano, M. 1962. Response of rat megakaryocytes and platelets to bleeding. Acta Haematol. 27: 171.

Schreiner, D. P., and Levin, J. 1970. Detection of thrombopoietic activity in plasma by stimulation of suppressed thrombopoiesis. J. Clin. Invest. 49: 1709.

Biochemical Events in Platelet-Collagen Adhesion

G. A. Jamieson

The primary event in hemostasis appears to be the adhesion of platelets to various components of connective tissue (Hughes, 1962; Kjaerheim and Hovig, 1962) such as collagen (Spaet and Zucker, 1964) or other subendothelial structures. This is followed by the platelet release reaction resulting in the aggregation of other platelets to those which have previously adhered to the damaged subendothelial elements. Thus, the sequence of platelet events in hemostasis involves a *recognition* phase between the platelet and collagen, and a subsequent *cybernetic* phase, in which the information regarding this recognition is transmitted to the interior of the platelet in order to initiate the events of platelet release. A knowledge of the mechanisms involved in these various steps is essential to the elucidation of an understanding of the hemostatic sequence and to the rational design of antithrombogenic drugs.

Over-all platelet reactions leading to aggregation have been studied by optical methods in the aggregometer, while studies on the biochemical steps involved in platelet adhesion, release, and aggregation have involved mainly nucleotide metabolism in the release reaction and the activities associated with metabolic maintenance in the platelets (for review see Johnson, 1971).

One approach to separating the recognition and cybernetic phases has been to isolate platelet membranes in order to distinguish the membrane-associated activities of adhesion from the intracellular events of release and aggregation.

ISOLATION OF PLATELET MEMBRANES

Platelet disruption has been effected by homogenization sonication, nitrogen cavitation, or by the use of the blender (Table 1). Comparison of these and other methods, both in the presence and absence of membrane-hardening agents (Barber *et al.*, 1971) showed wide variability in their effectiveness due, probably, to variation in the duration of the mechanical disruption techniques and in the conditions used for preliminary differential centrifugation after disruption. Their use for too short a time results in inadequate lysis while conditions favorable for adequate disrup-

Table 1. Methods used for platelet homogenization and separation of membranes

Method	Reference
Freeze-thaw/differential centrifugation	Schulz and Hiepler, 1959
Sonication/differential	Maupin, 1959
Sonication/differential	Buckingham and Maynert, 1964
Sonication/discontinuous gradient	Solantunturi and Paasonen, 1966
Tissue grinder/continuous	Marcus *et al.*, 1966
Tissue grinder/discontinuous	Weber and Mondt, 1967
Blender/discontinuous	Siegel and Lüscher, 1967
Modified blender and grinder methods	Day *et al.*, 1969

tion often result in membrane fragmentation and disruption of intracellular organelles.

A glycerol-lysis technique has recently been developed which appears to give a good yield of platelet membranes with minimum damage to the subcellular elements (Barber and Jamieson, 1970). This method involves the slow intracellular accumulation of glycerol into platelets by centrifugation through a continuous glycerol gradient (0–40 per cent) followed by lysis by an isotonic sucrose solution. Platelet membranes have a very slow transit time for glycerol, of the order of minutes, whereas the transit time for water is in microseconds. Hence, the net effect of the above treatment is for a rapid influx of water, and a slow efflux of glycerol, resulting in an "explosive" lysis from the interior of the platelet. The plasma membrane, cellular cytoplasm and cellular debris are then separated by density step (27 per cent sucrose; d, 1.106) centrifugation. This membrane fraction could be subfractionated on a continuous density gradient (15–40 per cent, d, 1.06–1.150). Two membrane subfractions were obtained in equal amounts; they were identical in their complement of enzymes and in their isoelectric points and carbohydrate content, but they differed in size, in protein and lipid analyses (Barber and Jamieson, 1970), and in the procoagulant activity of their extracted lipids (Barber *et al.*, 1972) (Table 2). The distribution of membrane glycoproteins and their accessibility to neuraminidase and to trypsin were identical in the two preparations (Barber and Jamieson, 1971a).

Table 2. Properties of platelet membrane fractions

Property	High density	Low density
Density	1.120	1.090
pI	3.9	3.9
Carbohydrate	7%	7%
Protein	36.3%	29.5%
Total lipid	43.7%	51.8%
Clotting time		
Membrane	6.9 sec	6.9 sec
Lipid extracts	10.4 sec	8.4 sec

The enzymes found in the platelet membranes were similar to those found in the plasma membranes of other cells. In particular, phosphodiesterase, acid phosphatase, and ATPase activity in the platelet membranes showed enrichments of 8-, 4-, and 2-fold, respectively, over the whole homogenate, compared with values of 15-, 4- (Lansing *et al.*, 1967), and 6-fold (Emmelot *et al.*, 1964) for plasma membranes of liver cells as compared with microsomes. In contrast, the low recoveries of glycosidase, esterase, and succinic dehydrogenase, which usually occur in intracellular membranes, indicated that both membranes isolated from the density step centrifugation and from the continuous gradient were free of contamination with intracellular membranes. Further studies have shown that adenyl cyclase activity is present in these purified platelet membranes, that the activity is stimulated by prostaglandin E_1, but that this stimulatory effect is markedly increased in the presence of guanosine triphosphate (Krishna *et al.*, 1972).

MECHANISM OF PLATELET-COLLAGEN ADHESION

Platelet membranes contain two enzymes which transfer galactose and glucose from the corresponding sugar nucleotides to a collagen acceptor. One of these, collagen galactosyltransferase, appears to be present on the inner surface of the membrane, since it cannot be detected on the intact platelets (Barber and Jamieson, 1971b), while the other, collagen glucosyltransferase, appears to be present on the outer aspect (Barber and Jamieson, 1971c,d), since it can be detected both in intact platelets and isolated membranes.

One of the mechanisms which has been proposed as the basis for intercellular adhesion is the interaction between glycosyltransferases and incomplete glycoproteins on the surface of the complementary aggregating cells (Roseman, 1970). Examination of the requirements for platelet-collagen adhesion and for collagen glucosyltransferase reaction showed that both were inhibited by sulfhydryl reagents and that both required free ϵ-amino groups in the lysine of the collagen substrate. Further studies showed that the collagen glucosyltransferase was inhibited by glucosamine, aspirin, and chlorpromazine, all drugs which have been considered to inhibit platelet-collagen adhesion. Since these results indicated a role for carbohydrate in the adhesion of platelets to collagen, an experiment was carried out in which glycopeptides were isolated from collagen and then added to platelet-rich plasma in the presence of collagen. Under these conditions there was an 85 per cent inhibition of adhesion in the presence of collagen glycopeptides but only a 15 per cent inhibition of adhesion in the presence of collagen peptides which were devoid of carbohydrate. The corresponding inhibitions of the collagen glucosyltransferase reaction were 40 and 10 per cent, respectively.

On the basis of these results it was proposed (Jamieson *et al.*, 1971) that platelet-collagen adhesion occurs by the formation of an enzyme-acceptor complex between the galactosyl residues present in collagen itself and the glucosyltransferase present on the platelet membrane. It is important to note that in platelet-collagen adhesion we are measuring only the first stage of the reaction, the formation of the enzyme-acceptor complex, while with the transferase we are measuring the over-all reaction, including the formation of the enzyme-acceptor complex, the interaction with uridine diphosphate glucose and Mn^{++}, and the transfer of glucose to the receptor site.

Confirmation of this idea has come from a series of elegant experiments on the effect of galactose oxidase on platelet aggregation (McI. Chesney *et al.*, 1972). Galactose oxidase converts the 6-hydroxymethyl group of galactose present in the terminal position of a heterosaccharide chain to an aldehyde group. Thus, treatment of collagen with galactose oxidase completely destroyed its ability to induce aggregation, while further treatment with sodium borohydride, which converts the 6-aldehydogalactose back to galactose, restored the ability to induce aggregation. Similarly, it has been found that treatment of collagen with galactose oxidase completely destroys its ability to act as a substrate for the collagen glucosyltransferase (Urban and Jamieson, unpublished results). These studies provide further support for a control role for galactose in the mechanism of platelet adhesion and aggregation.

SUGAR-LIPID INTERMEDIATE

Studies on the collagen glucosyltransferase reaction showed that significant radioactivity from glucose-labeled UDP-glucose was incorporated into a lipid intermediate involving retinol (vitamin A) or a derivative of it (De Luca *et al.*, 1972). A similar intermediate appears to be part of the corresponding mannosyltransferase which utilizes an endogenous acceptor present on the platelet membrane. Thus, the transferase reaction appears to proceed in two stages: in one stage the appropriate sugar nucleotide reacts to give a complex sugar-lipid involving retinol and in the second stage the monosaccharide is transferred to an appropriate endogenous or exogenous receptor. The collagen galactosyltransferase does not appear to involve a lipid intermediate. Although a direct role for vitamin A in platelet aggregation has not been demonstrated, it is known that retinol increases the adhesiveness to glass beads of platelets from vitamin A-deficient rats (McDonald, 1966) and reverses the retardation of wound healing caused by aspirin, a known inhibitor of platelet aggregation (Lee, 1968).

DIVALENT CATION EFFECTS

The collagen glucosyl- and galactosyltransferases, and the mannosyltransferase of platelet membranes, require Mn^{++} (15 m*M*) for full activity although they show limited activity in the presence of Cd^{++}. Moreover, each of these divalent cations causes flocculation of the membranes under the condition of assay. In view of this, and the possibility that the endogenous activities might play a role in aggregation similar to that suggested for intercellular adhesion (Roseman, 1970), a study was made of the effect of Mn^{++} and Cd^{++} on platelets (Urban *et al.*, 1972).

Both Cd^{++} and Mn^{++} ions induced aggregation in platelet-rich plasma with a maximum occurring at 15 m*M*. In neither case was aggregation accompanied by the release reaction, and a further phase of aggregation was induced by the addition of collagen. The aggregation induced by Mn^{++} and Cd^{++} did not appear to involve ADP since it was unaffected by apyrase at concentrations at which collagen-induced aggregation is completely inhibited (Eika, 1972). Higher concentrations of Mn^{++} had no further effect, but at concentrations of Cd^{++} above 25 m*M* there was a further wave of aggregation accompanied by the release reaction. Aggregation, accompanied by release, also occurred if the combined concentration of Mn^{++} and Cd^{++} exceeded 25 m*M*, provided a threshold concentration of Cd^{++} of about 3 m*M* had been reached.

These differences in response to Mn^{++} and Cd^{++} suggested that two types of binding site were involved. Binding studies with radioactive $^{54}Mn^{++}$ and $^{115}Cd^{++}$, using both intact platelets and isolated membranes, showed that bound $^{54}Mn^{++}$ was completely displaced by washing with a solution containing nonradioactive Cd^{++}, but that only 30 per cent of bound $^{115}Cd^{++}$ was displaced by a 10-fold excess of nonradioactive Mn^{++}.

MICROCALORIMETRY

In an attempt to obtain further information on the biochemical events occurring in platelet adhesion and aggregation we have made use of the microcalorimeter (Wadsö, 1968) to compare the heat changes resulting from the treatment of isolated (washed) platelets with ADP, collagen, divalent cations, or thrombin (Fletcher *et al.*, 1972).

Considerable differences exist in heat production in response to these reagents. With ADP or collagen heat production reached a maximum of 25 $\mu w/10^{10}$ platelets in 5 min and continued at a low level for at least 30 min. Quantitatively similar results were obtained with Mn^{++} and Cd^{++} although the kinetic form of heat production differed and was, in fact, different for each of the divalent cations. On the other hand, heat production in response to thrombin reached a maximum of about 300 $\mu w/10^{10}$ platelets in 5 min and totaled as high as 50 mcal over a period of 30–40 min.

Further study of the thrombin-induced aggregation showed that the early stages of the reaction were sensitive to antimycin, suggesting that oxidative phosphorylation is the principal source of energy production at this stage, while the later stages were sensitive to 2-deoxy-D-glucose, suggesting the importance of glycolysis. The effect of cyclic AMP was greatest in the early stages of the reaction but heat production was defocused throughout.

BIOCHEMICAL EVENTS IN PLATELET ADHESION AND AGGREGATION

These observations suggest certain possible speculations regarding the sequence of biochemical events in the recognition and cybernetic phases.

First, as postulated, platelet-collagen adhesion occurs via the formation of an enzyme-acceptor complex between galactosyl residues present on collagen and a collagen glucosyltransferase present on the platelet membrane.

Second, glucose is transferred from a retinol-phosphate-glucose intermediate present in the membrane to complete the collagen heterosaccharide chain. The source of the divalent cation required for this step has not yet been determined.

Third, the loss of glucose from the lipid intermediate changes the polarity and lipophilic nature of that molecule. This may initiate a sequence of biosynthetic events which leads eventually to the formation of more of the lipid intermediate from the intracellular pool of UDP-glucose, or it may initiate conformational changes in the platelet membrane. Either of these could be responsible for initiating the release reaction and for the activation of the sialyl (Mester *et al.*, 1972), mannosyl (Barber *et al.*, unpublished results), or other (Bosmann, 1971) transferases which may be involved in platelet aggregation.

While it must be emphasized that this sequence is purely speculative, the microcalorimeter studies with collagen and ADP suggest that the heat production associated with purely membrane events is small, although this may be a reflection more of the relatively small number of molecules interacting rather than the free energy changes as such.

The further definition of the biochemical events in platelet adhesion and aggregation will help in forming a sound basis for developing antithrombogenic drugs and controlling thromboembolic disease.

REFERENCES

Barber, A. J., and Jamieson, G. A. 1970. Isolation and characterization of plasma membranes from human blood platelets. J. Biol. Chem. 245: 6357.

Barber, A. J., and Jamieson, G. A. 1971a. Isolation of glycopeptides from high and low density platelet plasma membranes. Biochemistry 10: 4711.

Barber, A. J., and Jamieson, G. A. 1971b. Characterization of membrane-bound collagen: Galactosyltransferase of human blood platelets. Biochim. Biophys. Acta 252: 546.

Barber, A. J., and Jamieson, G. A. 1971c. Platelet collagen adhesion: Characterization of collagen glucosyltransferase of plasma membranes of human blood platelets. Biochim. Biophys. Acta 252: 533.

Barber, A. J., and Jamieson, G. A. 1971d. Collagen-glucosyltransferase of human blood platelets. Fed. Proc. 30: 540.

Barber, A. J., Pepper, D. S., and Jamieson, G. A. 1971. A comparison of methods for platelet lysis and the isolation of platelet membranes. Thromb. Diath. Haemorrh. 26: 38.

Barber, A. J., Triantaphyllopoulos, D. C., and Jamieson, G. A. 1972. Differing procoagulant activities in the extracted lipids of high and low density platelet plasma membranes. Thromb. Diath. Haemorrh. 28: 206.

Bosman, H. B. 1971. Platelet adhesiveness and aggregation: The collagen: glycosyl, polypeptide: N-acetylgalactosaminyl and glycoprotein: galactosyl transferases of human platelets. Biochem. Biophys. Res. Commun. 43: 1118.

Buckingham, S., and Maynert, E. W. 1964. The release of 5-hydroxytryptamine, potassium and amino acids from platelets. J. Pharmacol. Exp. Ther. 143: 332.

Day, H. J., Holmsen, H., Hovig, T. 1969. Subcellular particles of human platelets. Scand. J. Haemat., Suppl. 7:1.

De Luca, L., Barber, A. J., and Jamieson, G. A. 1972. Possible role of vitamin A in platelet collagen adhesion. Fed. Proc. 31: 242.

Eika, C. 1972. On the mechanism of platelet aggregation induced by heparin, protamine and polybrene. Scand. J. Haematol. 9: 248.

Emmelot, P., Bos, C. J., Benedetti, E. L., and Rumke, P. 1964. Studies on plasma membranes. I. Chemical composition and enzyme content of plasma membranes isolated from rat liver. Biochim. Biophys. Acta 90: 126.

Fletcher, A. P., Ross, P. D., and Jamieson, G. A. 1972. Calorimetry in the study of human blood platelets. Fed. Proc. 31: 241.

Hughes, J. 1962. Accolement des plaquettes aux structures conjoctives perivasculaires. Thromb. Diath. Haemorrh. 8: 241.

Jamieson, G. A., Urban, C. L., and Barber, A. J. 1971. An enzymatic basis for platelet:collagen adhesion. Nature New Biol. 234: 5.

Johnson, S. A. (ed.). 1971. The circulating platelet. Academic Press, New York.

Kjaerheim, A., and Hovig, T. 1962. The ultrastructure of haemostatic blood platelet plugs in rabbit mesenterium. Thromb. Diath. Haemorrh. 7: 1.

Krishna, G., Harwood, J., Barber, A. J., and Jamieson, G. A. 1972. Requirement for guanosine triphosphate in the prostaglandin activation of adenyl cyclase of platelet membranes. J. Biol. Chem. 247: 2263.

Lansing, A. I., Belkhode, M. L., Lynch, W. E., and Lieberman, I. 1967. Enzymes of plasma membranes of liver. J. Biol. Chem. 242: 1772.

Lee, K. H. 1968. Studies on the mechanisms of action of salicylate. II. Retardation of wound healing by aspirin. J. Pharm. Sci. 57: 1042.

Marcus, A. J., Zucker-Franklin, D., Safier, L. B., and Ullman, H. L. 1966. Studies on human platelet granules and membranes. J. Clin. Invest. 45: 14.

McDonald, T. P. 1966. Effects of vitamin A on mucopolysaccharides of rat blood platelets. Amer. J. Physiol. 210: 807.

McI. Chesney, C., Harper, E., and Colman, R. W. 1972. Critical role of the carbohydrate side chain of collagen in platelet aggregation. J. Clin. Invest. 51: 2693.

Maupin, B. 1959. Recherches sur les granules plaquettaires. Fraction sedimentable d'un lysat plaquettaire. Le Sang. 30: 114.

Mester, L., Szabados, T., Born, G. V. R., and Michal, F. 1972. Changes in the aggregation of platelets enriched in sialic acid. Nature New Biol. 236: 213.

Roseman, S. 1970. The synthesis of complex carbohydrates by multiglycosyltransferase systems and their potential function in intercellular adhesion. Chem. Phys. Lipids. 5: 270.

Schulz, H., and Hiepler, E. 1959. Über die Lokalisierung von gerinnungsphysiologischen Aktivitäten in submikroskopischen Strukturen der Thrombocyten. Klin. Wschr. 37: 273.

Siegel, A., and Lüscher, E. F. 1967. Non-identity of the α-granules of human blood platelets with typical lysosomes. Nature. 215: 745.

Solatunturi, E., and Paasonen, M. K. 1966. Intracellular distribution of monamine oxidase, 5-hydroxytryptamine and histamine in blood platelets of rabbis. Ann Med. Exp. Fenn. 44: 427.

Spaet, T. H., and Zucker, M. B. 1964. Mechanism of platelet plug formation and role of adenosine diphosphate. Amer. J. Physiol. 206: 1267.

Urban, C., Fletcher, A. P., and Jamieson, G. A. 1972. Divalent cation effects in platelet aggregation, p. 256. Abstracts, Third Congress of International Society on Thrombosis and Haemostasis, Washington, D. C.

Wadsö, I. 1968. Design and testing of a micro reaction calorimeter. Acta Chem. Scand. 22: 927.

Weber, E., and Mondt, H. 1967. Verteilung und Beeinflussung von Metabolites in fraktionierter Homogenaten aus Blüplättchen. Klin. Wschr. 45: 165.

Antiserotonin and Antihistamine Drugs as Inhibitors of Platelet Function

L. M. Aledort, S. Berger, B. Goldman, and E. Puszkin

Cyproheptadine and four other antiserotonin or antihistamine compounds, or both, were studied for their effects on platelet function. Inhibition of ^{14}C 5-HT [serotonin] uptake was correlated while antihistamine or antiserotonin effects of these drugs were not correlated well with inhibition of ADP-, epinephrine-, or collagen-induced platelet aggregation. These data suggest that membrane sites for 5-HT uptake may be important for some aspects of platelet function.

As early as 1947 (Zucker) platelet serotonin (5-HT) was implicated in hemostasis. Platelets do not synthesize serotonin but accumulate it from the argentaffin cells of the upper gastrointestinal tract. This uptake of 5-HT depends on intact platelet metabolism, an active transport mechanism at the platelet surface, and available storage sites (Stacey, 1961). A great many investigators have concerned themselves with the site of serotonin storage and the effect of platelet aggregation on its release. Little is known, however, of the relationship between 5-HT content and platelet function as it relates to uptake sites. Reserpinized platelets devoid of 5-HT are functionally intact (Baumgartner and Born, 1968). Patients with myeloproliferative disorders with decreased platelet 5-HT and functionally abnormal cells (Gilbert *et al.*, 1969) do not correct their aggregation defects when their 5-HT is returned to normal. Ouabain, an inhibitor of the platelet Na^{+}-K^{+}-dependent ATPase activity (Aledort *et al.*, 1968), inhibits 5-HT uptake (Mills and Roberts, 1967) without affecting function. In contrast to these observations are the findings that a large number of interrelated compounds affect 5-HT uptake and function (Stacey, 1961; O'Brien, 1961).

Antihistamines, phenothiazines, antimalarials, and local anesthetics are compounds that share the following characteristics: positive charge, a hydrocarbon, and lipophilic moieties. In addition they inhibit platelet functions, *i.e.* aggregation and retraction, and are capable of prolonging the bleeding time (O'Brien, 1961).

Cyproheptadine is a potent antihistamine and antiserotonin drug (Stone *et al.*, 1961). This compound has been useful to inhibit perfusion sequelae (Martin *et al.*, 1964), prevent renal necrosis (Selye *et al.*, 1967), and alter the platelet responses in renal allograft rejection (Aledort *et al.*, 1973). The studies to be presented deal with the evaluation of a series of antiserotonin and antihistaminic agents including cyproheptadine as inhibitors of platelet function.

MATERIALS AND METHODS

Cyproheptadine and four other compounds are listed in Fig. 1 with their structures and their ED_{50} for antihistamine and antiserotonin activities. The ED_{50} values for cyproheptadine and compounds A, B, and C were published by Engelhardt *et al.* (1965). Compound D was not studied under the same experimental conditions. According to Stone (personal communication), compound D effectively antagonized the pressor effects of serotonin in anesthetized dogs (CV dog) but at doses up to 7 mg/kg I.V. did not reduce the hypotensive effects of histamine. The chemical names of the compounds shown in Fig. 1 are as follows:

STRUCTURE	ANTISEROTONIN ED_{50}, mg/Kg RAT PAW	CV DOG	ANTIHISTAMINE ED_{50}, mg/Kg
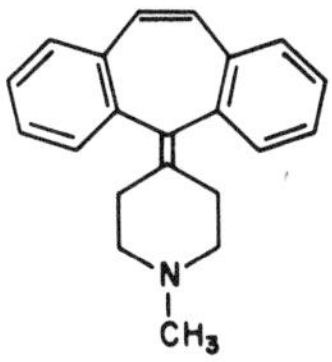 CYPROHEPTADINE (N–CH_3)	0.03	0.05	0.04
A 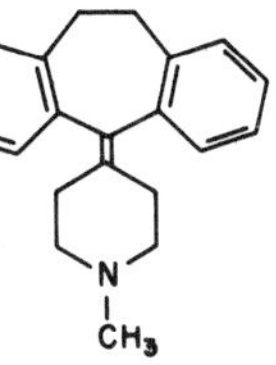 (N–CH_3)	0.1		0.04
B 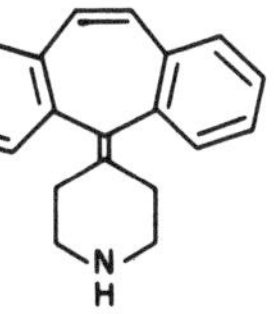 (N–H)	0.5		>12.5
C 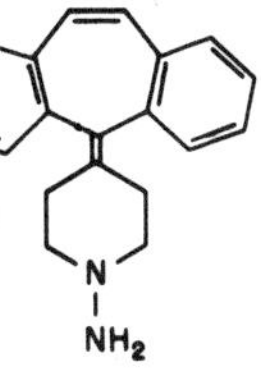 (N–NH_2)	3.6		2.8
D 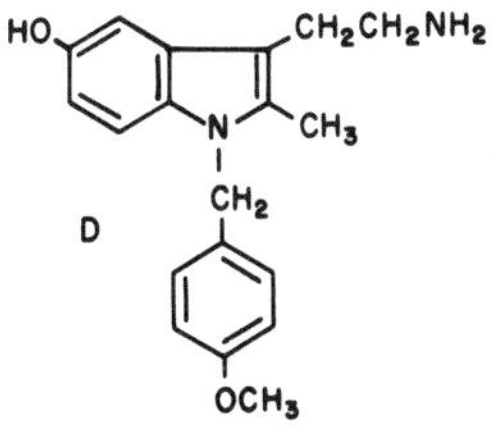 (HO, $CH_2CH_2NH_2$, CH_3, CH_2, OCH_3)		0.2	

Figure 1. Antiserotonin and antihistamine properties of cyproheptadine and four other compounds used in this study.

compound A, 4-(10,11-dihydro-5H-dibenzo[a,d]cyclohepten-5-ylidene)-1-methylpiperidine hydrochloride; compound B, 5-(5H-dibenzo[a,d]cyclohepten-5-ylidene)-piperidine hydrochloride; compound C, 4-(5H-dibenzo[a,d]cyclohepten-5-ylidene)-1-amino-piperidine hydrogen maleate; compound D, 1-(4-methoxybenzyl)-2-methyl-3-(β-aminoethyl)-5-hydroxyindole hydrochloride. All drugs were supplied as salts in the solid state (Merck Sharp and Dohme Research Laboratories). They were dissolved in distilled water to the desired final concentration and were used on the same day.

Antiserotonin activity was determined in rats by antagonism of serotonin-induced paw edema. Test drugs were administered subcutaneously. In anesthetized dogs, antiserotonin activity was evaluated by antagonism of pressor effects of serotonin. Test drugs were administered intravenously. Antihistamine activity was studied in guinea pigs by histamine-aerosol technique. Test drugs were administered intraperitoneally. For further details, see Engelhardt *et al.* (1965).

^{14}C-Cyproheptadine was labeled in positions 5, 10, and 11 of the middle ring (supplied by Merck Sharp and Dohme Research Laboratories).

Venous blood was collected in one-tenth its volume of 4 per cent sodium citrate from normal volunteers with no history of recent drug ingestion. The blood was centrifuged at 4°C for 20 min at 300 $\times$ g in an International Centrifuge to obtain platelet-rich plasma (PRP). The PRP was adjusted with autologous platelet-poor plasma so that the final platelet count for experiments was 300,000/μl.

Platelet aggregation was studied as previously described (Goldman and Aledort, 1972). The final concentration of ADP (used as the sodium salt supplied by Sigma) was 2×10^{-6} M. Epinephrine (Parke, Davis and Co.), stored in the dark and diluted just prior to its use, was used at a final concentration of 50 μM. Collagen tendon (Sigma) was prepared as follows: collagen, 250 mg, was mixed with 25 ml of buffered saline in a Waring Blendor and the supernatant was used for testing.

^{14}C 5-HT binoxalate (obtained from New England Nuclear) was added to aliquots of PRP. The final concentration of 5-HT-free base was 0.89 mg/ml. For measurement of 5-HT uptake, PRP was incubated with labeled material for 30 min at 37°C using the methods of Jerushalmy and Zucker (1966). Clot retraction was measured as previously described (Aledort *et al.*, 1968).

For studies of binding, or uptake of ^{14}C-cyproheptadine, or both, human platelet concentrates were prepared by the method of Aster and Jandl (1964). These concentrates which contained 5 to 7 $\times$ 10^9 platelets/ml were incubated at 37°C over a 30-min period with ^{14}C-cyproheptadine. Aliquots of the mixture were removed at varying intervals and the supernatants counted in a liquid scintillation counter. The amount of radioactivity associated with the platelets was then calculated from the plasma disappearance.

RESULTS

Cyproheptadine, over a concentration range of 2.5 to 10 mg/100 ml, inhibited both primary and secondary waves of ADP- and epinephrine-induced platelet aggregation (Fig. 2). Collagen-induced aggregation was similarly inhibited. The inhibition shown here

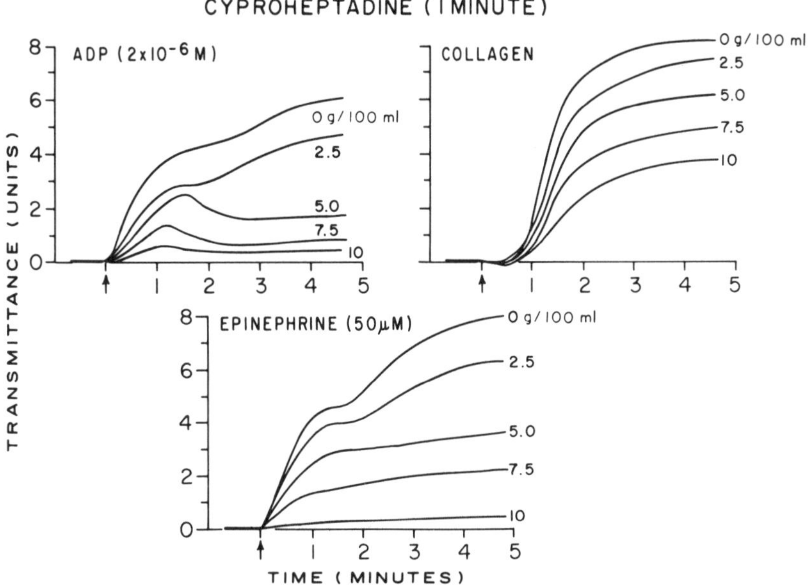

Figure 2. Effect of varying concentrations of cyproheptadine on ADP-, epinephrine-, and collagen-induced platelet aggregation.

after 1 min of preincubation with drug was minimal at lower concentrations but almost maximal at 10 mg/100 ml. Longer incubations up to 1 hr only slightly increased inhibition at any given concentration of cyproheptadine.

Figure 3 demonstrates the relative effectiveness of cyproheptadine (P) and four other compounds (A, B, C, and D) on ADP-, epinephrine-, and collagen-induced platelet aggregation at final drug concentrations of 5 mg/100 ml following a 5-min exposure to drug. Compounds B and D were the most effective inhibitors with cyproheptadine being intermediate in effectiveness.

5-HT uptake, followed over a 30-min period, was inhibited maximally by cyproheptadine at any given concentration after a 1-min incubation. The percentage of inhibition increased in a linear fashion with increasing concentrations of cyproheptadine (Fig. 4). When the four compounds were compared over a wide range of concentrations with cyproheptadine on ^{14}C 5-HT uptake, compounds B and D were the most potent inhibitors (Fig. 5).

The epinephrine- and collagen-induced release of ^{14}C 5-HT showed increasing inhibition with increasing doses of cyproheptadine. Inhibition was apparent after an exposure time of 1 min and increased minimally over a 30-min period.

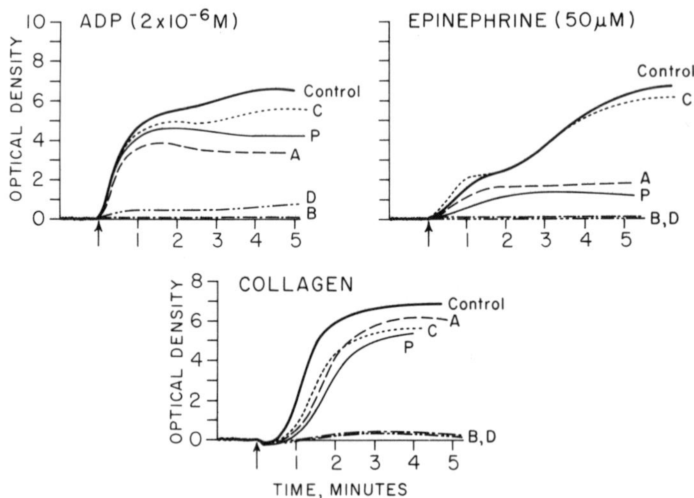

Figure 3. Relative effectiveness of cyproheptadine (P) and four related compounds (A, B, C, and D) on ADP-, epinephrine-, and collagen-induced platelet aggregation.

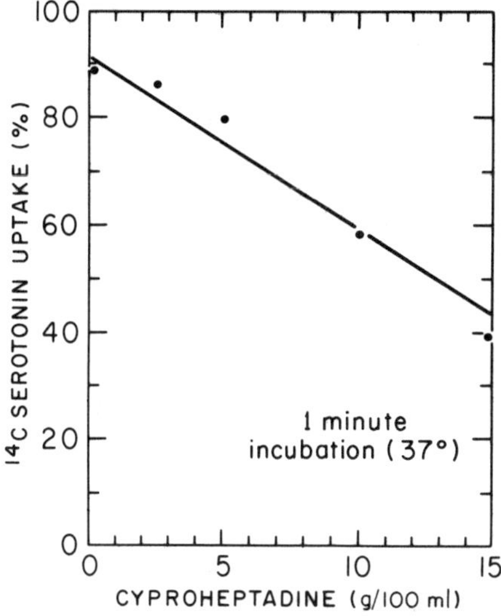

Figure 4. Effect of increasing concentrations of cyproheptadine on ^{14}C-serotonin uptake.

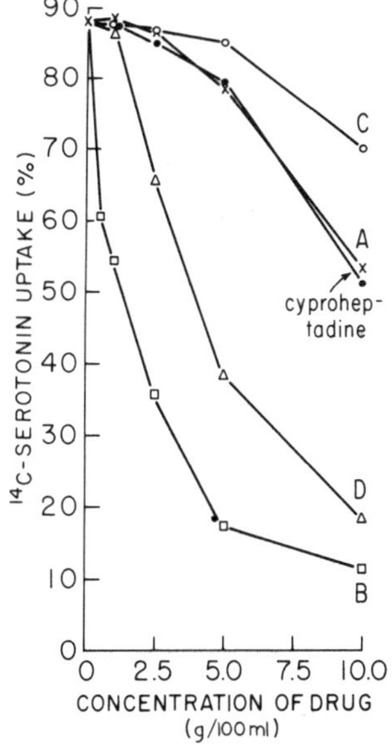

Figure 5. Relative effectiveness of increasing concentrations of cyproheptadine and four related compounds (A, B, C, and D) on ^{14}C-serotonin uptake. Average values for 4 experiments per drug.

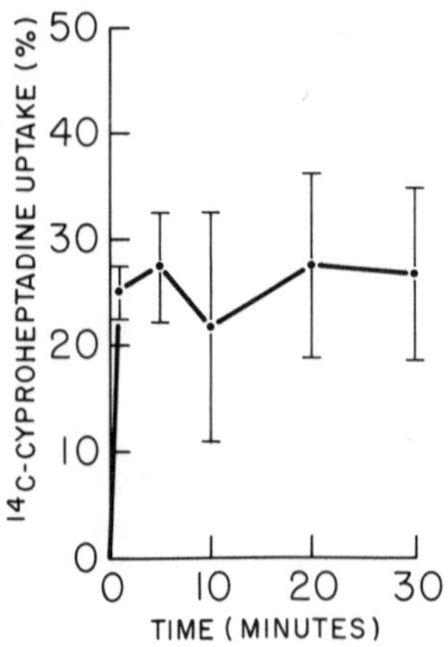

Figure 6. ^{14}C-Cyproheptadine uptake by human platelet concentrates over a 30-min. period. Average values for 5 experiments. Vertical bracket-like lines represent standard deviations of the mean.

When the five related compounds at a final drug concentration of 5 mg/100 ml were evaluated for their relative effects on epinephrine-induced ^{14}C 5-HT release, only compounds A and P showed a 60 per cent inhibition. Compounds B, C, and D had no appreciable effect. When collagen-induced ^{14}C 5-HT release was studied, each of the five compounds inhibited release by 30 per cent.

None of the five drugs inhibited clot retraction at concentrations up to 10 mg/100 ml.

The amount of radioactivity associated with platelet concentrates calculated from the plasma disappearance is demonstrated in Fig. 6. Binding reached a maximum of approximately 25 per cent of total radioactivity added after 1 min of incubation and then plateaued off, remaining essentially constant for 30 min.

DISCUSSION

Recently there has been great interest in finding an ideal platelet deaggregating agent for use as an antithrombogenic agent (Weiss, 1970). As a result, a large body of data has accumulated on platelet-deaggregating agents (Aledort, 1971). A large group of seemingly unrelated compounds, such as phenothiazines, anesthetics and antihistaminics, have been found to inhibit platelet function (O'Brien, 1961; Mitchell and Sharp, 1964; Aledort and Niemetz, 1968) as well as to inhibit the uptake of 5-HT by platelets (Mitchell and Sharp, 1964; Stacy, 1961). In contrast, depletion of platelet 5-HT did not alter platelet function (Mitchell and Sharp, 1964). Baumgartner and Born (1968) studying the role of 5-HT in platelets, suggested an interrelationship between 5-HT membrane receptor sites and function.

There is increasing evidence that cyproheptadine, an antiserotonin and antihistamine, is useful in preventing vascular occlusive disease via its effect on platelets (Martin *et al.*, 1964; Selye *et al.*, 1967; Aledort *et al.*, 1973). Cyproheptadine, three chemically related compounds and one chemically unrelated antiserotonin agent were, therefore, studied for their effects on platelet function.

No relationship was found between the antiserotonin or antihistamine activities of these five drugs and their effects on platelet function. These findings are in agreement with those published by Herrmann and Frank (1966). In contrast, there was a direct correlation between the inhibition of platelet aggregation and inhibition of 5-HT uptake. This finding extended further the observations of Baumgartner and Born (1968) who suggested the importance of 5-HT membrane binding sites in relation to platelet function.

The studies of platelet uptake, or binding of ^{14}C-cyproheptadine, or both, show a rapid binding, occurring almost immediately, without penetration into the cell. The time of maximal binding correlates well with the effect of this drug on aggregation and inhibition of 5-HT uptake. The lack of effect of sulfhydryl inhibitors (Berger *et al.*, 1972), cold, or metabolic inhibitors (Gaut, 1972) on the rapid uptake of cyproheptadine further suggests that the compound is bound by the platelet membrane rather than undergoing active transport.

The avidity of this drug for the cell membrane may explain its effectiveness in altering renal rejection and in producing remissions in patients with idiopathic thrombocytopenic purpura who did not respond to steroids (Pesse and Quappe, 1972). The success in these clinical settings warrants further study of cyproheptadine and its analogs.

ACKNOWLEDGMENTS

The authors would like to thank Mrs. Sadie Chu for technical assistance. This research was supported by a grant from Merck Sharp and Dohme Research Laboratories, Division of Merck and Co., Inc.

REFERENCES

Aledort, L. M. 1971. Platelet aggregation, pp. 259–281. *In* S. A. Johnson (ed.) The circulating platelet. Academic Press, New York.

Aledort, L. M., and Niemetz, J. 1968. Dissociation of platelet aggregation from clot retraction, potassium loss, and adenosine triphosphatase activity. Proc. Soc. Exp. Biol. Med. 128: 658.

Aledort, L. M., Taub, R., Burrows, L., Leiter, E., Glabman, S., Berger, S., Haimov, M., and Nirmul, G. 1973. Use of inhibitors of platelet function in renal rejection phenomena. (This symposium).

Aledort, L. M., Troup, S. B., and Weed, R. I. 1968. Inhibition of sulfhydryl-dependent platelet functions by penetrating and non-penetrating analogues of parachloromercuribenzene. Blood 31: 471.

Aster, R. H., and Jandl, J. H. 1964. Platelet-sequestration in man. I. Methods. J. Clin. Invest. 43: 843.

Baumgartner, H. R., and Born, G. V. R. 1968. Effects of 5-hydroxytryptamine on platelet aggregation. Nature 218: 137.

Berger, S., Puszkin, E., and Aledort, L. M. 1972. The effect of anti-serotonin and anti-histamine drugs on platelet function *in vitro*, p. 168. Abstract, Third Congress of International Society on Thrombosis and Haemostasis, Washington, D.C.

Engelhardt, E. L., Zell, H. C., Saari, W. S., Christy, M. E., Colton, C. D., Stone, C. A., Stavorski, J. M., Wenger, H. C., and Ludden, C. T. 1965. Structure-activity relationship in the cyproheptadine series. J. Med. Chem. 8: 829.

Gaut, Z. N. 1972. Binding of cyproheptadine—(N-Methyl. ^{14}C) by human blood platelets, p. 194. Abstract, Third Congress of International Society on Thrombosis and Haemostasis, Washington, D.C.

Gilbert, H. S., Aledort, L. M., Weiss, H. J., and Wasserman, L. R. 1969. Abnormalities of platelet function in polycythemia vera. Proc. Amer. Soc. Hematol. (abstr.), p. 181.

Goldman, B., and Aledort, L. M. 1972. Essential athrombia: a family study. Ann. Intern. Med. 76: 269.

Hermann, R. G., and Frank, J. D. 1966. Effect of adenosine derivatives and antihistaminics on platelet aggregation. Proc. Soc. Exp. Biol. Med. 123: 654.

Jerushalmy, Z., and Zucker, M. 1966. Some effects of fibrinogen degradation products (FDP) on blood platelets. Thromb. Diath. Haemorrh. 15: 413.

Martin, D. S., del Castillo, J., Martinez, M., Pickens, J., and Hudson, P. J. 1964. Beneficial influence of a serotonin-histamine antagonist on perfusion sequelae. Surgery 56: 1064.

Mills, D. C. B., and Roberts, G. C. K. 1967. Membrane active drugs and the aggregation of human blood platelets. Nature 213: 35.

Mitchell, J. R. A., and Sharp, A. A. 1964. Platelet clumping *in vitro*. Brit. J. Haematol. 10: 78.

O'Brien, J. R. 1961. Thc adhcsiveness of native platelets and its prevention. J. Clin. Pathol. 14: 140.

Pesse, F., and Quappe, G. 1972. Effecto de la cyproheptadina en el purpura thrombocitopenico idiopatico cronico en el nino. Rev. Med. Chile. 100: 417.

Selye, H., Pahk, U. S., and Somogyi, A. 1967. Prevention of renal necrosis by stress. J. Amer. Med. Assn. 201: 1026.

Stacey, R. S. 1961. Uptake of 5-hydroxytryptamine by platelets. Brit. J. Pharmacol. 16: 284.

Stone, C. A., Wenger, H. C., Ludden, C. T., Stavorski, J. M., and Ross, C. A. 1961. Anti-serotonin-antihistaminic properties of cyproheptadine. J. Pharmacol. Exp. Ther. 131: 73.

Weiss, H. J. 1970. Aspirin ingestion compared with bleeding disorders—search for a useful platelet antiaggregant. Blood 35: 333.

Zucker, M. B. 1947. Platelet agglutination and vasoconstriction as factors in spontaneous hemostasis in normal, thrombocytopenic, heparinized and hypothrombinemic rats. Amer. J. Physiol. 148: 275.

Inhibition of Platelet Aggregation by Cyproheptadine

D. H. Minsker, P. T. Jordan, and A. MacMillan

Cyproheptadine inhibited *in vitro* platelet aggregation induced by antigen-antibody complex, collagen, ADP, thrombin, or serotonin. Cyproheptadine administered systemically inhibited collagen- or ADP-induced aggregation of guinea pig platelets and antagonized thrombosis induced by electric stimulation of venules in the hamster cheek pouch. Cyproheptadine did not prevent formation of antigen-antibody complex consisting of human γ-globulin (Ag) and anti-human γ-globulin prepared from goats (Ab). Cyproheptadine in subthreshold concentrations *in vitro* enhanced the inhibitory effect of dipyridamole or acetylsalicylic acid on collagen-induced aggregation of guinea pig platelets.

Our observations suggest that cyproheptadine may be of benefit in the management or prevention of thrombosis.

Vessel lesions, bacteria, viruses, prosthetic surfaces, and antigen-antibody complexes are some of the many initiators of blood platelet aggregation that have been described in the literature and recently reviewed by Mustard and Packham (1970). Platelet aggregation is destructive if it results in occlusion of critical vessels. Platelet aggregation *in vivo* can be harmful even if damaging thrombosis does not occur because blood will not clot normally when large numbers of platelets adhere to the vessel walls and are sequestered from the circulating blood.

Currently available anticoagulant drugs such as heparin are generally ineffective in prevention of platelet aggregation and arteriol thrombosis (Salzman, 1965). Presented in this paper are the results of testing cyproheptadine (Periactin®), a commonly used drug which is a potent serotonin and histamine antagonist (Stone *et al.*, 1961). Previous reports have shown that cyproheptadine inhibits platelet aggregation and release reaction (Goldman *et al.*, 1971; Minsker, 1972). Another inhibitor of platelet aggregation, acetylsalicylic acid (ASA), was also studied.

The following information and rationale were used in designing our tests. Platelet aggregation can be observed *in vitro* by challenging platelet-rich plasma (PRP) with such naturally occurring compounds as collagen, thrombin, serotonin, and adenosine diphosphate (ADP). ADP is the nucleotide mainly responsible for self-propagating platelet aggregation in physiological situations (Mustard and Packham, 1970). Collagen may be a more physiological *initiator* of aggregation in that the first reaction of platelets in injured tissue seems to be to adhere to subendothelial connective tissue; furthermore, collagen causes platelet release of ADP (Hovig, 1963), thereby furthering aggregation. Thrombin releases platelet constituents (Grette, 1962) and by this means may contribute to arterial thrombosis. Platelet aggregation induced by connective tissue is associated with serotonin release (Zucker and Peterson, 1967) and aggregation in many species can be induced by serotonin (Mills, 1970). Cyproheptadine reduces platelet trapping in dog renal xenografts or allografts and extends graft survival; it has been reported to delay the onset of acute rejection in human renal transplants (Rattazzi *et al.*, 1970). In light of these findings, we studied the effects of cyproheptadine on the formation of antigen-antibody complex *in vitro;* we also evaluated cyproheptadine as an inhibitor of platelet aggregation induced by antigen-antibody complex. To evaluate the antithrombotic properties of cyproheptadine *in vivo*, hamster cheek pouch venules were damaged, and the subsequent occlusive thrombi were observed before and after administration of the drug. We also investigated the possibility that cyproheptadine might enhance the activity of other drugs that are known to inhibit platelet aggregation.

MATERIALS AND METHODS

Collagen suspension was prepared by adding 50 mg of bovine collagen (Worthington Biochemical, Freehold, N.J.) to 150 ml of physiological saline and homogenizing in a Virtis "45" homogenizer at highest speed for 20 min. The suspension was kept at approximately 40°C during homogenization. The suspension was filtered through four loose layers of cheesecloth four times and refrigerated at 4°C. Four to ten microliters were used to induce aggregation in each standard sample, 0.6 ml of human or guinea pig PRP.

Thirty milligrams of ADP base (34.8 mg of ADP monosodium 2½ hydrate, Calbiochem, Los Angeles, Calif.) were dissolved in 50 ml of water and stored in the refrigerator for no longer than 4 months. On the day of use, 1 1:20 dilution was made from a sample of the stock solution. An average of 5 μl/0.6-ml sample of PRP (0.25 μg ADP/ml PRP) were used to induce aggregation of guinea pig platelets.

Five thousand units of dry topical thrombin (Parke, Davis and Co., Detroit) were dissolved in 83.3 ml of water, divided into 2-ml samples, and frozen (−10°C). Samples were thawed on the day of use. Twenty to fifty microliters per 0.6-ml sample of PRP (2–5 units/ml PRP) were used to induce aggregation of guinea pig platelets.

Ten milligrams of serotonin (22 mg of serotonin creatinine sulfate, K & K Co., Plainview, N.Y.) were dissolved in 16.7 ml of water; a 1:10 dilution was used for aggregation tests and discarded at the end of the day. An average of 10 μl/0.6-ml sample of human PRP (1 μg/ml PRP) were used to induce aggregation in human PRP.

Cyproheptadine was used as the hydrochloride sesquihydrate, which contains 81.9 per cent cyproheptadine base. For incubation studies, 10 mg of cyproheptadine hydrochloride sesquihydrate (N.F.) were dissolved in 2 ml of water with the aid of gentle boiling. To each milliliter of PRP, 0.025 ml of recently dissolved drug was added, giving a final concentration of 100 μg/ml. Lower concentrations were obtained by appropriate dilution of the stock solution with water. Higher concentrations of drug in PRP were obtained by adding more stock solution to PRP. The use of diluents containing salts, particularly sodium chloride, may result in precipitation of cyproheptadine. To administer cyproheptadine orally, the drug was dissolved in water and given by gavage, at 2 ml/kg.

The sodium salt of ASA was used for incubation studies. The concentrations prepared were such that, during incubation, the drug solution occupied 1 per cent of the volume of drug-PRP mixture. In studies that required oral administration, a water suspension of ASA, particle size 100 mesh, was used at 2 ml/kg.

Methysergide (Sandoz Pharmaceutical, Hanover, N.J., courtesy of Dr. J. H. Trapold) was dissolved in water and mixed with PRP in such a concentration that the drug solution occupied 1 per cent of the total drug-PRP volume.

Dipyridamole (Ciba-Geigy Corp., Ardsley, N.Y., courtesy of Dr. A. J. Plummer) was dissolved in 2–3 ml of dilute (0.05 *N*) hydrochloric acid and brought to the desired final concentration with water.

Concentrations and dose levels of all drugs were expressed as base weights.

Platelet Aggregation Tests

Platelet aggregation was studied by the turbidometric method of Born (1962). For *in vitro* incubation, blood was withdrawn from unanesthetized male English Short-Hair guinea pigs that weighed 500–1000 g, via cardiac puncture into plastic syringes containing 3.5 per cent sodium citrate (9 volumes of blood + 1 volume of citrate), and PRP was prepared by centrifugation (200 × *g*, 10 min). Human PRP was prepared similarly by taking blood from the antecubital vein. Pooled PRP was divided into 3-ml samples and incubated at room temperature in capped plastic test tubes for 30–45 min with drug solution or appropriate control. Samples of control PRP, 0.6 ml each, were stirred at 1200 rpm and simultaneously warmed to 37°C in a Chronolog aggregometer. The least amount of aggregating agent required to induce consistent aggregation responses in the samples was determined. A Chronolog strip-chart recorder (paper speed, 1 inch/min) was used to record aggregation as a curve that described the rate and amount of increase in light transmittance through PRP as aggregation proceeded.

The optimal amount of aggregating agent required to aggregate control platelets was added to drug-treated platelets in the aggregometer and aggregation responses were recorded. Percentage of inhibition was calculated from the formula:

$$\% \text{ inhibition} = \frac{100X}{Y},$$

where X = light transmittance of control PRP minus light transmittance of drug-treated PRP, and Y = light transmittance of control PRP. Either the value for *rate* of increase in light transmittance (curve slope) or the value for *amount* of increase (curve height) was used in the formula, depending on which was the more sensitive indicator of inhibition of platelet aggregation. When aggregation was induced by collagen, serotonin, or antigen-antibody complex, the most sensitive indicator of inhibition of platelet aggregation was the slope of the aggregation curve. When ADP or thrombin was used, the height of the aggregation curve was the most sensitive indicator of inhibitory drug effect. The effect of drugs administered orally was studied by giving either drug or appropriate control solution to guinea pigs and preparing PRP. PRP from control animals was pooled and samples were challenged with collagen or ADP in the aggregometer; the optimal amount required to induce aggregation was added to samples of pooled PRP from animals that received the drug, and the percentage of inhibition was calculated.

Antigen-antibody complex was prepared and used in a series of experiments. Human γ-globulin (Ag) (Cutter, Berkeley, Calif.) and anti-human γ-globulin prepared from goats (Ab) (Bioquest, Cockeysville, Md.) were combined as follows to form Ag-Ab complex: 44 mg of Ab were dissolved in 1 ml of water, 0.05 ml of Ag was diluted with 17 ml of physiological saline, and 1-ml samples of each solution were combined. After incubation at 37°C for 45 min, each sample of the Ag-Ab complex suspension was centrifuged at 900 $\times g$ for 4 min and resuspended three times in 2 ml of physiological saline. The effect of cyproheptadine on the formation of Ag-Ab complex was studied by incubating both Ag and Ab separately with cyproheptadine at room temperature for 5 min. The final concentrations of cyproheptadine were 2, 25, and 50 μg/ml. After combining Ag and Ab as above, volumes of centrifuged precipitate from each test were recorded. To be aggregated by Ag-Ab complex, guinea pig platelets required the presence of calcium. PRP samples were titrated in the aggregometer with 1.25 per cent $CaCl_2$ to determine the minimum amount of calcium required to induce aggregation; 70 per cent of the amount required for calcium-induced aggregation was added to each PRP test sample, which was then stirred in the aggregometer for 1 min before addition of 10–20 μl of Ag-Ab complex. PRP was challenged in the aggregometer with Ag-Ab complex that had been formed either in the absence of cyproheptadine ("control" complex) or in the presence of cyproheptadine ("treated" complex); the amount of "control" complex required to induce aggregation of guinea pig platelets was compared with the amount of "treated" complex required to induce aggregation.

A series of experiments was conducted to determine whether cyproheptadine enhanced ASA- or dipyridamole-caused inhibition of aggregation. First, ASA (1.25, 2.5, 5.0, and 10 μg/ml) or dipyridamole (5, 10, 20, and 40 μg/ml) was incubated with guinea pig PRP for 30–45 min and the inhibitory effects on collagen-induced aggregation were recorded. Next, the maximum concentration of cyproheptadine that did not inhibit collagen-induced platelet aggregation was determined (concentration referred to as "subthreshold"). Finally, the amount of cyproheptadine required to produce a subthreshold concentration was added to the solution of ASA or dipyridamole used in the first part of the test. ASA + cyproheptadine or dipyridamole + cyproheptadine was incubated with PRP, and the effects on collagen-induced aggregation were recorded.

Hamster Cheek Pouch Preparation

A modification of a technique used by Callahan *et al.* (1960) was used. Male hamsters that weighed 45–65 g were anesthetized with vinbarbital (50 mg/kg) given intraperitoneally. The microcirculation of the everted cheek pouch was surgically exposed, and excessive connective tissue was removed. After a light coat of mineral oil was applied to the preparation, an Emerson micromanipulator was used to touch the tip of a unipolar platinum-glass electrode (approximately 10 μ in diameter) to a 40-μ venule. A 50-VDC, stimulus 100 msec from a type of 161 Tektronix stimulator was applied to the vessel. The percentage of venule lumen remaining free of obstruction caused by platelet aggregation was recorded after thrombus growth reached maximum (in approximately 3–5 min). The test was repeated, using another venule in the same preparation. Cyproheptadine was then administered subcutaneously to the same animal, and, 30 min later, two more lesions were created using two other venules.

RESULTS

The EC_{50} (estimated concentration required to produce 50 per cent inhibition), ED_{50} (estimated dose required to produce 50 per cent inhibition), and 95 per cent confidence limit values were determined.

Cyproheptadine and ASA inhibited *in vitro* platelet aggregation induced by a variety of agents (Figs. 1 through 4).

The EC_{50} of cyproheptadine as an inhibitor of collagen-induced aggregation was 9.4 μg/ml, with 95 per cent confidence limits of

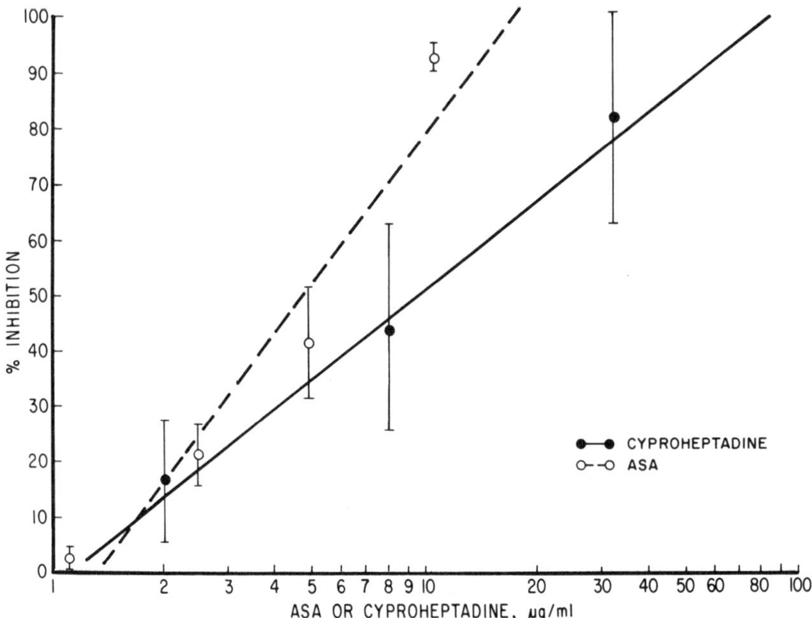

Figure 1. Effect of cyproheptadine or ASA on the rate of collagen-induced aggregation of guinea pig platelets. Values are averages ± standard error of the mean (SEM) for six experiments at each concentration of each drug.

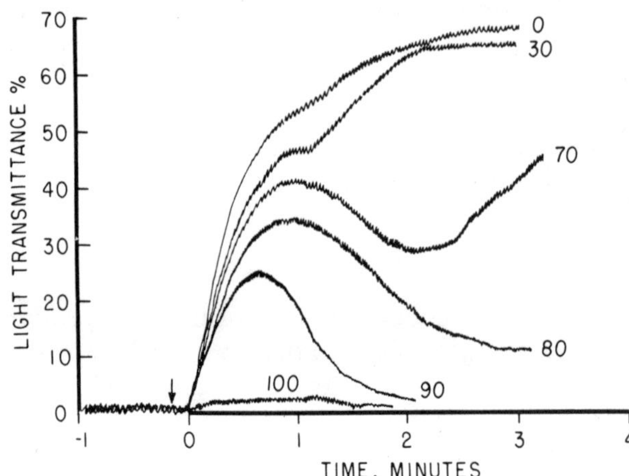

Figure 2. Effect of cyproheptadine on ADP-induced aggregation of guinea pig platelets. Concentration of ADP, 0.12 μg/ml. Concentration of cyproheptadine during incubation is shown (in micrograms per milliliter at end of each curve.

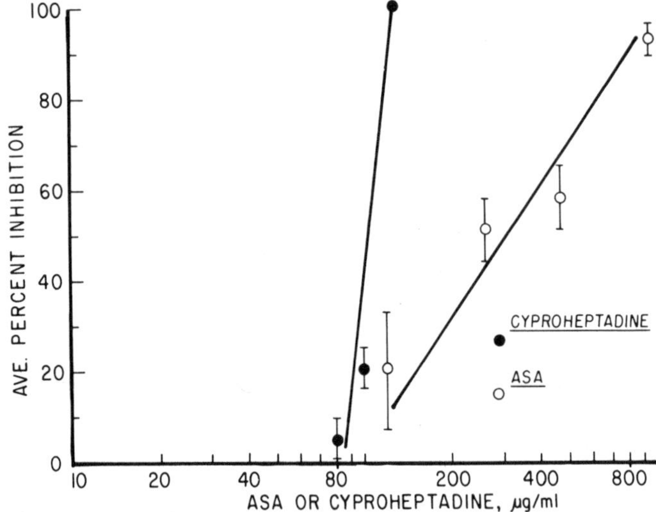

Figure 3. Effect of ASA or cyproheptadine on thrombin-induced aggregation of guinea pig platelets. Values are averages (±SEM) of four experiments at each concentration of cyproheptadine and of three experiments at each concentration of ASA. Peak amplitude of aggregation curves (degree of aggregation) was used in calculating results.

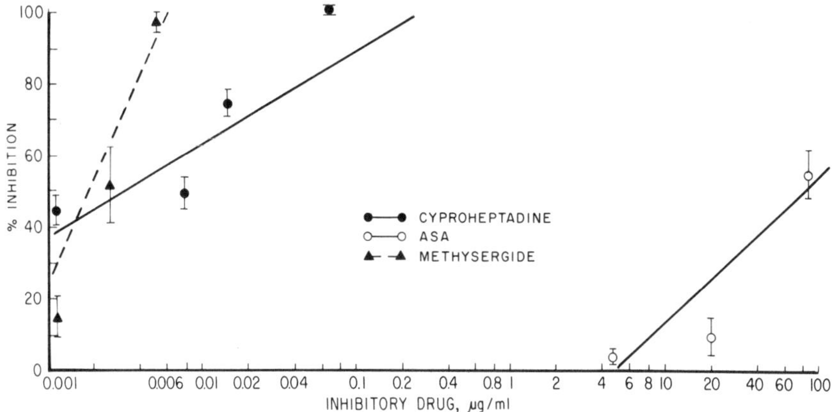

Figure 4. Effect of cyproheptadine, ASA, or methysergide on serotonin-induced aggregation of human platelets. Values are averages (±SEM) of five experiments at each concentration of cyproheptadine and ASA and of four experiments at each concentration of methysergide.

2.4 and 78.8; the EC_{50} of ASA was 4.6 µg/ml, with 95 per cent confidence limits of 3.9 and 5.7.

The experiments with ADP-induced aggregation showed that cyproheptadine abolished secondary aggregation at 80 µg/ml and primary aggregation at 100 µg/ml. ASA, at concentrations up to 1000 µg/ml, had no effect on the first phase of ADP-induced aggregation. Five tests were performed at each concentration of cyproheptadine; at concentrations of 30–100 µg/ml, the amount of aggregation was significantly less than that in controls ($p < 0.05$).

Thrombin-induced aggregation was inhibited by cyproheptadine or ASA. The EC_{50} of cyproheptadine was 94.2 µg/ml, with 95 per cent confidence limits of 84.2 and 101.6; the EC_{50} of ASA was 272.3 µg/ml, with 95 per cent confidence limits of 195.1 and 357.5.

Serotonin-induced aggregation of human PRP was markedly inhibited by cyproheptadine or methysergide. The EC_{50} of cyproheptadine was 0.003 µg/ml, with 95 per cent confidence limits of 0.0002 and 0.007; the EC_{50} of methysergide was 0.002 µg/ml, with 95 percent confidence limits of 0.0002 and 0.003; the EC_{50} of ASA was 88.5 µg/ml, with 95 per cent confidence limits of 45 and 427.9.

As seen in Fig. 5, the effect of cyproheptadine on collagen-induced aggregation increased markedly as the incubational period increased from 1–10 min. Suppression of thrombin-induced aggregation became more pronounced as the incubational period increased to 45 min. The effect of length of incubation on serotonin-induced aggregation was minimal; inhibition at 1 min of incubation was slightly less than the inhibition measured at 45 min or longer. The effect of cyproheptadine on ADP-induced aggregation was maximal at 1 min of incubation.

The ED_{50} of cyproheptadine administered orally was 3.2 mg/kg, with 95 percent confidence limits of 2.3 and 4.2; the ED_{50} of ASA was 2.2 mg/kg with 95 per cent confidence limits of 1.3 and 3.3. The effect of cyproheptadine was evident at 0.5 through 6 hr after drug administration; there was no activity at 24 hr (Fig. 6).

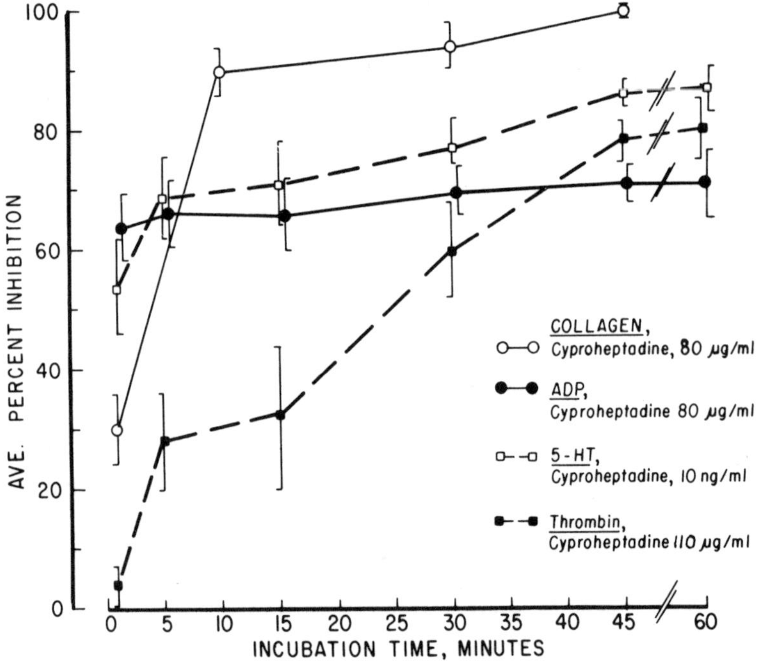

Figure 5. Effect of cyproheptadine on collagen-, ADP-, serotonin-, or thrombin-induced aggregation; effect of length of incubational period. Values are averages (±SEM) for five experiments. Aggregating agents and minimal concentrations of cyproheptadine required to produce 60–100 per cent inhibition of aggregation are listed in the lower right.

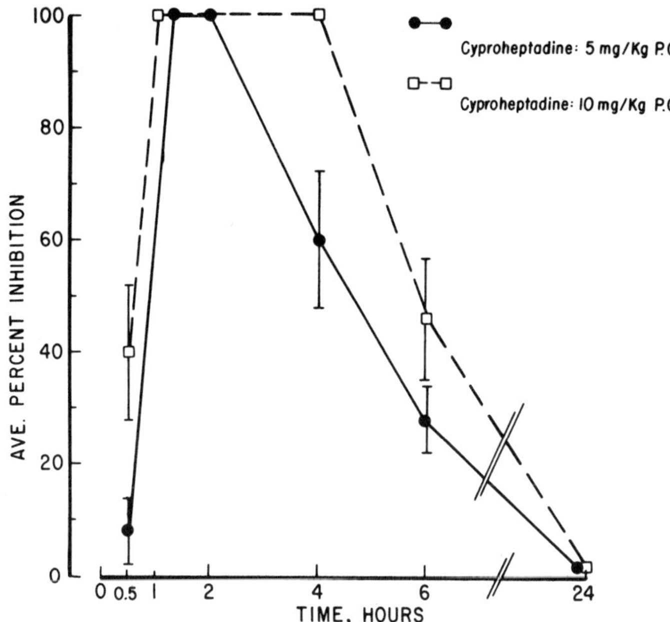

Figure 6. Duration of action of orally administered cyproheptadine on collagen-induced aggregation of guinea pig platelets. Values are averages (±SEM) for five animals at the lower dose and four animals at the higher dose. Each of the values was obtained from a different group of animals.

Neither rate nor amount of ADP-induced aggregation was significantly altered by cyproheptadine at 10 or 40 mg/kg, but *deaggregation* occurred readily after the dose of 40 mg/kg. The results shown in Fig. 7 are examples of what we consistently observed in control and treated animals.

In vivo tests using damaged venules in the hamster cheek pouch revealed that cyproheptadine was effective in maintaining patency of damaged vessels (Fig. 8) at 10 and 20 mg/kg, but not at 5 mg/kg, subcutaneously. The results from each animal are displayed and, despite considerable variability in the effect of cyproheptadine from one experiment to another, the beneficial effect of the drug can be seen at 10 and 20 mg/kg.

Cyproheptadine had no apparent effect on the quantity of Ag-Ab complex formed after the mixing of Ag with Ab. Eight trials were conducted at each concentration of cyproheptadine. The concentrations of cyproheptadine used and the average centri-

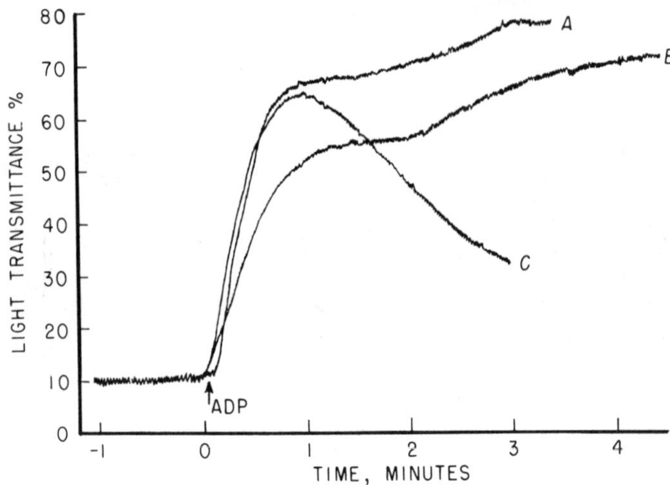

Figure 7. Effects of orally administered cyproheptadine on ADP-induced aggregation of guinea pig platelets. Concentration of ADP, 0.09 μg/ml. A, control (water), 2 ml/kg; B, cyproheptadine, 10 mg/kg; C, cyproheptadine, 40 mg/kg.

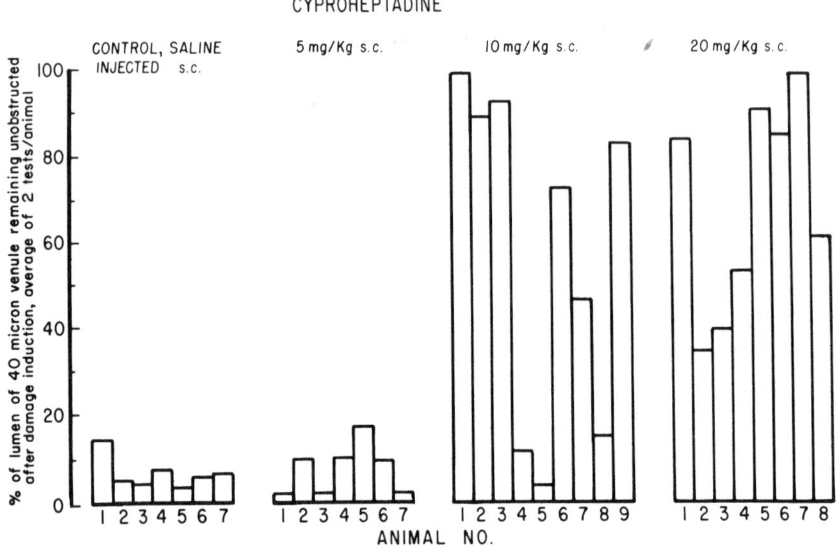

Figure 8. Effect of cyproheptadine on thrombus formation after electric stimulation of hamster cheek pouch venules.

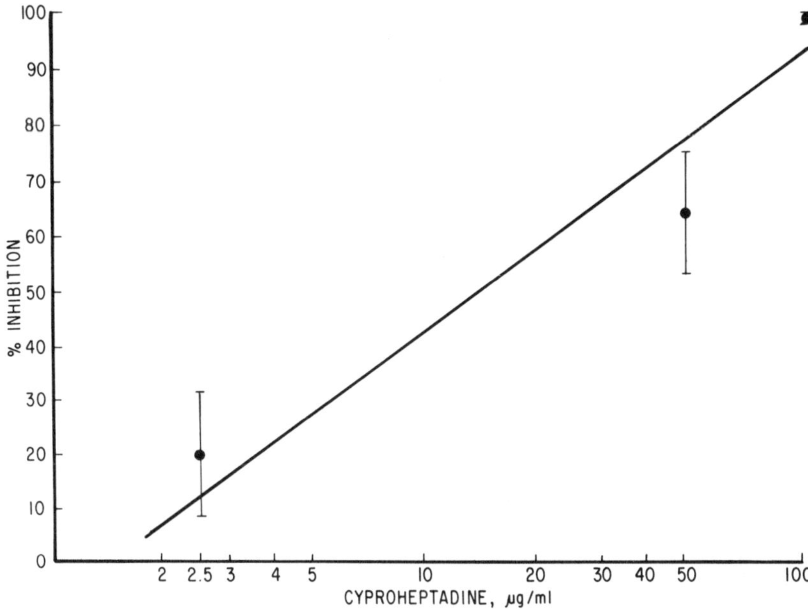

Figure 9. Effect of cyproheptadine on aggregation of guinea pig platelets induced by Ag-Ab complex. Values are averages (±SEM) of four experiments.

fuged (900 × *g*, 4 min) volumes (±SEM) of Ag-Ab complex formed at each concentration were: 2 μg/ml, 0.18 ml (±0.06); 25 μg/ml, 0.20 ml (±0.05); 50 μg/ml, 0.19 ml (±0.07). The average centrifuged volume (±SEM) of Ag-Ab complex formed in the absence of cyproheptadine (nine trials) was 0.20 ml (±0.06).

It required 10–15 μl of "treated" Ag-Ab complex to aggregate partially recalcified guinea pig platelets; the same volumetric range of "control" Ag-Ab complex was required for aggregation. The presence of cyproheptadine during formation of Ag-Ab complex apparently had no effect on the aggregation-inducing property of the complex. Cyproheptadine inhibited Ag-Ab complex-induced platelet aggregation (Fig. 9); the EC_{50} was 33.2 μg/ml, with 95 per cent confidence limits of 28.2 and 49.1.

The inhibition of collagen-induced aggregation of guinea pig platelets by ASA or dipyridamole was enhanced by subthreshold concentrations of cyproheptadine (Figs. 10 and 11). The subthreshold concentration of cyproheptadine varied daily from 2.5 to 6.0 μg/ml and had to be determined before each test. The EC_{50}

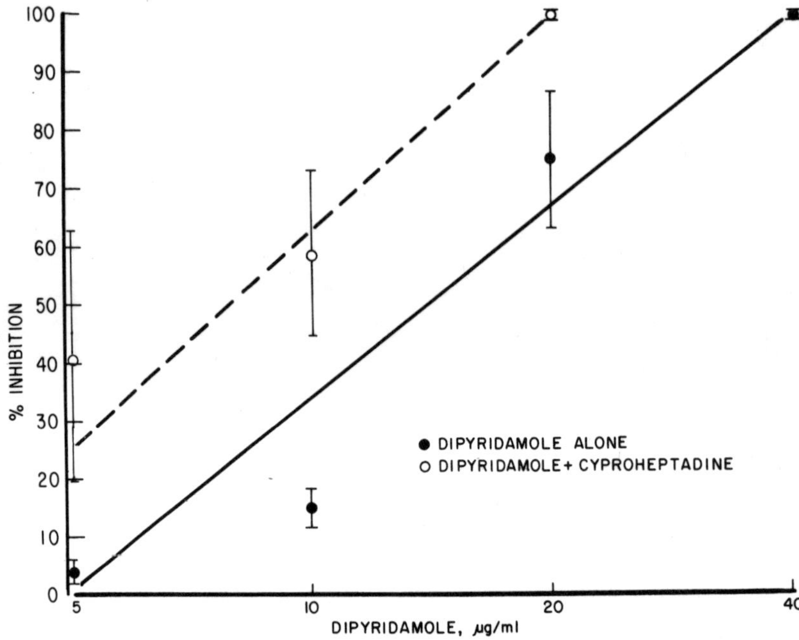

Figure 10. Enhancement of ASA effect on collagen-induced aggregation of guinea pig platelets by cyproheptadine at subthreshold concentrations. Average values (±SEM) for 11 experiments at each concentration of ASA alone and for four experiments at each concentration of ASA + cyproheptadine.

of ASA alone was 4.8 μg/ml, with 95 per cent confidence limits of 4.1 and 5.8; EC_{50} of ASA + cyproheptadine was 2.5 μg/ml, with 95 per cent confidence limits of 1.6 and 3.5. The EC_{50} of dipyridamole alone was 14.4 μg/ml, with 95 per cent confidence limits of 10.4 and 19.9; EC_{50} of dipyridamole + cyproheptadine was 6.9 μg/ml, with 95 per cent confidence limits of 0.03 and 11.9.

DISCUSSION

Cyproheptadine differs from nonsteroid anti-inflammatory drugs and dipyridamole in that it is a highly potent inhibitor of serotonin-induced aggregation. It also differs from the nonsteroid anti-inflammatory drugs in that it blocks both phases of ADP-induced aggregation. Platelet uptake and release of serotonin are concomitantly inhibited by cyproheptadine with no effect on clot

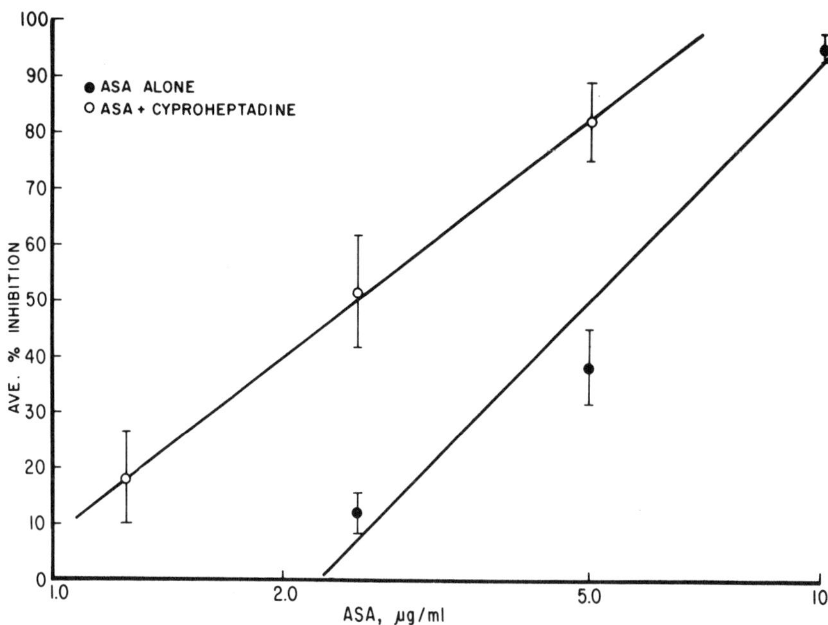

Figure 11. Enhancement of dipyridamole effect on collagen-induced aggregation of guinea pig platelets by cyproheptadine at subthreshold concentrations. Average values (±SEM) for four experiments.

retraction (Goldman *et al.*, 1971). Our work with cyproheptadine shows the drug to be effective in preventing platelet aggregation induced by different agents *in vitro* and by vessel lesions *in vivo*. It is therefore likely that cyproheptadine may prevent thrombosis. Our studies on the effects of ASA or dipyridamole in combination with cyproheptadine suggested that cyproheptadine may enhance the activity of other antithrombotic drugs.

The beneficial effects of cyproheptadine in kidney transplants has been described by Rattazzi *et al.* (1970) and by Aledort in this symposium. It is currently believed that, in a transplanted kidney during the rejection process, Ag-Ab complexes adhering to the vessel wall, or lesions exposing subendothelial connective tissue, may initiate platelet aggregation and vessel occlusion. Cyproheptadine inhibits platelet aggregation induced *in vitro* by both collagen and Ag-Ab complex. It seems plausible, therefore, to suggest that one of the ways in which cyproheptadine may help to prevent renal transplant rejection is by inhibiting platelet aggregation.

On the basis of its effect on platelet aggregation *in vitro* and *in vivo* and the relative safety of the drug, further clinical evaluation of cyproheptadine as a potential antithrombotic drug is recommended.

ACKNOWLEDGMENT

The authors would like to thank Dr. Neeti Bohidar for providing assistance in the statistical evaluation of data.

REFERENCES

Born, G. V. R. 1962. Quantitative investigations into the aggregation of blood platelets. J. Physiol. (London) 162: 67P.

Callahan, A. B., Lutz, B., Fulton, G., and Degelman, J. 1960. Smooth muscle and thrombus thresholds to unipolar stimulation of small blood vessels. Angiology 11: 35.

Goldman, B., Aledort, L. M., Puszkin, E., and Burrows, L. 1971. Cyproheptadine, a new platelet deaggregating agent. Circulation 44(2): 68.

Grette, K. 1962. Studies on the mechanism of thrombin-catalyzed hemostatic reactions in blood platelets. Acta Physiol. Scand. 56(195): 5.

Hovig, T. 1963. Release of platelet-aggregating substance (adenosine diphosphate) from rabbit blood platelets induced by saline "extract" of tendons. Thromb. Diath. Haemorrh. 9: 264.

Mills, D. C. B. 1970. Platelet aggregation and platelet nucleotide concentration in different species. Symp. Zool. Soc. London 27: 99.

Minsker, D. H. 1972. Inhibition of platelet aggregation by cyproheptadine (C); dependency upon incubation time. Fed. Proc. 31(2): 599.

Mustard, J. F., and Packham, M. A. 1970. Factors influencing platelet function: adhesion, release, and aggregation. Pharmacol. Rev. 22: 97.

Rattazzi, L., Haimov, M. N., Glabman, S., Papatestas, A., Gelernt, I. M., and Burrows, L. 1970. Role of the platelet in the obliterative vascular transplant rejection phenomenon. Surg. Forum 21:241.

Salzman, E. W., 1965. The limitations of heparin therapy after arterial reconstruction. Surgery 57: 131.

Stone, C. A., Wenger, H. C., Ludden, C. T., Stavorski, J. M., and Ross, C. A. 1961. Antiserotonin-antihistaminic properties of cyproheptadine. J. Pharmacol. Exp. Ther. 131: 73.

Zucker, M. B., and Peterson, J. 1967. Serotonin, platelet factor 3 activity and platelet aggregating agent released by adenosine diphosphate. Blood 30: 556.

Inhibition of Nicotinic Acid Metabolism in Human Blood Platelets by Nicotinic Acid Analogs and Nonsteroidal Anti-inflammatory Drugs

Zane N. Gaut

Human platelets incubated for 1 hr at 37°C with (7-^{14}C)nicotinic acid (10 μM) accumulate radioactivity with a gradient (disintegrations per min per ml intraplatelet water)/(disintegrations per min per ml incubation medium) of approximately 20. The uptake process involved incorporation of the isotope into compounds such as nicotinamide adenine dinucleotide (NAD) which do not readily diffuse from the cell. Of the total radioactivity inside, nicotinic acid represented approximately 1.7 per cent; nicotinamide, 3.1 per cent; NAD, 22.0 per cent; and nicotinic acid mononucleotide (NMN), 35.0 per cent. Such synthesis and accumulation of radioactivity were variously inhibited by a number of analogs of nicotinic acid as well as by 2,4-dinitrophenol, NaF, salicylate, and NaCN. Of the analogs studied, 2-hydroxynicotinic acid was the most potent. It reduced the gradient of radioactivity to 1.4 at 1 mM

Portions of this chapter were taken from the following journals with permission of the publishers: Journal of Pharmaceutical Sciences, Biochemical Pharmacology, Research Communications in Chemical Pathology and Pharmacology, and Biochimica et Biophysica Acta.

and inhibited isotopic incorporation into the compounds previously described. These data suggest that 2-hydroxynicotinic acid inhibits nicotinate phosphoribosyltransferase. (7-^{14}C)Nicotinamide was neither accumulated nor metabolized by the platelet.

Nicotinate phosphoribosyltransferase was then studied in platelet lysate wherein various nicotinic acid analogs and salicylate competed with nicotinic acid for the enzyme. These data suggested that the free carboxyl group, its position on the pyridine ring, and the pyridine nitrogen of nicotinic acid were particularly apposite to interaction with nicotinate phosphoribosyltransferase.

The steric similarities between 2-hydroxynicotinic acid and salicylic acid led to the studies involving inhibition of niacin metabolism in the intact platelet as well as its lysate by other nonsteroidal anti-inflammatory drugs. Such drugs were also competitive with nicotinic acid for nicotinate phosphoribosyltransferase. The apparent inhibition of the same enzyme in the human erythrocyte and rat liver slice further substantiate the hypothesis that niacin antagonism may be a fundamental property of anti-inflammatory drugs. Nicotinic acid mononucleotide is common to the interrelationships of anti-inflammatory activity, nicotinic acid antagonism by anti-inflammatory drugs, augmentation of platelet aggregation by nicotinic acid, and inhibition of platelet aggregation by anti-inflammatory drugs.

In conclusion, it would appear worthwhile to explore the possibility that NMN has some physiological and biochemical role in the cell and may be involved in platelet aggregation, the inflammatory process, and the mechanism of anti-inflammatory compounds.

The human blood platelet accumulates radioactivity by a saturable process when incubated with (7-^{14}C)nicotinic acid. Such accumulation is due to incorporation of (7-^{14}C)nicotinic acid into nicotinamide adenine dinucleotide (NAD), nicotinamide adenine dinucleotide phosphate (NADP), and their precursors which do not readily diffuse from the cell (Gaut and Solomon, 1970a). This is a review of data involving the inhibition of such incorporation by nicotinic acid analogs and various nonsteroidal anti-inflammatory drugs (Dietrich *et al.*, 1958; Gaut *et al.*, 1970; Gaut and Solomon, 1970b,c, 1971a,b; Seifert *et al.*, 1966).

MATERIALS AND METHODS

Except for the nicotinic acid analogs (supplied by Dr. O. Neal Miller of Hoffmann-La Roche, Inc.) compounds were either purchased from commercial sources or were gifts from the pharmaceutical company manufacturing the respective drug. Nicotinic acid mononucleotide (NMN) was synthesized from nicotinamide mononucleotide by the method of Wagner (1968).

For experiments with the intact platelet, approximately 30 mg (wet weight) of the washed cells were suspended in 0.8 ml of Ca^{++}- and Mg^{++}-free, Krebs-Ringer bicarbonate buffer. (7-^{14}C)Nicotinic acid solution (0.1 ml) and 0.1 ml of solution of inhibitor or buffer were added to each suspension. Incubation was then carried out in a Dubnoff metabolic shaker under 95 per cent O_2–5 per cent CO_2 at 37°C. After incubation, the platelets were sedimented at 22,000 $\times$ *g* for 5 min, the supernatants decanted, and the tubes swabbed with a cotton-tipped applicator. The samples were weighed and then lysed in 1 ml of distilled water. Aliquots of 0.5 ml of each supernatant and lysate were added to 10 ml of scintillation medium and the radioactivity determined. The distribution ratio ([I]/[O]) of radioactivity is expressed as the ratio of disintegrations per min per ml intracellular platelet water to disintegrations per min per ml incubation medium. The concentration of radioactivity in the intraplatelet water was corrected for that trapped within the extracellular space of the platelet pellet by the formulation of Helmreich and Kipnis (1962). Duplicate controls accompanied each experiment.

After incubation, "carrier" nicotinic acid, NMN, NAD, NADP, and nicotinamide were added to the platelet lysate and medium prior to chromatographic separation according to the method of Hagino *et al.* (1968). The compounds were visualized by UV light, scraped from the plates, suspended in gelled scintillation medium (Bollinger *et al.*, 1967), and the radioactivity determined as previously described (Gaut and Solomon, 1970a).

For inhibitory constant (K_i) determinations in disrupted cells, approximately 200 mg of platelets, isolated as described above, were lysed in 10 volumes of distilled water. Aliquots of the lysate (0.2 ml) were incubated in Ca^{++}-free, Krebs-Ringer bicarbonate buffer modified to contain: Mg^{++}, 3.3 m*M;* the Mg^{++} salt of phosphorylribose-1-pyrophosphate (PRPP), 1.5 m*M;* and various concentrations of (7-^{14}C)nicotinic acid and inhibitors. Such incubations were carried out in total volumes of 0.5 ml in a metabolic shaker under 95 per cent O_2–5 per cent CO_2 for 1 hr at 37°C. The reaction was stopped by immersing the tubes in a solid CO_2-acetone mixture. Subsequently, "carrier" nicotinic acid and NMN were added to the lysate and the compounds separated on thin layers of cellulose (Hagino *et al.*, 1968). The compounds were visualized by UV light, scraped from the plates, suspended in gelled scintillation medium (Bollinger *et al.*, 1967), and the radioactivity was determined. Velocity was expressed as moles of NMN formed per mg of platelets per hr. Parallel K_m determinations accompanied each K_i determination. Under these conditions, more than 98 per cent of the radioactivity migrated with nicotinic acid and NMN. Since the yield of platelets from human blood is small, purification of the enzyme was not feasible.

Human erythrocytes were obtained by differential centrifugation, washed twice with saline, and approximately 50 mg suspended in 0.8 ml of Krebs-Ringer bicarbonate buffer. (7-^{14}C)Nicotinic acid (0.1 ml) and 0.1 ml of solution of inhibitor or buffer were added to each suspension. Incubation was then carried out as described above in Krebs-Ringer bicarbonate buffer modified to contain Mg^{++}, 3.3 m*M*. The cells were then separated by centrifugation, disrupted in distilled water, and the lysate analyzed by thin layer chromatography (TLC) as described for platelets.

Rat liver slices were similarly incubated, homogenized in 10% trichloroacetic acid and homogenates analyzed by TLC. ATP levels were measured with the Biochemica Test kit from Boehringer Mannheim GmbH.

In experiments characterizing prostaglandin F_{2a} (PGF_{2a}) release, platelet-rich plasma (PRP) was incubated at 37°C for various times in the presence of thrombin (5.0 units/2 ml), or nicotinic acid (2.0 m*M*, final concentration), or both. Duplicate controls accompanied each experiment. PGF_{2a} was quantitated by the immunoassay technique of Caldwell *et al.* (1971).

RESULTS

Inhibition of (7-^{14}C)Nicotinic Acid Metabolism in the Intact Platelet by Nicotinic Acid Analogs

When incubated with (7-^{14}C)nicotinic acid, human platelets accumulated radioactivity against a gradient. At an initial concentration of 10 μM nicotinic acid, the distribution ratio ([I]/[O]) increased linearly with time and reached a value of approximately 20 within 1 hr (Fig. 1). Increasing the initial concentration of nicotinic acid diminished the steady state distribution so that the process was saturated at approximately 50 μM. Chromatographic data indicated that platelets also incorporate labeled nicotinic acid

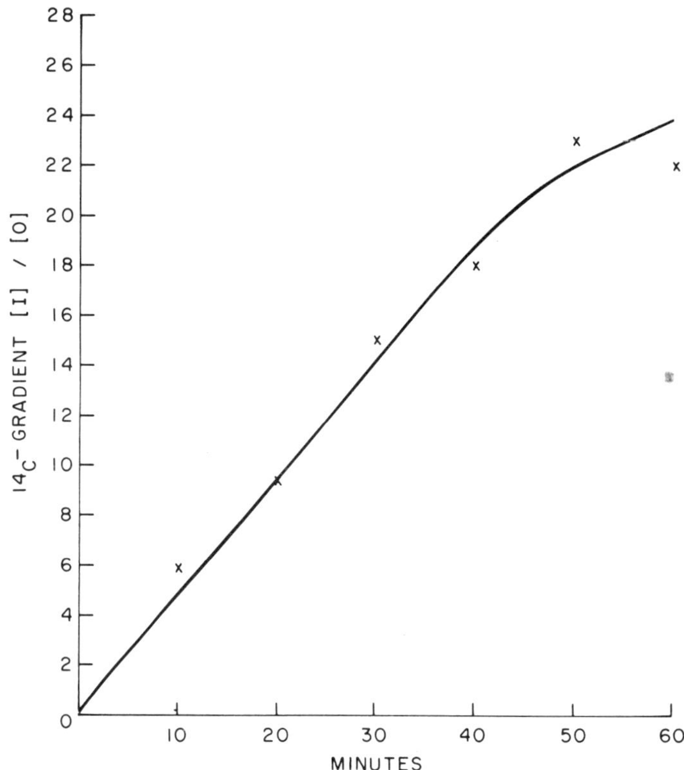

Figure 1. Rate of isotopic accumulation by the human platelet, expressed as [I]/[O] when incubated with (7-^{14}C)nicotinic acid (10 μM). Results of a representative experiment are shown.

into NAD, nicotinamide, and unidentified compounds progressively with time (Fig. 2). The unidentified material presumably represents intermediates in the biosynthesis of NAD since the radioactivity on the chromatograms had R_F values identical with those previously reported for such intermediates (Hagino *et al.*, 1968). At the end of 1 hr of incubation, with an initial concentration of 10 μM nicotinic acid, nicotinic acid represented 1.7 per cent, NAD, 22.0 per cent, nicotinamide, 3.1 per cent, NMN, 35.0 per cent, and NADP, 10.0 per cent of the total intraplatelet radioactivity. The steady state distribution ratio of nicotinic acid was approximately 0.8 after this period. Since there was efflux of (7-^{14}C)nicotinamide from the platelet, the radioactivity expressed

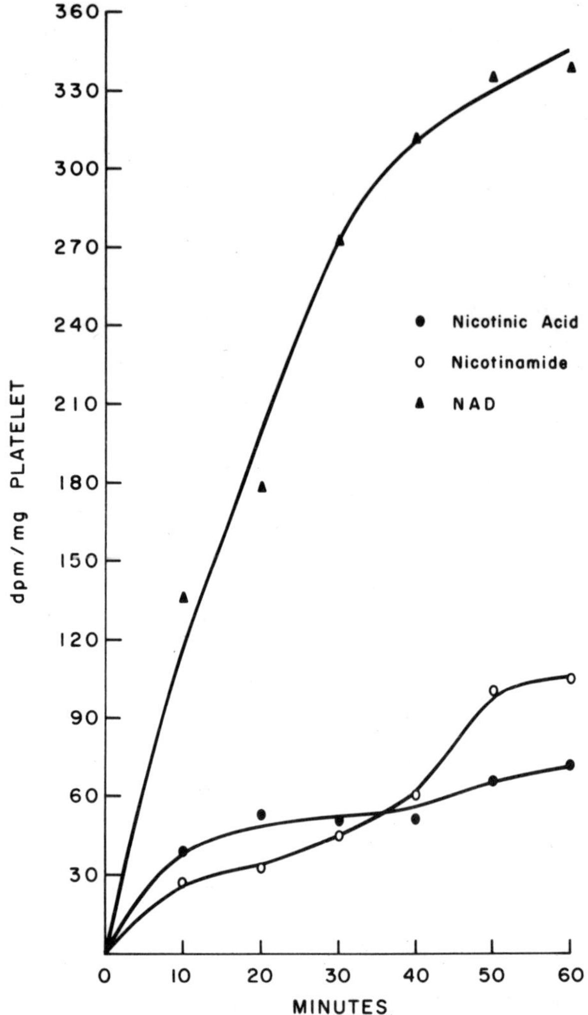

Figure 2. Rate of appearance of (7-^{14}C)nicotinic acid (10 μM) into various compounds of the human platelet. Points represent disintegrations per min per mg platelet. Results of a representative experiment are shown.

in Fig. 1 and Table 1 for this compound is the summation of that in the incubation medium and platelet lysate. Such efflux amounted to about 25 per cent of the total nicotinamide formed within the platelet during 1 hr of incubation but represented less than 1 per cent of total intraplatelet radioactivity; hence, such

Table 1. Effect of various concentrations of 2-hydroxy-nicotinic acid on the incorporation of (7-^{14}C)nicotinic acid (10 μM) into other compounds by the human platelet

Concentration of inhibitor (M)	Compound		
	Nicotinic acid	Nicotinamide	NAD
0	52.0	51.0	238
10^{-5}	62.1	44.5	220
5×10^{-5}	74.0	35.0	183
10^{-4}	81.3	31.6	136
5×10^{-4}	95.6	14.1	47.5
10^{-3}	109	12.5	25.4

Incubation was carried out for 1 hr. Numbers expressed as disintegrations per min per mg platelet. Results of a representative experiment are shown.

radioactivity was neglected in calculating the isotopic accumulation. According to the rates of appearance of the label into NAD and nicotinamide, the minimum rates of incorporation expressed as micromoles of nicotinic acid per mg of platelet per hr into NAD and nicotinamide were 15.1 and 5.07, respectively. An attempt was made to delineate the half-life of NAD by preincubation of the platelets for 1 hr with (7-^{14}C)nicotinic acid (10 μM) followed by incubation with unlabeled nicotinic acid (10 μM) for a 2nd hr. However, the exchange between the intra- and extraplatelet pools of nicotinic acid, under these conditions, was so slow that isotopic incorporation continued into the 2nd hr. Therefore, the half-life of NAD could not be accurately established. (7-^{14}C)Nicotinamide was neither accumulated nor metabolized by the platelet at a concentration of 10 μM owing, presumably, to absence of the requisite deamidase. The steady state distribution ratio for this compound at 10 μM after 60 min of incubation was 1.1.

Various metabolic inhibitors including CN^-, 2,4-dinitrophenol, F^-, iodoacetate, and salicylate suppressed accumulation of radioactivity (Table 2). Further evaluation of salicylate revealed inhibition in direct relation to its concentration with 90 per cent

Table 2. Effect of metabolic inhibitors and salicylate on the isotopic accumulation by the human platelet when incubated for 1 hr with (7-^{14}C)nicotinic acid (10 μM)

Inhibitor	Concentration of inhibitor (M/l)	Gradient [I]/[0]	Inhibition (%)
Control	0	24.4	0
Cyanide	10^{-4}	21.0	14
Dinitrophenol	10^{-4}	9.0	63
Fluoride	10^{-3}	18.5	24
Iodoacetate	5×10^{-4}	4.1	83
Salicylate	10^{-6}	4.9	80

Results of a representative experiment are shown.

inhibition at 50 μM. *p*-Chloromercuribenzoate was inactive as an inhibitor at a concentration of 0.1 mM. Theophyllin, which in other cells (Alivisatos *et al.*, 1956) inhibits nicotinamide adenine dinucleotidase, did not influence accumulation at a concentration of 5 mM.

A number of nicotinic acid congeners were also assessed as inhibitors of isotopic accumulation (Table 3). Of the compounds studied, 2-hydroxynicotinic acid was the most potent and 2-hydroxynicotinamide among the least. The former compound inhibited 26 per cent at 10 μM and 95 per cent at 1 mM in the presence of 10 μM of nicotinic acid, and the extent of inhibition was directly related to the concentration of the analog. Furthermore, 2-hydroxynicotinic acid restricted the incorporation of (7-^{14}C)nicotinic acid into NAD, nicotinamide, and unidentified compounds, where, again, the extent of restriction was directly related to its concentration (Table 1). At initial concentrations of 1 mM of this inhibitor and 10 μM of nicotinic acid, the intraplatelet level of nicotinic acid was twice that of controls after 1 hr of incubation such that the distribution ratio was approximately 1.4 (Table 1). The following compounds were inactive as inhibitors at a concentration of 1 mM in the presence of 10 μM of nicotinic acid: 2-aminonicotinic acid, 2-bromonicotinic acid, 2-chloronicotinic acid, 2,6-dichloronicotinic acid, 2,6-dihydroxynicotinic acid,

Table 3. Effect of various nicotinic acid analogs (1 mM) on the isotopic accumulation by the human platelet when incubated for 1 hr with (7-^{14}C)nicotinic acid (10 μM)

Compound	Inhibition (%)
2-Hydroxynicotinic acid	90
2-Pyridylcarbinol	86
4-Hydroxynicotinic acid	74
2-Fluoronicotinic acid	71
3,5-Pyridyldicarboxylic acid	58
4-Chloronicotinic acid	26
5-Hydroxynicotinic acid	26
6-Chloronicotinic acid	24
2,3-Pyridyldicarboxylic acid	23
3-Pyridylcarbinol	22
Pyridine	21
5-Chloronicotinic acid	19
Nicotinuric acid	18
Nicotinic acid-N-oxide	17
Ethyl-2-hydroxynicotinate	16
2-Hydroxynicotinamide	8
Nicotinamide	0

Results of representative experiments are shown.

2-hydroxy-*n*-propylnicotinate, 2-methylnicotinic acid, nicotinamide, nicotinamide-N-oxide, 3-pyridylaldoxime, 3-pyridylsulfonamide, and 3-pyridylsulfonic acid.

Inhibition of Nicotinate Phosphoribosyltransferase in Platelet Lysate by Nicotinic Acid Analogs

When incubated with (7-^{14}C)nicotinic acid and PRPP, human platelet lysate incorporates radioactivity into NMN. Such incorporation was linear up to 3 hr at nicotinic acid concentrations of 6.8, 14, 17, and 34 μM (Fig. 3). Kinetics were evaluated according to the method of Lineweaver and Burke (1934) in which velocity was expressed as moles of NMN formed per mg platelet per hr (Fig. 4). The intercepts for calculation of the apparent K_m and K_i values were obtained by the method of least squares. Figure 4 reveals the apparent K_m for nicotinic acid to be 24 μM where PRPP and Mg^{++} were in excess. Incubation in Mg^{++}-free buffer diminished the

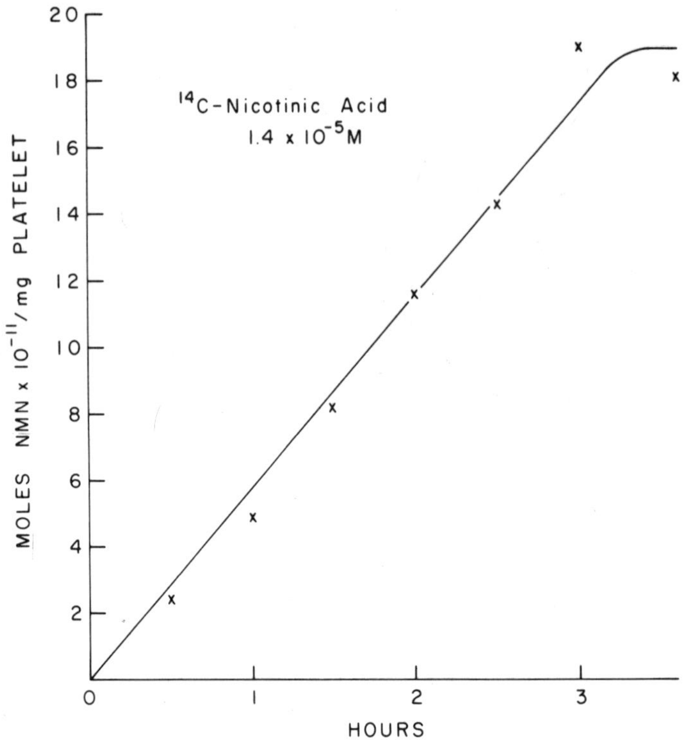

Figure 3. Incorporation of (7-^{14}C)nicotinic acid (14 μM) into NMN by human platelet lysate with time. Velocity expressed as moles of NMN formed $\times$ 10^{-11} per mg platelet. Results of a representative experiment are shown. See text for composition of incubation medium.

velocity approximately 50 per cent but left the apparent K_m unchanged. Although EDTA (3.3 mM) diminished the velocity by 50 per cent in the presence of Mg^{++} (3.3 mM), no further reduction occurred with EDTA in the absence of Mg^{++}. Addition of NaF (1.0 mM) and ATP (0.5 mM) both separately and together did not change the K_m or velocity. NAD, NADP, and NADH also had no effect at 0.5 mM.

Of the several nicotinic acid analogs studied, 2-pyrazinoic acid was the most potent inhibitor with an apparent K_i of 0.075 mM. 2-Hydroxynicotinic acid was the second most potent with an apparent K_i of 0.23 mM; however, its structural congener, salicylic acid, had a slightly lower value of 0.16 mM (Fig. 4). Apparent K_i

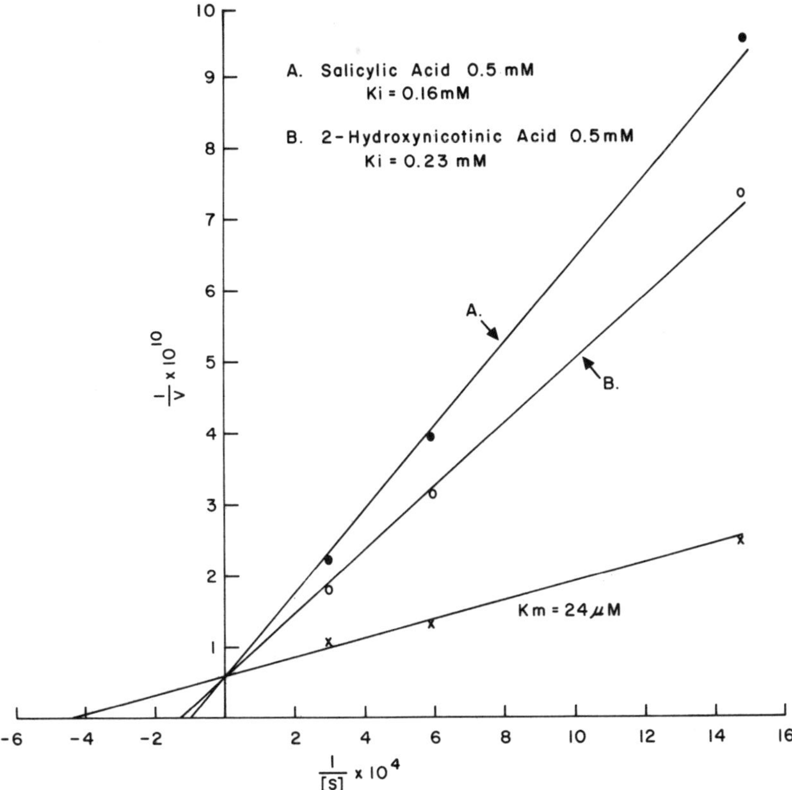

Figure 4. **Inhibition of nicotinate phosphoribosyltransferase in human platelet lysate by 2-hydroxynicotinic acid and salicylic acid.** Velocity is expressed as moles of NMN formed per mg platelet per hr; substrate concentration, moles per liter.

values for other analogs are listed in Table 4. Inactive as inhibitors at 0.5 m*M* were: 2-Cl-, 2-Br-, 2-methyl-, 2,6-dihydroxy-, 2-hydroxymethyl-, 4-hydroxy-, 5-hydroxy-, 5-Cl-, and 6-hydroxynicotinic acid; 3-pyridylsulfonamide; nicotinamide; and ethyl-2-hydroxynicotinate.

Nicotinate phosphoribosyltransferase catalyzes the first reaction in the pathway of Preiss and Handler (1958a,b) for NAD biosynthesis (Fig. 5). The enzyme, in the main, is Mg^{++}-dependent and, in some preparations, is stimulated allosterically by ATP (Smith and Gholson, 1969). Likewise, the velocity of the reaction

Table 4. Apparent inhibitory constants (K_i) of various competitive inhibitors of nicotinate phosphoribosyltransferase in human platelet lysate

Compound*	Apparent K_i (mM)
2-Pyrazinoic acid	0.075
Salicylic acid	0.16
2-Hydroxynicotinic acid	0.23
2-Fluoronicotinic acid	0.28
6-Chloronicotinic acid	0.56
Isonicotinic acid	0.75
3-Pyridylsulfonic acid	0.75
Pyridine	0.78
2-Aminonicotinic acid	0.82
Picolinic acid	1.16
3-Pyridylacetic acid	1.28
Benzoic acid	1.90

* Parallel studies were carried out at (7-^{14}C)nicotinic acid concentrations of 34, 17, 14, and 6.8 μM in the presence and absence of the above compounds. See text for composition of incubation medium.

catalyzed by this enzyme in human platelet lysate is stimulated by magnesium without alteration of the apparent K_m. Its apparent K_m of 24 μM agrees closely with that reported by Smith and Gholson (1969) for partially purified enzyme from bovine liver. However, unlike the enzyme from bovine liver, neither the velocity nor K_m is changed by the addition of ATP.

1. Nicotinic acid + PRPP $\rightleftharpoons$ Nicotinic acid mononucleotide + PP_i

2. Nicotinic acid mononucleotide + ATP $\rightleftharpoons$ Nicotinic acid adenine dinucleotide (N_aAD) + PP_i

3. N_aAD + ATP + glutamine $\longrightarrow$ NAD + glutamate + AMP + PP_i

4. NAD $\xrightarrow{\text{NADase}}$ Adenosine diphosphate ribose + Nicotinamide

Figure 5. Preiss-Handler pathway of NAD biosynthesis and degradation.

Inhibition of (7-^{14}C)Nicotinic Acid Metabolism in the Intact Platelet by Various Nonsteroidal Anti-inflammatory Drugs

Table 5 depicts the concentrations of various anti-inflammatory agents which inhibit, by 50 per cent, isotopic accumulation by the platelet when incubated with (7-^{14}C)nicotinic acid (1.7 μM). Table 6 reveals the influence of acetylsalicylic and flufenamic acids on the incorporation of (7-^{14}C)nicotinic acid into NAD, NADP, nicotinamide, and their precursor, NMN. The amount of radioactivity incorporated into the intermediates and products of the pathway of Preiss and Handler (1958a,b) was diminished in the presence of these drugs and, at the same time, intraplatelet concentrations of (7-^{14}C)nicotinic acid increased.

Table 5. Concentrations of various anti-inflammatory agents that inhibit, by 50 per cent, isotopic accumulation in human platelet when incubated with (7-^{14}C)-nicotinic acid (1.7 μM) for 30 min

Compound	Concentration (M/l)
Flufenamic acid	1.0×10^{-5}
Mefenamic acid	5.0×10^{-5}
Phenylbutazone	1.0×10^{-4}
Indomethacin	1.5×10^{-4}
Oxyphenbutazone	3.0×10^{-4}
Acetylsalicylic acid	5.0×10^{-4}
Sulfinpyrazone	5.0×10^{-4}
Acetanilide	1.0×10^{-3}
Aminopyrine	1.0×10^{-3}
Antipyrine	1.0×10^{-3}

Results of representative experiments are shown.

Table 6. Effect of acetylsalicylic acid (0.5 m*M*) and flufenamic acid (10 μM) on the metabolism of (7-^{14}C)nicotinic acid (1.7 μM) by the human platelet

Inhibitor	Compound				
	Nicotinic acid	NMN	NAD	NADP	Nicotinamide
None	31.0	640	400	180	56.0
Acetylsalicylic acid	44.3	290	184	84	34.0
Flufenamic acid	56.1	251	188	76	26.0

Results of representative experiments expressed as disintegrations per min per mg platelet.

Inhibition of Nicotinate Phosphoribosyltransferase in Platelet Lysate by Various Nonsteroidal Anti-inflammatory Drugs

Along with nicotinic acid analogs, various nonsteroidal anti-inflammatory drugs were competitive with (7-^{14}C)nicotinic acid for nicotinate phosphoribosyltransferase. The formation of NMN was competitively inhibited by flufenamic acid, mefenamic acid, salicylic acid, phenylbutazone, and indomethacin (Fig. 6; Table 7).

Inhibition of (7-^{14}C)Nicotinic Acid Metabolism in the Human Erythrocyte and Rat Liver Slice

Although not depicted in detail but similar to data derived from the platelet, nicotinic acid analogs and various nonsteroidal anti-inflammatory agents inhibited (7-^{14}C)nicotinic acid metabolism in the human erythrocyte (Gaut, unpublished data) and rat liver slice (Gaut and Costanza, unpublished data). Such hindrance occurred at concentrations of the inhibitors which did not suppress tissue levels of ATP. While there were decreases in the incorporation of (7-^{14}C)nicotinic acid into NMN, NAD, NADP, and nicotinamide, in the presence of these compounds, the tissue content of (7-^{14}C)nicotinic acid increased. Such data suggest, concordantly with those derived from the platelet, inhibition of NAD biosynthesis early in the pathway, probably at the step catalyzed by nicotinate phosphoribosyltransferase.

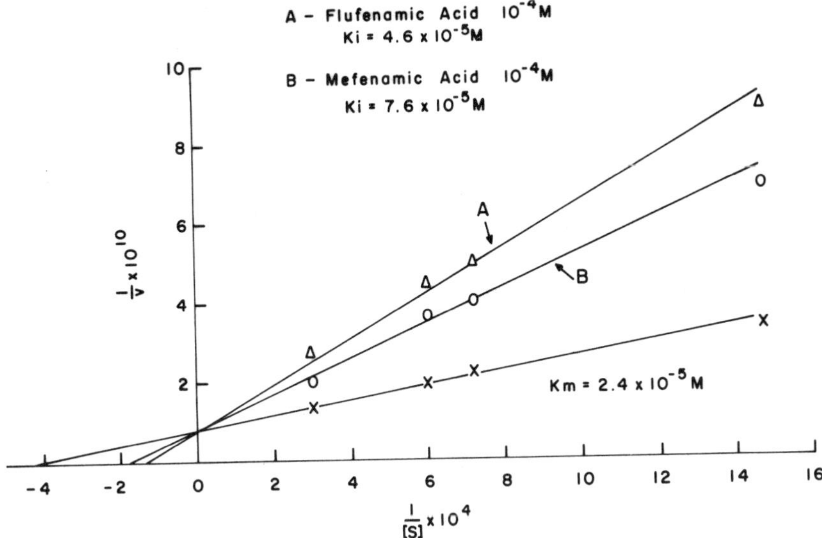

Figure 6. Inhibition of nicotinate phosphoribosyltransferase in human platelet lysate by flufenamic and mefenamic acids. Velocity is expressed as moles NMN formed per mg platelet per hr; substrate concentration is expressed as moles per liter. Results of representative experiments are shown.

Table 7. Apparent inhibitory constants (K_i) of various nonsteroidal anti-inflammatory drugs and 2-hydroxynicotinic acid as competitive inhibitors of nicotinate phosphoribosyltransferase in human platelet lysate

Compound*	Apparent K_i (mM)
2-Hydroxynicotinic acid	0.23
Flufenamic acid	0.046
Mefenamic acid	0.076
Salicylic acid	0.16
Phenylbutazone	0.16
Indomethacin	0.42

* Parallel studies were carried out at (7-^{14}C)nicotinic acid concentrations of 34, 17, 14, and 6.8 μM, in the presence and absence of the above compounds.

Stimulation of $PGF_{2\alpha}$ Production in Platelets by Thrombin and Nicotinic Acid

After incubation of PRP for 10 min in the presence of nicotinic acid, thrombin, and thrombin plus nicotinic acid, $PGF_{2\alpha}$ production increased 39, 120, and 270 per cent, respectively, above controls. Such enhancement of $PGF_{2\alpha}$ production was hindered by anti-inflammatory drugs at concentrations which also inhibit niacin metabolism and restrain platelet aggregation (J. Paulsrud, personal communication).

DISCUSSION

Inhibition of (7-^{14}C)Nicotinic Acid Metabolism in the Intact Platelet by Nicotinic Acid Analogs

The uptake of nicotinic acid in the rat and human erythrocyte (Lan and Henderson, 1968; Preiss and Handler, 1958a) consisted of two processes, diffusion and enzyme-catalyzed conversion to nucleotides, which do not readily diffuse from the cell. Such uptake was inhibited in the cold and by F^-, arsenate, 2-deoxyglucose, and iodoacetate.

The present study demonstrates that the human platelet also accumulates radioactivity when incubated with (7-^{14}C)nicotinic acid. Such accumulation is not due to nicotinic acid itself, whose concentration in cellular water approaches that in the medium, but rather to incorporation of (7-^{14}C)nicotinic acid into compounds such as NAD, which do not readily diffuse from the cell. In this regard, the human platelet resembles the rat erythrocyte. However, unlike the erythrocyte, the platelet neither metabolizes nor accumulates nicotinamide. The slower incorporation of label into nicotinamide relative to NAD and other products and the preference for nicotinic acid over nicotinamide, by the human platelet, are consistent with the pathway of Preiss and Handler (1958a,b). The presence of nicotinamide in the platelet lysate and medium suggests that the platelet contains nicotinamide adenine dinucleotidase.

Since the metabolism of nicotinic acid is energy-dependent, it was expected and confirmed, in the platelet, that incorporation into other compounds was hindered by such metabolic inhibitors as CN^-, iodoacetate, 2,4-dinitrophenol, and F^-. Suppression by salicylate was remarkably great in that 90 per cent inhibition occurred at a concentration as low as 50 μM in the presence of 10 μM nicotinic acid. Salicylate is structurally similar to the potent inhibitor, 2-hydroxynicotinic acid, and also uncouples oxidative phosphorylation (Brody, 1956). Therefore, its total inhibitory capacity in the intact platelet may be the sum of direct competition with nicotinic acid as well as uncoupling.

Since 6-aminonicotinamide has been shown to be a powerful antagonist of niacin, *in vivo* and *in vitro* (Johnson and McColl, 1955; Dietrich *et al.*, 1958), other congeners of nicotinamide and nicotinic acid were assessed as antagonists of isotopic accumulation of (7-^{14}C)nicotinic acid by the human platelet. Of those studied, precise structure-activity relations were not apparent. The differences in effect among these compounds (Table 2) could be allied to inhibitor-enzyme affinity as well as to their rates of penetration into the platelet. The data do indicate that inhibition by 2-hydroxynicotinic acid was strong whereas 2-hydroxynicotinamide was weak. Furthermore, inhibition of isotopic accumulation was either absent or trivial for nicotinamide and its congeners and for the esters of nicotinic acid derivatives. For example, amidation or esterification of 2-hydroxynicotinic acid, the most potent inhibitor, resulted in compounds virtually devoid of inhibitory activity. These data suggest that a free carboxyl group is necessary for an inhibitory effect. Relative to substituents in position 2 of nicotinic acid, arrangement in decreasing order of potency is OH and F $\gg$ Cl and Br. Such an arrangement roughly approximates the increases in size and electron-withdrawing properties of these substituents; therefore, data relative to this particular series of compounds could be explained on the basis of steric hindrance of the pyridine nitrogen, electron withdrawal therefrom, or increases in acidity, or both. The lack of inhibition by 3-pyridylsulfonic acid further substantiates the hypothesis related to acidity. Reasonably, increases in acidity and, therefore, polarity, would deter their entry into the platelet by passive diffusion so that inhibition of nicotinic acid metabolism would not occur.

While there were decreases in the incorporation of (7-^{14}C)nicotinic acid into NAD, nicotinamide, and other compounds under the influence of 2-hydroxynicotinic acid, the intraplatelet level of (7-^{14}C)nicotinic acid increased. Such data are consistent with inhibition of NAD and nicotinamide synthesis early in the pathway. The decreased isotopic incorporation into nicotinamide in the intact platelet is probably due to such early inhibition rather than suppression of nicotinamide adenine dinucleotidase. It is not known whether these inhibitors are metabolized to form their respective NAD and NADP analogs.

Inhibition of Nicotinate Phosphoribosyltransferase in Platelet Lysate by Nicotinic Acid Analogs

The data relative to competitive inhibition by nicotinic acid analogs reveal marked specificity of the enzyme, since any substitution on the substrate greatly increases the apparent K_i relative to the apparent K_m. The same is true for purely isomeric changes as in picolinic and isonicotinic acids. Even so, general patterns, based on chemical structure of the analogs, emerge from the data.

Large substituents in position 2 of nicotinic acid, *e.g.* $-NH_2$, $-Cl$, $-Br$, $-CH_3$, and $-CH_2OH$, result in compounds virtually devoid of inhibitory activity; therefore, data relative to this series of compounds could be explained on the basis of steric hindrance of the pyridine nitrogen. This hypothesis is further substantiated by the lack of inhibition by 2,6-dihydroxy- and 2,6-dichloronicotinic acid as well as the weak inhibitory capacity of 6-chloronicotinic acid. Positions 4 and 5 appear vulnerable to steric effects, since 4-hydroxy-, 5-chloro-, and 5-hydroxynicotinic acids are not inhibitory at 0.5 m*M*. Such data are consistent with a size-restricted hydrophobic region at the binding site of the enzyme to accommodate carbon atoms 4, 5, and perhaps 6 of the pyridine ring. This type of bonding was hypothesized by Mares-Guia and Shaw (1965) for the active center of trypsin in which its substrate apparently was bound in a hydrophobic slit or crevice.

The keto-tautomer of 2-hydroxynicotinic acid is probably not the active form, since the apparent K_i of this compound is very close to that of 2-fluoronicotinic acid. The fluorinated species is of course incapable of this configuration.

The pyridine nitrogen of nicotinic acid is important for interaction with the enzyme for several reasons. Substitution of a carbon for this nitrogen atom, as in benzoic acid, greatly diminishes inhibitory activity. Substantial activity is retained, as in pyridine, even though the carboxyl group is deleted. Further support lies in the loss of activity in compounds where this nitrogen atom is sterically hindered and in the relatively large inhibitory capacity of 2-pyrazinoic acid.

A major difference, structurally, between benzoic acid, a poor inhibitor, and nicotinic acid is the unshared pair of electrons in the sp^2 orbital of the pyridine-nitrogen. Hence the profound divergence between the apparent K_i of benzoic acid and the apparent K_m of nicotinic acid may be explained on the basis of nucleophilic interaction of this sp^2 orbital with carbon- 1 of PRPP. The relatively low apparent K_i values of 2-hydroxynicotinic acid and *o*-hydroxybenzoic acid (salicylic acid) lend further credence to this possibility. The position of these nucleophilic hydroxyl groups would also favor such interaction at the enzyme's catalytic site.

The carboxyl group of nicotinic acid is also important since its deletion, as in pyridine, diminished activity. Amidation, as in nicotinamide, and esterification, as in ethyl-2-hydroxynicotinate, results in compounds virtually devoid of inhibitory activity. The size of this acidic substituent is critical as well, since replacement by the larger sulfonic group, as in 3-pyridylsulfonic acid, resulted in an apparent K_i, much higher than the apparent K_m of nicotinic acid.

The proximity of the carboxyl group to the pyridine ring is salient, since interposition of a methylene group, as in 3-pyridylacetic acid, results in a compound of weak inhibitory capacity. The positional relationship of the carboxyl group to the pyridylnitrogen is also meaningful, since isonicotinic and picolinic acids are quite weak inhibitors.

Although this discussion is mainly concerned with relating steric effects to the extent of inhibition, other possibilities remain. Resonance and induction influences of various substituents on the pyridine ring in general and of the pyridine nitrogen in particular could also be implicated in structure-activity relations.

In summary, the data suggest that the free carboxyl group, its position on the pyridine ring, and the pyridine nitrogen of nicotinic acid are particularly apposite to interaction with nicotinate phosphoribosyltransferase.

Inhibition of (7-^{14}C)Nicotinic Acid Metabolism in the Intact Platelet by Various Nonsteroidal Anti-inflammatory Drugs

Isotopic accumulation and metabolism of (7-^{14}C)nicotinic acid is inhibited in the platelet by various nonsteroidal anti-inflammatory agents. While there were decreases in the incorporation of

(7-^{14}C)nicotinic acid into NMN, NAD, NADP, and nicotinamide, in the presence of these drugs, the intraplatelet content of (7-^{14}C)nicotinic acid increased. Such data suggest inhibition of NAD biosynthesis early in the pathway, probably at the step catalyzed by nicotinate phosphoribosyltransferase.

Inhibition of platelet aggregation is apparent within 15 min of exposure to various anti-inflammatory agents (O'Brien, 1968). Even though NAD and NADP biosynthesis is restrained by such drugs, significant depletion of these cofactors is unlikely within so short a time since their rates of degradation are relatively slow. Hence, the inhibition of NAD biosynthesis by these drugs is probably not related to their influence on platelet aggregation. On the other hand, the rapid appearance and accumulation of ^{14}C-NMN in the platelet during incubation with (7-^{14}C)nicotinic acid and inhibition thereof by anti-inflammatory drugs (anti-aggregants) and the fact that nicotinic acid augments platelet aggregation (Salzman, 1972) imply that NMN may be involved in aggregation.

Anti-inflammatory drugs also inhibit a number of enzymes such as uridine-5′-diphosphoglucose dehydrogenase (Lee and Spencer, 1969), esterase activity of α-chymotrypsin, and serotonin formation *in vitro* (Skidmore and Whitehouse, 1966; Whitehouse, 1966). Salicylate also inhibits numerous dehydrogenases by a mechanism involving reversible competition with the appropriate pyridine-nucleotide coenzyme (Smith and Smith, 1966). These data reveal yet another common feature of such drugs, suppression of nicotinic acid metabolism in the human platelet.

Inhibition of Nicotinate Phosphoribosyltransferase in Platelet Lysate by Various Nonsteroidal Anti-inflammatory Drugs

Since data derived from the intact platelet suggested that anti-inflammatory drugs inhibited nicotinate phosphoribosyltransferase, this hypothesis was tested and confirmed using platelet lysate. Although such drugs, like niacin, are acidic, further structure-activity relationships were not apparent as compared with the niacin analogs.

Platelet aggregation, a precursor of blood coagulation, is inhibited by various nonsteroidal anti-inflammatory drugs (Zucker and Peterson, 1970); hence, O'Brien (1968) postulated a connection between inflammation and platelet function. This review describes another common feature of these drugs in the platelet: inhibition of nicotinate phosphoribosyltransferase by reversible competition with nicotinic acid. Such inhibition again suggests that NMN may participate in the aggregation process in addition to those listed by Salzman (1972) such as cAMP, serotonin, ADP, and catecholamines.

Another hypothesis relating niacin antagonism by these drugs to their anti-inflammatory activity is as follows. Such drugs also inhibit the oxidation of uridine-5′-diphosphoglucose, competitively with nicotinamide adenine dinucleotide and noncompetitively with uridine-5′-disphosphoglucose. Therefore, Lee and Spencer (1969) theorized that mucopolysaccharide biosynthesis is restrained and inflammatory responsiveness is reduced. It follows that inhibition of nicotinamide adenine dinucleotide biosynthesis by anti-inflammatory agents would exert the same restraint on this pathway since tissue concentrations of the cofactor would be diminished.

Imsande and Handler (1961) and Imsande (1961) suggested that the reaction catalyzed by nicotinate phosphoribosyltransferase was rate-limiting for NAD and NADP formation. Therefore, such inhibition of this enzyme may explain the decreases in NADP content of rat liver after administration of salicylate, as reported by Slater and Sawyer (1966).

The concentrations of nicotinic acid employed in the present study were greater than those in human serum and within the range of those in human whole blood (Altman, 1961); also, the apparent K_i values of the inhibitory drugs are within the range of therapeutic blood levels (Hucker *et al.*, 1966; Burns *et al.*, 1953). Hence, this antagonism of niacin at the cellular and enzyme level may be involved in the pharmacological activity and, particularly, the toxicity of anti-inflammatory drugs.

Inhibition of (7-^{14}C)Nicotinic Acid Metabolism in the Human Erythrocyte and Rat Liver Slice

The apparent inhibition of nicotinate phosphoribosyltransferase in the human erythrocyte and rat liver slice by nicotinic acid analogs and nonsteroidal anti-inflammatory drugs further substantiates the hypothesis that niacin antagonism may be a fundamental property of such drugs. Again NMN is central and common to the interrelationships of anti-inflammatory activity, nicotinic acid antagonism by anti-inflammatory drugs, augmentation of platelet aggregation by nicotinic acid, and inhibition of platelet aggregation by anti-inflammatory drugs.

Concluding Discussion and Relevant Questions

The question obtrudes: how may salicylate, so readily available and commonly abused, strike at biochemical reactions so fundamental to the cellular economy? First, up to 75 per cent of NAD, in tissues, exists in the oxidized state implying a "surplus" under physiological conditions. Second, the maximal capacity of the cell to synthesize NMN, the apparent rate-limiting step toward the synthesis of this cofactor, exceeds its rate of degradation. Furthermore, the apparent K_i of salicylate is 7 to 8 times the K_m for nicotinic acid; *i.e.* nicotinate phosphoribosyltransferase clearly "prefers" nicotinic acid. Even at high blood levels of salicylate, 50–80 per cent of the drug is bound to plasma protein (Woodbury, 1970), thus reducing the drug's availability for enzymic inhibition. Finally, like the enhancement of erythrocytic dihydrofolic acid reductase during administration of folate reductase inhibitors to man (Calabresi and Parks, 1970), it is reasonable that inhibitors of nicotinate phosphoribosyltransferase, such as salicylate, may act analogously. This would result in an increased capacity of the cell to generate NMN. These factors and theoretical expectations would tend to ameliorate the metabolic impact of these drugs relative to their inhibition of nicotinate phosphoribosyltransferase.

Assuming niacin antagonism by nonsteroidal anti-inflammatory drugs to be related to anti-inflammatory and anti-aggregant activities, does 2-hydroxynicotinic acid exhibit these properties?* To the author's knowledge, 2-hydroxynicotinic acid has not been tested for anti-aggregant activity; however, its rapid metabolism and excretion as the riboside (plasma $t_{1/2}$ approximately 30 min), in the dog and man (A. S. Leon, S. Kaplan, and M. Schwartz, personal communication), may explain its apparent lack of activity in the adjuvant arthritic animal at doses comparable to salicylate (L. O. Randall, personal communication) which has a plasma

* Recently, niflumic acid, a nicotinic acid derivative (Fig. 7), was reported to be useful as an anti-inflammatory drug in man (Palmer *et al.*, 1972).

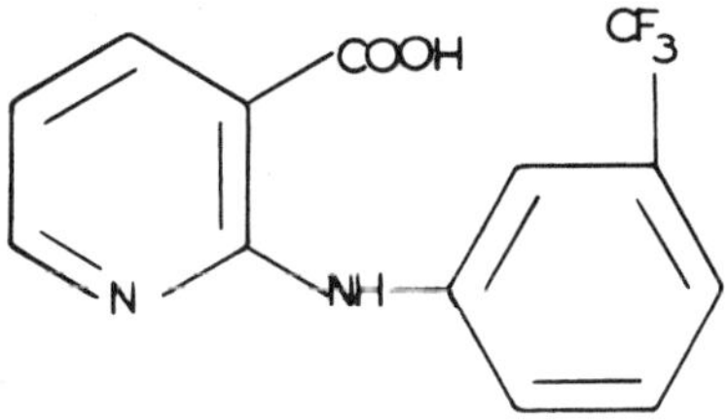

Figure 7. Structural formula of niflumic acid.

$t_{1/2}$ of 3–5 hr (Woodbury, 1970). Also, nothing is known of its tissue distribution, or penetration into inflamed tissue. Hence, at higher and frequently administered doses, anti-inflammatory activity might be manifest. The compound does increase the acute toxicity of aspirin (W. Pool and D. Hane, personal communication).

As implied previously in the discussion, does NMN have some function in cells other than serving as a convenient intermediate in the biosynthesis of nicotinamide adenine dinucleotides? Could NMN act as a mediator analogous to cAMP or in hydrogen transfer correspondent to flavin mononucleotide? Interestingly, concentrations of nicotinamide adenine dinucleotides in the erythrocytes of pellagrins do not differ from the normal (Raghuramulu *et al.*, 1965); therefore, is the concentration of NMN diminished and, if so, would this deficiency explain the clinical syndrome? Are pellagrins more susceptible to the toxicity of anti-inflammatory drugs? Would NMN induce platelet aggregation as does ADP, or explain the enhancement of $PGF_{2\alpha}$ production in the platelet by nicotinic acid, or both? Is NMN involved in PG production which could then mediate the "flush reaction" induced by nicotinic acid administration? Could the anti-bacterial activity of salicylate and the anti-aggregant properties of anti-inflammatory drugs be reversed by niacin? Could niacin antagonism in the platelet be a useful pharmacological screen for anti-aggregant and anti-inflammatory compounds? Would niacin administration be a specific treatment for salicylism?

In conclusion, it would appear worthwhile to explore the possibility that NMN has some physiological and biochemical role in the cell and may be involved in platelet aggregation, the inflammatory process, and the mechanism of anti-inflammatory compounds.

ACKNOWLEDGMENTS

Appreciation is expressed to Dr. James G. Hamilton, Dr. John Paulsrud, and Mrs. Catharine Schemm for help in preparing this review.

REFERENCES

Alivisatos, S. G. A., Kashnet, S., and Denstedt, O. F. 1956. The metabolism of erythrocytes. IX. Diphosphopyridine nucleotidase of erythrocytes. Can. J. Biochem. Physiol. 34: 56.

Altman, P. L. 1961. Blood, vitamins, hormones, enzymes, p. 89. *In* D. S. Dittmer (ed.) Blood and other body fluids. FASEB, Washington, D.C.

Bollinger, J. N., Mallow, W. A., Register, J. W., and Johnson, D. E. 1967. A simple gelation procedure for liquid scintillation counting. Anal. Chem. 39: 1508.

Brody, T. M. 1956. Action of sodium salicylate and related compounds on tissue metabolism *in vitro.* J. Pharmacol. Exp. Ther. 117: 39.

Burns, J. J., Rose, R. K., Chenkin, T., Goldman, A., Schulert, A., and Brodie, B. B. 1953. The physiological disposition of phenylbutazone (butazolidin) in man and a method for its estimation in biological material. J. Pharmacol. Exp. Ther. 109: 346.

Calabresi, P., and Parks, R. E., Jr. 1970. Alkylating agents, antimetabolites, hormones, and other anti-proliferative agents, pp. 1348–1395. *In* L. S. Goodman and A. Gilman (eds.) The pharmacological basis of therapeutics, 4th Ed. MacMillan Co., New York.

Caldwell, B. V., Burstein, S., Brock, W. A., and Speroff, L. 1971. Radioimmunoassay of the F Prostaglandins. J. Clin. Endocrinol. Metab. 33: 171.

Dietrich, L. S., Friedland, I. M., and Kaplan, L. A. 1958. Pyridine nucleotide metabolism: Mechanism of action of the niacin antagonist, 6-aminonicotinamide. J. Biol. Chem. 233: 964.

Gaut, Z. N., Ashley, C. J., and Wiggan, E. B. 1970. The effect of various anti-inflammatory agents on the metabolism of 7-^{14}C-nicotinic acid in the human platelet. Fed. Proc. 29: 419.

Gaut, Z. N., and Solomon, H. M. 1970a. Uptake and metabolism in nicotinic acid by human platelets: Effects of structure analogs and metabolic inhibitors. Biochim. Biophys. Acta 201: 316.

Gaut, Z. N., and Solomon, H. M. 1970b. Inhibition of 7-^{14}C-nicotinic acid metabolism in the human platelet by some 2-arylbenzo(b)-thiophen-3(2H)-one-1,1-dioxides possessing anti-inflammatory activity. Clin. Res. 18: 598 (abstr.).

Gaut, Z. N., and Solomon, H. M. 1970c. Inhibition of 7-^{14}C-nicotinic acid metabolism in the human blood platelet by anti-inflammatory drugs. Res. Commun. Chem. Pathol. Pharmacol. 1: 547.

Gaut, Z. N., and Solomon, H. M. 1971a. Inhibition of nicotinate phosphoribosyltransferase in human platelet lysate by nicotinic acid analogs. Biochem. Pharmacol. 20: 2903.

Gaut, Z. N., and Solomon, H. M. 1971b. Inhibition of nicotinate phosphoribosyltransferase by nonsteroidal anti-inflammatory drugs: A possible mechanism of action. J. Pharm. Sci. 60: 1887.

Hagino, Y., Lan, S. J., Ng, C. Y., and Henderson, L. M. 1968. Metabolism of pyridinium precursors of pyridine nucleotides in perfused rat liver. J. Biol. Chem. 243: 4980.

Helmreich, E., and Kipnis, D. M. 1962. Amino acid transport in lymph node cells. J. Biol. Chem. 237: 2582.

Hucker, H. B., Zacchei, A. G., Cox, S. V., Brodie, D. A., and Cantwell, N. H. R. 1966. Studies on the absorption, distribution and excretion of indomethacin in various species. J. Pharmacol. Exp. Ther. 153: 237.

Imsande, J. 1961. Pathway of diphosphopyridine nucleotide biosynthesis in *Escherichia coli.* J. Biol. Chem. 236: 1494.

Imsande, J., and Handler, P. 1961. Biosynthesis of diphosphopyridine nucleotide. III. Nicotinic acid mononucleotide pyrophosphorylase. J. Biol. Chem. 236: 525.

Johnson, W. J., and McColl, J. D. 1955. 6-Aminonicotinamide. A potent nicotinamide antagonist. Science 122: 834.

Lan, S. J., and Henderson, L. M. 1968. Uptake of nicotinic acid and nicotinamide by rat erythrocytes. J. Biol. Chem. 243: 3388.

Lee, K. H., and Spencer, M. R. 1969. Studies on the mechanism of action of salicylates. VII. Effect of a few anti-inflammatory agents on uridine-5′-diphosphoglucose dehydrogenase. J. Pharm. Sci. 58: 1152.

Lineweaver, H., and Burke, D. 1934. The determination of enzyme dissociation constants. J. Amer. Chem. Soc. 56: 658.

Mares-Guia, M., and Shaw, E. 1965. Studies on the active center of trypsin: The binding of amidines and guanidines as models of the substrate side chain. J. Biol. Chem. 240: 1579.

O'Brien, J. R. 1968. Effect of anti-inflammatory agents on platelets. Lancet 1: 894.

Palmer, D. G., Moller, P. W., and Highton, T. C. 1972. Niflumic acid in rheumatoid arthritis: A pilot study. N. Z. Med. J. 75: 351.

Preiss, J., and Handler, P. 1958a. Biosynthesis of diphosphopyridine nucleotide. I. Identification of intermediates. J. Biol. Chem. 233: 488.

Preiss, J., and Handler, P. 1958b. Biosynthesis of diphosphopyridine nucleotide. II. Enzymatic aspects. J. Biol. Chem. 233: 493.

Raghuramulu, N., Srikantia, S. G., Narasinga Rao, B. S., and Gopalan, C. 1965. Nicotinamide nucleotides in the erythrocytes of patients suffering from pellagra. Biochem. J. 96: 837.

Salzman, E. W. 1972. Cyclic AMP and platelet function. N. Engl. J. Med. 286: 358.

Seifert, R., Kittler, M., and Hilz, H. 1966. Purification and characterization of nicotinate phosphoribosyltransferase from Ehrlich ascites carcinoma cells, pp. 413–431. *In* N. O. Kaplan and E. P. Kennedy (eds.) Current aspects of biochemical energetics. Academic Press, New York.

Skidmore, I. F., and Whitehouse, M. W. 1966. Biochemical properties of anti-inflammatory drugs. X. The inhibition of serotonin formation *in vitro* and inhibition of the esterase activity of α-chymotrypsin. Biochem. Pharmacol. 16: 737.

Slater, T. F., and Sawyer, B. C. 1966. Nicotinamide-adenine dinucleotides in acute liver injury induced by ethionine, and a comparison with the effects of salicylate. Biochem. J. 101: 24.

Smith, L. D., and Gholson, R. K. 1969. Allosteric properties of bovine liver nicotinate phosphoribosyltransferase. J. Biol. Chem. 244: 68.

Smith, M. J. H., and Smith, P. K. 1966. The salicylates, pp. 63–66. Interscience Publishers, John Wiley and Sons, New York.

Wagner, C. 1968. A simple method for the synthesis of nicotinic acid mononucleotide. Anal. Biochem. 25: 472.

Whitehouse, M. W. 1966. Biochemical properties of anti-inflammatory drugs. XI. Structure-action relationship for the uncoupling of oxidative phosphorylation and inhibition of chymotrypsin by N-substituted anthranilates and related compounds. Biochem. Pharmacol. 16: 753.

Woodbury, D. M. 1970. Antipyretics, anti-inflammatory agents, and inhibitors of uric acid synthesis, pp. 314–329. *In* L. S. Goodman and A. Gilman (eds.) The pharmacological basis of therapeutics, 4th Ed. MacMillan Co., New York.

Zucker, M. B., and Peterson, J. 1970. Effect of acetylsalicylic acid, other nonsteroidal anti-inflammatory agents and dipyridamole on human blood platelets. J. Lab. Clin. Med. 76: 66.

Effect of Antithrombotic Drugs on *in Vivo* Experimental Thrombosis

R. G. Herrmann and W. B. Lacefield

Platelets play a major role in thrombus formation and in the production of hemostasis. Several inhibitors of platelet function were examined in various test systems for their effect on *in vivo* thrombus formation and on hemostasis in small blood vessels. In the mouse mesentery bleeding time (BT) was increased by several amines which inhibit ADP-induced platelet aggregation (chloroquine, nortriptyline, methapyrilene, methdilazine), by several nonsteroidal anti-inflammatory agents (aspirin, phenylbutazone, fenoprofen sodium, but not sulfinpyrazone), by clofibrate, and by two hydrocinnamic acid relatives. On the other hand, in the guinea pig no increase in BT was observed with these agents. In the dog extracorporeal shunt heparin and phenylbutazone decreased the thrombotic deposit. In the rabbit extracorporeal shunt fenoprofen sodium significantly reduced the thrombotic deposit, but phenylbutazone, aspirin, and VK 744 did not. *In vivo* thrombus formation induced in the carotid artery of the rabbit by an electrical stimulus was investigated. It was found that the composition of the electrode was important for thrombus production and that the current and voltage were of lesser importance as long as the potential applied to the artery was positive.

Thrombosis is the pathological exaggeration of that portion of the bio-defense system responsible for the maintenance of hemostasis. It is responsible for more deaths and morbidity in the United States than any other single condition. It is toward this objective that the search for therapeutic and prophylactic antithrombotic agents is directed.

Intravascular thrombus formation involves the vessel wall, the blood platelets, and the coagulation system. The relative importance of the individual constituents depends on the particular situation. In arterial thrombosis platelets play a major role and perhaps represent the trigger mechanism. Fibrin formation stabilizes the platelet mass and leads to progressive growth of the thrombus. In venous thrombosis fibrin formation is a major event while the platelets play a more secondary and supporting role.

The adherence of platelets to the vessel wall and to each other certainly is a basic phenomenon involved in thrombosis. Consequently, inhibition of platelet function should decrease the tendency of thrombus formation. With this reasoning, several agents which inhibit platelet aggregation *in vitro* have been tested in both man and the experimental animal for antithrombotic activity. The anticoagulant drugs, heparin and the coumarins, have been used for this purpose for some time. They are effective in decreasing venous thrombosis and pulmonary embolism but are of lesser value in arterial thrombosis (Wessler *et al.*, 1966). This is not surprising in view of the primary importance of fibrin formation on the venous side.

Many methods for the production of experimental thrombosis have been published. Henry (1962) lists 219 such methods with a short description of each and more have been published since. This large variety of methods illustrates the uncertainty which exists regarding the correlation of experimental results to the human counterpart. It may be that different factors are involved in different clinical situations, so that one method may relate to one situation but not the other.

In 1910 Duke published a method for determination of bleeding time and presented evidence for involvement of platelets in hemostasis (Duke, 1910). Using Duke's method, Quick (1966) studied the effect of aspirin on bleeding time in normal human volunteers and found that 2 hr after a single oral dose of 1.3 g the bleeding time increased from a normal of about 3 min to about 4.5 min. It is now well established (Mustard *et al.*, 1970) that the nonsteroidal anti-inflammatory drugs inhibit collagen-induced platelet aggregation *in vitro* but have relatively little effect on that induced by ADP. This presumably is due to their effect on the platelet release reaction. Collagen-induced platelet aggregation proceeds via the release reaction and ADP has a direct effect.

Aspirin, in doses of 1–1.5 g/day, was found to decrease the incidence of thromboembolic complications after hip surgery (Salzman *et al.*, 1971; Hey, 1972). In another study aspirin had no effect on the incidence of venous thrombosis after surgery (O'Brien, 1972). In the rabbit, at a dose of 200 mg/kg, aspirin decreased the thrombotic deposit in an extracorporeal shunt (Evans *et al.*, 1968) but was without effect on thrombus formation in a section of polyethylene tubing chronically implanted into the abdominal aorta (Weigensberg *et al.*, 1972). In an extracorporeal flow chamber in the dog, intravenous heparin, 30 units/kg, reduced the deposition of thrombotic material by 57 per cent and intravenous aspirin, 50 mg/kg, produced a 24 per cent reduction (Benis *et al.*, 1972). These findings indicate that aspirin may have some antithrombotic potential but its activity varied with the experimental conditions employed.

Phenylbutazone, at a dose of 50 mg/kg iv, decreased the amount of thrombus deposition in the extracorporeal shunt in the rabbit by about 40 per cent (Mustard *et al.*, 1967). In rats both phenylbutazone and sulfinpyrazone, at a dose of 100 mg/kg orally, decreased hepatic thrombosis initiated by intravenous endotoxin administration (Renaud *et al.*, 1970). Sulfinpyrazone given intravenously at a dose of 125 mg/kg increased the survival time of renal allografts in dogs (Sharma *et al.*, 1972). There is good evidence implicating platelet thrombi with the kidney graft rejection episode (Mustard *et al.*, 1970).

In injury-induced platelet thrombosis in exposed cerebral arteries of the rabbit, dipyridamole, 2.6 mg/kg iv, and prostaglandin E_1, 25 μg iv, were effective inhibitors of thrombus formation (Emmons *et al.*, 1965, 1967). On the other hand, RA433, a more active pyrimido-pyrimidine agent than dipyridamole *in vitro*, had no effect on thrombus formation in this experimental model (Elkeles *et al.*, 1968).

Laser-induced platelet thrombosis in the rabbit ear chamber was inhibited by aspirin, phenylbutazone, and a new anti-inflammatory agent, 5-cyclohexylindan-1-carboxylic acid (Fleming *et al.*, 1972). The monoamine oxidase inhibitor nialamide, at 3 mg/kg iv, was found significantly to inhibit thrombus formation on the intimal injury of the rabbit ear artery produced with a dental burr (Shimamoto *et al.*, 1962).

The studies mentioned above are samples of the many publications on this subject that have appeared in the literature. In spite of the variable, even contradictory, results, it is clear that agents which inhibit platelet function have some inhibitory effect on thrombus formation. It is apparent that different methods yield different results and possibly, as more knowledge is acquired, the appropriate method for a particular clinical situation can be found.

In this study various agents were treated for antithrombotic activity using several experimental methods.

METHODS

The mouse mesentery micropuncture wound bleeding time technique (Herrmann *et al.*, 1968) was used in this study. It involves the production of a standardized micropuncture wound in a fat-free section of a venule in the mouse mesentery. Bleeding time (BT) was measured in seconds from five such wounds in each mouse and averaged. Using four control and six experimental mice, it was found that a 10-sec increase in BT over the controls is usually significant at $p = 0.05$ or less. The same technique was used for determination of mesentery bleeding time in guinea pigs.

The extracorporeal shunt was constructed from Tygon tubing as shown in Fig. 1. The shunt was inserted between the carotid artery and jugular vein by coupling to polyethylene tubing cannulas. The inside diameter of the 2-inch centerpiece containing the tared silk thread was 1/8 inch for the rabbit and 3/16 inch for the dog experiments. For the experiments with dogs a small piece of collagen was tied at the end in contact with the flowing blood. The duration of blood flow was either 30 or 60 min, after which time the carotid end was clamped and 5 ml of saline were injected into the tubing to wash away the blood and visualize the thrombus. The thread with thrombus was removed for dry weight determination.

In the experiments with rabbits it was not possible to prepare identical pieces of collagen for each shunt; the surface area of the collagen exposed to the blood flow was variable. Collagen was,

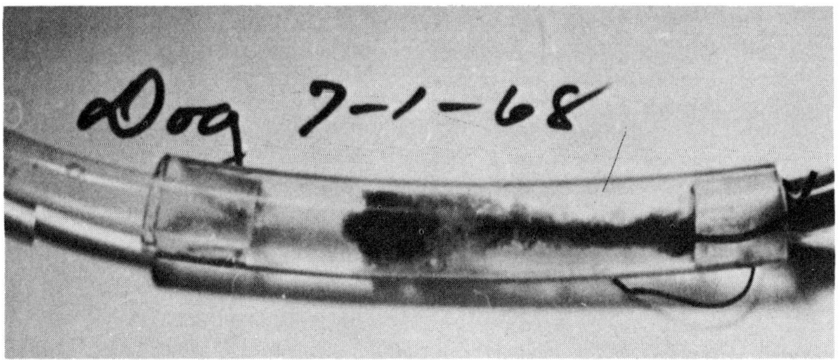

Figure 1. Extracorporeal shunt.

therefore, replaced with a triple knot to induce turbulence and promote thrombus formation (Herrmann *et al.*, 1972).

To study thrombosis induced by electrical stimulation the carotid arteries of the rabbit were isolated and laid across the U-shaped end of an electrode. A second electrode was attached to the surrounding tissue at a distance of about 1–2 inches from the carotid electrode. A Trygon constant current power supply unit (Trygon Electronics, Inc., Roosevelt, N.Y.) was used to provide the electric stimulus. Thirty minutes after stimulation, the stimulated section of the carotid artery was excised and the thrombus was graded as shown in Fig. 2. Using a paper clip for the carotid electrode, it was found that a current of 2 ma consistently produced a thrombus only when a + potential was applied. No thrombus was formed with a − potential. This agrees with the findings of Sawyer (Sawyer *et al.*, 1972).

In the carotid artery of rabbits thrombus formation was induced with a No. 50 white cotton thread which was introduced transversely through the center of the artery and tied snugly causing a 50 per cent constriction. Blood was allowed to flow for 1 hr, after which time the tied section was excised, opened lengthwise, and spread on a glass microscope slide to dry. When dry, the thrombus was carefully removed under × 100 magnification and weighed.

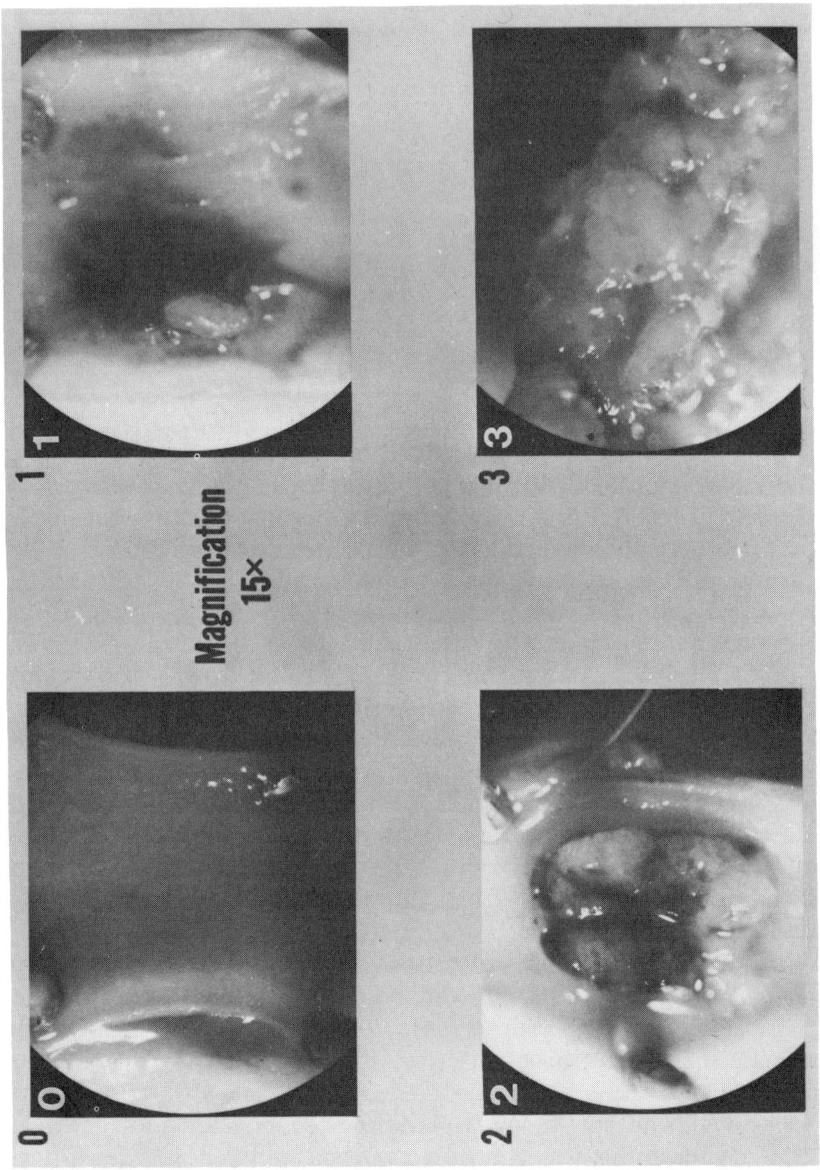

Figure 2. Carotid artery thrombi produced by electrical stimulation, grades 0–3. × 9.

RESULTS AND DISCUSSION

Table 1 summarizes the results obtained with several amines which had previously been shown to inhibit ADP-induced platelet aggregation *in vitro*. The *in vitro* relative potency with respect to inhibition of ADP-induced aggregation is given in the last column. Methapyrilene was one-third as potent as 66533 *in vitro* as an inhibitor of platelet aggregation. *In vivo*, however, in respect to bleeding time, it was only slightly less potent than 66533. Methdilazine was slightly more potent than 66533 as an *in vitro* inhibitor of platelet aggregation, but considerably less potent *in vivo* in prolonging the bleeding time. Heparin affected bleeding time only at the high dose even though at the low dose it rendered the blood incoagulable in a glass test tube for at least 3 hr. This agrees with the observation that a high dose of heparin is required partially to inhibit collagen-induced platelet aggregation *in vitro* (Herrmann *et al.*, 1966) and appears to indicate that fibrin formation is of lesser consequence in this assay. Both chloroquine and nortriptyline showed good activity in this assay.

Clofibrate has been shown to decrease platelet adhesiveness to latex particles (Glynn *et al.*, 1967; Robinson, 1966) and to increase bleeding time in six out of seven patients without any effect on adhesiveness of platelet to glass (O'Brien *et al.*, 1966). The results obtained with clofibrate, two closely related compounds, and several anti-inflammatory drugs are presented in Table 2. The first three compounds show a good dose-response relationship with compound 3 being the most potent. Compound 1 (*a*-(4-chlorophenylmercapto)-*a*-methylhydrocinnamic acid, sodium salt (PMC)) was tested in man without showing any effect on platelet function. This may possibly be due to a difference in metabolism since this agent has no effect on platelet aggregation *in vitro*. The nonsteroidal anti-inflammatory compounds 4, 6, and 8 produced an increase in bleeding time at 20, 5, and 10 mg/kg, respectively. No activity was observed with sulfinpyrazone even when fed in the diet at the 0.1 per cent level for 8 weeks.

The mouse mesentery micropuncture bleeding time technique was adapted to the guinea pig. The average control bleeding time of 21 guinea pigs was found to be 34.8 sec. In contrast to the results in mice, none of the compounds tested had any effect on the bleeding time of guinea pigs (Table 3). Immediately after

Table 1. Effect of heparin and some amines on bleeding time (BT) of the mouse mesentery

Compound	No. of mice	Dose/kg	Route	Time after dosing (min)	BT↑* (sec)	R_p†
Normal controls	92				45	
Heparin	7	1000 units	iv	5	18.8‡	
	6	100 units	iv	5	0.2	
No. 66533						
$Cl-C_6H_3(C_6H_5)-O-(CH_2)_2-CH(CH_3)-N(CH_3)_2 \cdot HCl$	6	20 mg	Oral	30	36.6‡	1
	6	10 mg	Oral	30	24.3‡	
	8	5 mg	Oral	30	0	
	6	0.05 % in diet for 7 days			141.2‡	
Methapyrilene HCl						
(thienyl)$-CH_2-N$(2-pyridyl)$-(CH_2)_2-N(CH_3)_2 \cdot HCl$	6	20 mg	Oral	30	18.7‡	
	6	10 mg	Oral	30	10.0‡	0.33
	6	5 mg	Oral	30	0.3	
	6	0.05 % in diet for 7 days			50.3‡	

Methdilazine HCl						
S, $N{-}CH_2{-}$, $N{-}CH_3 \cdot HCl$	6	20 mg	Oral	30	9.6‡	1.2
	6	10 mg	Oral	30	0.7‡	
Chloroquine						
Cl, N, $NH{-}CH{-}(CH_2)_3{-}N(C_2H_5)_2$	6	25 mg	Oral	30	69.6‡	1.4
Nortriptyline						
$CH{-}(CH_2)_2{-}N(H)(CH_3)$	16	10 mg	Oral	30	52.4‡	
	6	0.05 % in diet for 7 days			92.4‡	0.7
	6	0.05 % in diet for 14 days			143.2‡	

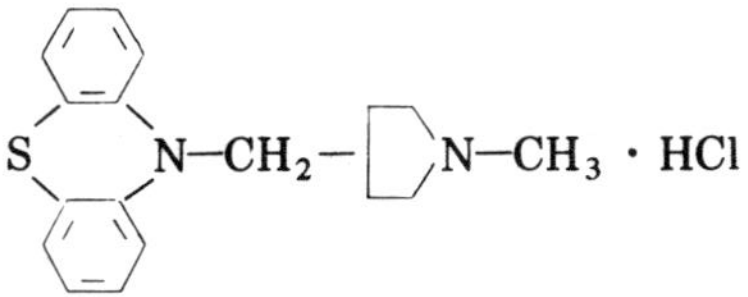

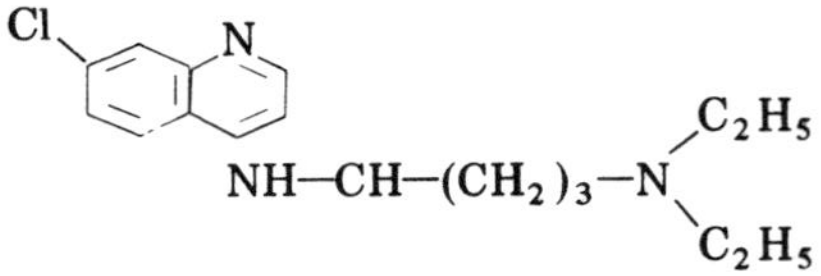

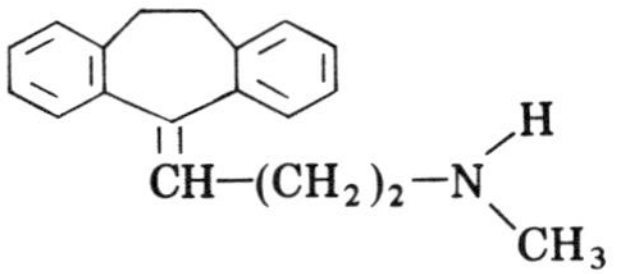

* Bleeding time increase over controls.

† Relative potency of *in vitro* inhibition of ADP-induced platelet aggregation, R_p, of 1 = 50 per cent inhibition of 1×10^{-4} *M*.

‡ $p > 0.05$.

Table 2. Effect of nonsteroidal anti-inflammatory agents and clofibrate and related derivatives on bleeding time (BT) of the mouse mesentery

Compound	No. of mice	Oral dose (mg/kg)	Time after dosing (min)	BT increase over controls (sec)
1. PMC†				
PMC $C_6H_5-CH_2$; $Cl-C_6H_4-S-C(CH_3)-C(=O)-ONa$	8	20	30	34.8*
	8	10	30	23.0*
	14	5	30	10.5*
	12	2.5	30	6.3
2. Clofibrate				
$Cl-C_6H_4-O-C(CH_3)_2-C(=O)-O-C_2H_5$	6	20	30	73.9*
	8	10	30	18.6*
	6	5	30	0.9
3. $C_6H_5-CH_2$; $Cl-C_6H_4-S-C(CH_3)-C(=O)-O-C_2H_5$	11	1.25	30	27.0*
	7	0.625	30	1.1
4. Aspirin	6	20	30	11.6*
	6	10	30	0
5. Sodium salicylate	6	40	30	22.2*
	6	20	30	1.9
6. Phenylbutazone	14	5	30	14.0*
	6	2.5	30	4.3
7. Sulfinpyrazone	6	40	30	0
	6	0.1% in diet for 56 days		4.6
8. Fenoprofen, sodium	8	10	30	14.5*
$C_6H_5-O-C_6H_4-CH(CH_3)-COONa$	8	5	30	2.2

* $p \leq 0.05$.

† PMC = α-(4-chlorophenylmercapto)-α-methylhydrocinnamic acid, sodium salt.

Table 3. Effect of heparin and several platelet aggregation inhibitors on guinea pig mesentery micropuncture bleeding time (BT)

Compound	No. of animals	Dose/kg	Route	Time after dosing (min)	BT (sec)
Control, saline	21	1 ml	Oral	60	34.8
Heparin	5	100 units	iv	5	34.3
	6	1000 units	iv	5	39.8
No. 66533*	4	50 mg	Oral	30	31.8
	5	50 mg	Oral	60	34.1
Aspirin	5	50 mg	Oral	120	38.9
	14	100 mg	Oral	120	37.8
	4	500 mg	Oral	120	34.4
Phenylbutazone	7	200 mg	Oral	60	30.0
	6	400 mg	Oral	120	31.2
Chloroquine	5	100 mg	Oral	120	37.6
	6	200 mg	Oral	120	31.1
Methapyrilene	3	100 mg	Oral	60	31.2

* See Table 1 for structure.

determination of bleeding time, blood samples were obtained from animals treated with aspirin and phenylbutazone. Platelet-rich plasma was prepared for assessment of platelet aggregation induced by a standard collagen challenge. Nearly complete inhibition of aggregation was observed. There was no correlation between the effects of aspirin and phenylbutazone on bleeding time and inhibition of collagen-induced platelet aggregation.

The results obtained in dogs are shown in Table 4. Each dog served as his own control. Saline produced no significant change in thrombus formation. Phenylbutazone, at 25 mg/kg, produced a 41 per cent inhibition of thrombus deposition. For a similar reduction of thrombus weight 100 mg/kg of phenylmercaptohydrocinnamic acid was required, while in the mouse mesentery micropuncture assay PMC and phenylbutazone were of equal potency. At 100 units/kg heparin produced a 71 per cent reduction of thrombus weight. The deposit was presumably a platelet thrombus because it was white and showed no visible evidence of red cell incorporation.

Table 4. Effects of phenylbutazone, PMC, and heparin on thrombus weight in dog, shunt with collagen*

No. of dogs	Drug/kg	Dose/kg	Thrombus dry wt (mg) Before drug	After drug	Inhibition (%)
	Saline				
24		1 ml	24.2 ± 1.8†	21.6 ± 2.1	11
	Phenylbutazone				
5		25 mg	22.0 ± 3.7	13.0 ± 1.3	41‡
6		10 mg	24.0 ± 5.0	15.2 ± 2.7	37
	PMC §				
7		100 mg	19.1 ± 2.1	11.6 ± 0.7	39‡
7		50 mg	27.6 ± 5.2	22.4 ± 3.1	19
	Heparin				
4		1000 units	25.2 ± 2.1	2.2 ± 0.3	91‡
4		100 units	20.6 ± 0.2	6.0 ± 1.6	71‡
4		10 units	26.1 ± 7.0	21.6 ± 1.6	17

* Intravenous dosing 5 min prior to drug, 30-min blood flow.

† Average ± SE.

‡ $p \leq 0.05$.

§ PMC = α-(4-chlorophenylmercapto)-α-methylhydrocinnamic acid, sodium salt.

Table 5. Effects of fenoprofen, aspirin, phenylbutazone, and VK-744 on thrombus weight in rabbit, shunt with knot

No. of rabbits	Drug (amount orally)	Time dosed before shunt (hr)	Thrombus formation		Inhibition (%) of *in vitro* platelet aggregation; aggregation inducer		
					Collagen suspension		ADP
			Dry wt (mg)	Inhibition (%)	Undiluted	1:4 diluted	$2.1 \times 10^{-5}\ M$
	Saline						
32	1 ml	1	9.1		1.12	0.66	22.2
	Fenoprofen, sodium salt						
6	200 mg	1	4.8	46*	59*	93*	0
6	100 mg	1	5.5	40*	43*	80*	4
7	50 mg	1	9.3	0	31	63*	1
3	100 mg	3	8.8	3			
	Aspirin						
6	200 mg	1	6.9	24	43*	81*	0
7	100 mg	1	7.7	15	63*	96*	0
	Phenylbutazone						
4	200 mg	1	7.0	23	43*	91*	0
4	100 mg	1	7.0	23	22	83*	7
6	50 mg	1	6.4	30	0	0	18
	VK-744†						
4	100 mg	1	7.3	20	39*	90*	5
5	50 mg	1	7.0	23	47*	83*	20

* $p \leq 0.05$.

† The chemical name of VK-744 is 2-[(2-aminoethyl)amino]-4-morpholinothieno[3,2d]pyrimidine dihydrochloride.

The results obtained in rabbit shunt preparations with knot are presented in Table 5. Fenoprofen (sodium salt of *dl*-2-(3-phenoxyphenyl)propionic acid) at 200 and 100 mg/kg orally produced about 40 per cent reduction in thrombus weight and significant inhibition of collagen-induced platelet aggregation. The duration of action was less than 3 hr. Aspirin, phenylbutazone, and the pyrimido-pyrimidine VK744 had no significant effect on thrombus formation even though collagen-induced platelet aggregation was inhibited to the same degree as that produced by fenoprofen.

The results obtained in rabbit shunt preparations with thread are presented in Table 6. The average thrombus weight of 20 saline control rabbits was 920 μg. Aspirin at 200 mg/kg orally produced a 31 per cent reduction in thrombus weight. This effect was not significant at the 95 per cent confidence level. Fenoprofen sodium at a dose as low as 50 mg/kg orally produced a 73 per cent reduction of thrombus weight. This was significant statistically.

Composition of the electrode was found to be important for thrombus formation induced by electrical stimulation. This is illustrated in Table 7. Both carotid arteries of each rabbit were used yielding twice the number under "Grade of Thrombus." The only electrodes which produced thrombi were the paper clip, stainless steel and iron, with iron being the common denominator. During stimulation dissociation of the electrode occurred at the anode (+ electrode) (Getman *et al.*, 1940) and therefore suggested that the ionic iron liberated was responsible for thrombus formation rather than the current or voltage. This finding of the importance of the electrolyte for thrombus formation agrees with the study of Cowan *et al.* (1966). They observed that the electrolytic dissociation products were important since by removal of these dissociation products thrombus formation was prevented. Their interpretation was that the pH change to 2 or less at the anode was responsible for thrombus formation.

Using the carbon electrode, which is slightly porous, we investigated the effect of ionic iron. These results are presented in Table 8. As indicated in Table 7, the carbon electrode did not promote thrombus formation with the 2 ma and +6-volt stimulus. Increasing the stimulus to 5 ma and +19 volts also was without effect. The electrode was impregnated with either $FeCl_2$ or $FeCl_3$ by placing it into a tube containing the respective aqueous solutions for the specified duration of time. The electrode was then removed and allowed to dry before use. A new piece of carbon rod was used for

Table 6. Effects of aspirin and fenoprofen on thrombus weight in rabbit, shunt with thread*

No. of rabbits	Drug (ml or mg/kg orally)	Time dosed before thread introduced (hr)	Thrombus dry wt (μg)	Inhibition (%)
	Saline			
20	1	2	920 ± 128†	
	Aspirin			
6	200	2	633 ± 92	31
	Fenoprofen, sodium salt			
8	200	2	338 ± 96	63‡
2	150	2	300 ± 100	67‡
6	50	2	250 ± 129	73‡

* No. 50 white cotton thread tied transverse through carotid artery, 1-hr blood flow.

† Average ± SE.

‡ $p \leq 0.05$.

Table 7. Effect of electrode composition on thrombus formation using a 2-ma current of 3-min duration

Wire	Volts	No. of rabbits*	Grade of thrombosis (No. in each grade)			
			0	1	2	3
Paper clip	+5	12		2	7	15
Paper clip	−5	3	6			
Stainless steel	+6	2		2	2	
Iron	+6	2				4
Copper	+5	2	4			
Silver	+5	2	3	1		
Nichrome	+6	2	4			
Platinum	+8	6	11	1		
98% Magnesium-2% Aluminum	+5	2	3	1		
Carbon	+6	4	8			
Carbon	−6	2	4			

* Right and left carotid artery of each rabbit.

each experiment. As may be observed, the electric stimulus in the presence of ionic iron induced thrombus formation and the ferrous ion was more effective than the ferric ion. Since we were not able to induce platelet aggregation *in vitro* by the addition of either $FeCl_3$ or $FeCl_2$, it appears that the ionic iron produces some effect or change in the vessel wall which leads to thrombus formation.

On the basis of our studies, it may be stated that inhibitors of platelet aggregation possess antithrombotic properties. Since antithrombotic therapy deals with a multicomponent system which may vary with different clinical conditions, any one experimental model probably does not apply to all thrombotic situations.

Table 8. Effect of ferric and ferrous iron on thrombus formation

Carbon electrode presoak solution	Current (ma)	Volts	Stimulus duration (min)	No. of rabbits*	Grade of thrombosis (No. in each grade)			
					0	1	2	3
No presoak	2	+6	3	4	8			
No presoak	5	+19	3	2	3	1		
$FeCl_3$ (1440 mg/ml, 3 hr)	2	+8	3	2				4
$FeCl_3$ (144 mg/ml, 1 hr)	2	+6	3	2	4			
$FeCl_3$ (1440 mg/ml, 1 hr)	2	+6	3	2	4			
$FeCl_2$ (500 mg/ml, 1 hr)	2	+6	3	2				4
$FeCl_2$ (100 mg/ml, 1 hr)	2	+6	3	2		1	1	2
$FeCl_2$ (50 mg/ml, 1 hr)	2	+8	3	4	8			

* Right and left carotid artery of each rabbit.

REFERENCES

Benis, A. M., Nossel, H. L., Aledort, L. M., and Leonard, E. F. 1972. Thrombus formation in flow chambers studied with dogs having long term extracorporeal shunts, p. 352. Abstract, Third Congress of International Society on Thrombosis and Haemostasis, Washington, D.C.

Cowan, C. R., and Monkhouse, F. C. 1966. Studies on electrically induced thrombosis and related phenomena. Can. J. Physiol. Pharmacol. 44: 88.

Duke, W. W. 1910. The relation of blood platelets to hemorrhagia disease. J. Amer. Med. Ass. 55: 1185.

Elkeles, R. S., Hampton, J. R., Honour, A. J., and Mitchell, J. R. A. 1968. Effect of a pyrimido-pyrimidine compound on platelet behavior *in vitro* and *in vivo*. Lancet 2: 751.

Emmons, P. R., Hampton, J. R., Harrison, J. G., Honour, A. J., and Mitchell, J. R. A. 1967. Effect of prostaglandin E_1 on platelet behavior *in vitro* and *in vivo*. Brit. Med. J. 2: 468.

Emmons, P. R., Harrison, J. G., Honour, A. J., and Mitchell, J. R. A. 1965. Effect of a pyrimidopyrimidine derivative on thrombus formation in the rabbit. Nature 208: 255.

Evans, G., Packham, M. A., Nishizawa, E. E., Mustard, J. F., and Murphy, E. A. 1968. The effect of acetylsalicylic acid on platelet function. J. Exp. Med. 128: 877.

Fleming, J. S., King, S. P., Buchanan, J. O., and Bierwagen, M. E. 1972. Antithrombotic potential of a new, synthetic, non-steroidal anti-inflammatory agent, 5-cyclohexylindan-1-carboxylic acid (BL-2365), p. 420. Abstract, Third Congress of International Society on Thrombosis and Haemostasis, Washington, D.C.

Getman, F. H., and Daniels, F. 1940. Outlines of theoretical chemistry. 6th Ed., p. 360. John Wiley and Sons, New York.

Glynn, M. F., Murphy, E. A., and Mustard, J. F. 1967. Effect of clofibrate on platelet economy in man. Lancet 2: 447.

Henry, R. L. 1962. Methods for inducing experimental thrombosis. Angiology 13: 554.

Herrmann, R. G., and Frank, J. D. 1966. Effect of adenosine derivatives and antihistaminics on platelet aggregation. Proc. Soc. Exp. Biol. Med. 123: 654.

Herrmann, R. G., Frank, J. D., and Marlett, D. L. 1968. An *in vivo* technique for assessing the formation of a hemostatic platelet plug. Proc. Soc. Exp. Biol. Med. 128: 960.

Herrmann, R. G., Marshall, W. S., Crowe, V. G., Frank, J. D., Marlett, D. L., and Lacefield, W. B. 1972. Effect of a new anti-inflammatory drug, fenoprofen, on platelet aggregation and thrombus formation. Proc. Soc. Exp. Biol. Med. 139: 548.

Hey, D. M., Burckhardt, H., Heinrich, D., and Roka, L. 1972. Antithrombotic treatment by means of ASA (aspirin) in patients with major hip joint operations, p. 426. Abstract, Third Congress of International Society on Thrombosis and Haemostasis, Washington, D.C.

Mustard, J. F., Glynn, M. F., Nishizawa, E. E., and Packham, M. A. 1967. Platelet-surface interactions: relationship to thrombosis and hemostasis. Fed. Proc. 26: 106.

Mustard, J. F., and Packham, M. A. 1970. Factors influencing platelet function: adhesion, release, and aggregation. Pharmacol. Rev. 22: 98.

O'Brien, J. R. 1972. A trial of aspirin in postoperative venous thrombosis, p. 42. Abstract, Third Congress of International Society on Thrombosis and Haemostasis, Washington, D.C.

O'Brien, J. R., and Heywood, J. B. 1966. A comparison of platelet stickiness tests during an atromid-S trial. Thromb. Diath. Haemorrh. 16: 768.

Quick, A. J. 1966. Salicylates and bleeding: the aspirin tolerance test. Amer. J. Med. Sci. 252: 265.

Renaud, S., and LeCompte, F. 1970. Thrombosis prevention by coagulation and platelet aggregation inhibitors in hyperlipemic rats. Thromb. Diath. Haemorrh. 24: 577.

Robinson, R. W. 1966. Platelet adhesiveness with chlorophenoxyisobutyric ester. J. New Drugs 6: 126.

Salzman, E. W., Harris, W. H., and DeSanctis, R. W. 1971. Reduction in venous thromboembolism by agents affecting platelet function. New Engl. J. Med. 284: 1287.

Sawyer, P. N., and Srinivasan, S. 1972. The role of electrochemical surface properties in thrombosis at vascular interfaces: cumulative experience of studies in animals and man. Bull. N. Y. Acad. Med. 48: 235.

Sharma, H. M., Moore, S., Merrick, H. W., and Smith, M. R. 1972. Platelets in early hyperacute allograft rejection in kidneys and their modification by sulfinpyrazone (Anturan) therapy. Amer. J. Pathol. 66: 445.

Shimamoto, T., Ishioka, T., and Fujita, T. 1962. Antithrombotic effect of monamine oxidase inhibitor (Nialamide), comparison with prothrombinopenic anticoagulants. Circ. Res. 10: 647.

Weigensberg, B. I., Senikas, V., Mok, A., and Pawliwec, W. 1972. Effect of acetylsalicylic acid on aortic thrombosis induced in rabbits by polyethylene tubing, p. 446. Abstract, Third Congress of International Society on Thrombosis and Haemostasis, Washington, D.C.

Wessler, S., and Gaston, L. W. 1966. Anticoagulant therapy in coronary artery disease. Circulation 34: 856.

Use of a Rabbit Extracorporeal Shunt in the Assay of Antithrombotic and Thrombotic Drugs

F. J. Rosenberg, P. G. Phillips, and P. R. Druzba

A carotid-jugular extracorporeal shunt has been devised for use in rabbits to assay the effects of drugs on thrombus formation. Actual thrombus weights were determined along with estimates of platelet consumption and bleeding time. Ancillary measurements of blood pressure and flow were made to determine their participation in thrombus formation and their possible relation to the effects of drugs on thrombus formation.

Acetylsalicylic acid inhibited thrombus formation without affecting blood pressure or flow. Platelet consumption was reduced in relation to the reduction of thrombus weight.

Hydroxychloroquine inhibited thrombus formation without affecting blood pressure or flow. It reduced platelet consumption but not in direct relationship to thrombus formation.

The estrogens, ethynylestradiol and mestranol, increased thrombus weights and decreased bleeding time in a dose-dependent fashion. Contraceptive drug combinations containing these estrogens had less effect on thrombus weights than the pure estrogens. This protective effect could not be related to an antithrombotic effect of the progestins.

As early as 1882, Bizzozero (1882) suggested that platelets were involved in the formation of thromboses, and Welch (1887) and Eberth and Schimmelbusch (1888) extended this hypothesis. The role of platelet adherence and aggregation, in thrombi, has been recently reviewed by Mustard *et al.* (1966, 1967), Packham *et al.* (1968), and Mustard and Packham (1970).

Screening of compounds for inhibition of platelet aggregation and adhesiveness may have utility in predicting antithrombotic activity in man. The inhibition of platelet aggregation by acetylsalicylic acid has been demonstrated by Weiss *et al.* (1968), O'Brien (1968), and Rosenberg *et al.* (1971).

Similarly, Carter *et al.* (1971) demonstrated that hydroxychloroquine inhibited platelet aggregation, and reduced the incidence of postoperative deep vein thrombosis and pulmonary embolism in man.

Observations on platelet aggregation, however, are performed *in vitro*, although the drug may be administered directly to the species under study at specific intervals before preparation of the platelet-rich plasma required for the assay. It would be desirable to have available an *in vivo* system wherein formation of a thrombus can be evaluated quantitatively.

Murphy *et al.* (1962) and Downie *et al.* (1963) used a carotid-jugular extracorporeal shunt to induce and quantify thrombus formation in pigs. The pig is an inconvenient animal to use when large numbers of compounds are to be screened or when extensive dose-response and duration of action data must be obtained. This report describes the modification of the technique for use in rabbits, a species used earlier for this purpose by Rowntree and Shionoya (1972) for morphological observations of thrombus formation.

METHODS

Rabbits weighing 1.5–3.0 kg were anesthetized with intravenous pentobarbital and secured to a dissecting board. The right femoral artery was cannulated and connected to a pressure transducer for continuous measurement of arterial blood pressure. The right jugular vein and carotid artery were exposed and cannulated as shown in Fig. 1. The Y-connectors were polypropylene while the arterial and venous catheters were polyethylene.[1] Tygon tubing

1 Intramedic® Luer-End tmCatheters supplied by Clay-Adams Inc., New York, N.Y.

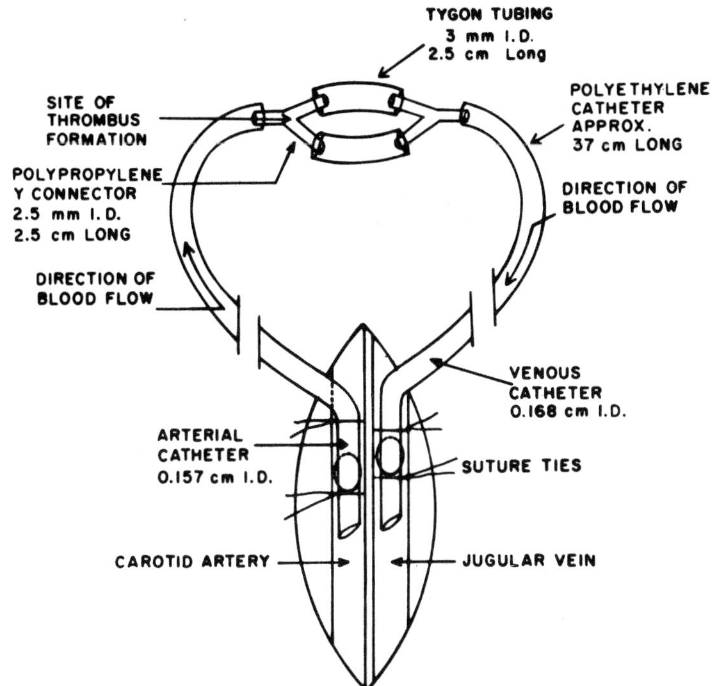

Figure 1. Schematic diagram of a rabbit extracorporeal shunt.

was used for the connections between the two Y-connectors. All components of the shunt were siliconized except for the Y-connector on the arterial side of the shunt. The arterial Y-connectors were weighed prior to the experiments. The entire shunt was filled with Tyrode's solution at the time of insertion.

A blood sample was withdrawn from the femoral artery to provide a base-line platelet count. The animal was allowed 10–12 min to attain a stable blood pressure level after which the shunt was opened and blood permitted to flow. The time for the first appearance of blood in the arterial catheter until its re-entry into the body on the venous side, was measured and recorded as flow time. If circulation through the shunt was not complete in less than 5 sec the animal was discarded. Actual blood flow was measured in several animals in each group with a Carolina Medical Electronics Flowmeter and a flow probe of appropriate size on the carotid artery just below the arterial catheter.

The shunt remained open for a period of 20 min. One minute before terminating the experiment a second femoral arterial blood sample was taken for determination of the final platelet count. The shunt was then disconnected, arterial catheter first, and the whole Y-connector segment removed and gently flushed with 10 ml of normal saline. The arterial Y-connector was separated, dried overnight at 50°C, and reweighed. Its initial weight subtracted from the final weight was recorded as thrombus weight.

Platelet counts were obtained by phase microscopy as described by Davidsohn (1966). Platelet consumption was calculated as the initial platelet count minus the final platelet count for each animal.

Inhibition or stimulation of thrombus formation was determined by comparing the thrombus weights of medicated animals with those of concurrently run controls.

Bleeding time was recorded during the operation of the shunt. An area of the inner thigh was prepared by gently clipping the hair with scissors and swabbing the area with saline. A magnifying lens and light were positioned over the area to be examined and a small quick incision, 1 cm long, was made in the skin. A stop watch was started as the severed subcutaneous vessels started bleeding. Normal saline was slowly dripped onto the incision at the rate of 1 drop every 2 sec to gently wash away the blood from the cut vessels. Cessation of bleeding was clearly visible. Duplicate readings, one from each thigh, were obtained from all animals.

Drugs[2] were administered by gastric intubation. Acetylsalicylic acid was dissolved in 1 *N* Na_2CO_3. Hydroxychloroquine was dissolved in water. Mestranol and 17-ethynylestradiol were administered in cottonseed oil. The commercially available forms of Demulen®, Enovid-E®, and Norinyl-2® were finely ground and put into cottonseed oil. Concentrations of all drugs were adjusted so that the desired doses were always administered in 1 ml/kg.

Acetylsalicylic acid and hydroxychloroquine were studied at various time intervals after a single dose but the estrogens and contraceptives were given once each day for 3 days, the shunt being run 24 hr after the last dose. Five rabbits were used in each group except for the contraceptives where three to five animals were used per group. Only female rabbits were used for the estrogen and contraceptive studies.

2 Mestranol, Organon Inc., West Orange, N.J.; 17-ethynylestradiol, Sigma Chemical Co., St. Louis, Mo.; Demulen, Searle and Co., San Juan, Puerto Rico; Enovid-E, G. D. Searle Co., Chicago, Ill.; Norinyl-2, Syntex Laboratories, Palo Alto, Calif.

RESULTS

Thrombus weight, hemodynamic, and platelet consumption data for 40 control rabbits are presented in Table 1. The mean thrombus weight of 1.88 mg was accompanied by a platelet consumption of 95,000 cells/mm^3 over the 20-min period. Acetylsalicylic acid significantly ($p < 0.01$) inhibited thrombus formation in a dose-dependent fashion (Table 2). Inhibition persisted, unabated, for 72 hr after a single oral dose. Platelet consumption appeared to be related to thrombus weight. Similarly, there was a dose-related increase in bleeding time. Administration of acetylsalicylic acid did not affect initial platelet counts, blood pressure, or blood flow.

Hydroxychloroquine also significantly inhibited ($p \leq 0.01$) thrombus formation as a function of dose (Table 3), without affecting initial platelet count, blood pressure, or blood flow. The inhibition decreased from 66 to 26 per cent over the first 48 hr after a single dose of 25 mg/kg. Hydroxychloroquine reduced platelet consumption, but, as opposed to acetylsalicylic acid, the reduction seemed unrelated to dose or the actual weight of the thrombus.

The action of hydroxychloroquine is also different from that of acetylsalicylic acid in that it did not increase bleeding time significantly at any of the doses studied.

Table 1. Extracorporeal shunt values for 40 control rabbits

Thrombus weight (mg ± SE)	1.88 ± 0.007
Initial platelet count (cells $\times$ 10^3/mm^3 ± SE)	233 ± 11
Final platelet count (cells $\times$ 10^3/mm^3 ± SE)	137 ± 8
Platelet consumption (initial-final $\times$ 10^3/mm^3 ± SE)	95 ± 10
Bleeding time (min, sec ± SE)	2′11″ ± 5″
Initial blood pressure (mm Hg ± SE)	96 ± 6
Final blood pressure (mm Hg ± SE)	92 ± 5
Arterial blood flow* (ml/min ± SE)	40 ± 4

* Five rabbits only.

Table 2. Dose- and time-related effects of acetylsalicylic acid as an inhibitor of thrombus formation in the rabbit extracorporeal shunt

		Thrombus weight		Platelet consumption		
Time (hr)	Dose (mg/kg p.o.)*	Mean thrombus wt (mg ± SE)	Decrease in thrombus wt (%)	Platelet consumption (cells × 10^3/mm^3 ± SE)	As percentage of initial platelet count	Bleeding time (min, sec ± SE)
3	Control	1.84 ± 0.02		100 ± 16	37	2′08″ ± 15″
	10	1.52 ± 0.03	17	51 ± 18	18	5′28″ ± 14″
	25	1.27 ± 0.02	30	34 ± 7	14	6′13″ ± 27″
	50	0.94 ± 0.02	49	26 ± 3	10	7′56″ ± 13″
24	Control	1.86 ± 0.03		95 ± 6	39	1′57″ ± 10″
	5	1.60 ± 0.01	14	67 ± 3	23	4′18″ ± 8″
	10	1.40 ± 0.01	25	44 ± 4	18	5′41″ ± 19″
	25	1.28 ± 0.02	31	31 ± 5	15	8′00″ ± 30″
	50	1.00 ± 0.05	46	32 ± 5	13	8′06″ ± 27″
48	Control	1.88 ± 0.01		90 ± 8	37	2′09″ ± 26″
	10	1.53 ± 0.04	19	39 ± 7	16	4′16″ ± 9″
	50	0.58 ± 0.04	69	25 ± 2	10	9′12″ ± 29″
72	Control	1.86 ± 0.02		104 ± 16	39	2′12″ ± 14″
	25	1.31 ± 0.01	30	42 ± 8	17	6′40″ ± 19″
	50	0.61 ± 0.02	67	36 ± 5	15	9′33″ ± 18″
96	Control	1.84 ± 0.02		110 ± 12	44	2′21″ ± 8″
	25	1.78 ± 0.02	NS*	83 ± 10	37	2′50″ ± 8″
	50	1.40 ± 0.03	24	43 ± 5	17	3′22″ ± 12″

* p.o., per os; NS, not significant.

Table 3. Dose- and time-related effects of hydroxychloroquine as an inhibitor of thrombus formation in the rabbit extracorporeal shunt

		Thrombus weight		Platelet consumption		
Time (hr)	Dose (mg/kg p.o.)*	Mean thrombus wt (mg ± SE)	Decrease in thrombus wt (%)	Platelet consumption (cells × 10^3/mm^3 ± SE)	As percentage of initial platelet count	Bleeding time (min, sec ± SE)
1	Control	1.86 ± 0.02		90 ± 17	32	2′26″ ± 22″
	5	1.54 ± 0.01	17	39 ± 9	15	2′25″ ± 8″
	10	1.14 ± 0.04	39	38 ± 8	17	2′21″ ± 20″
	50	0.74 ± 0.04	60	39 ± 6	16	2′28″ ± 12″
3	5	1.62 ± 0.02	13	74 ± 19	25	2′09″ ± 9″
	10	1.28 ± 0.06	31	43 ± 9	15	2′28″ ± 8″
	50	1.04 ± 0.02	44	30 ± 4	12	2′19″ ± 7″
1	Control	1.94 ± 0.02		95 ± 14	35	2′40″ ± 51″
	25	0.66 ± 0.02	66	45 ± 10	15	2′12″ ± 8″
3	25	0.94 ± 0.02	52	31 ± 4	13	2′21″ ± 6″
24	25	1.06 ± 0.03	45	54 ± 5	17	2′55″ ± 7″
48	25	1.42 ± 0.02	26	33 ± 6	12	2′16″ ± 9″
72	25	1.44 ± 0.02	25	23 ± 5	10	2′28″ ± 12″

* p.o., per os.

Mestranol, 2 or 3 μg/kg, and ethynylestradiol, 1 or 3 μg/kg, were given as single oral daily doses for 3 days. These doses were chosen to be at or just above the doses ingested by human females taking oral contraceptives containing these estrogens. Twenty-four hours after the last medication the thrombi in the medicated animals were heavier than those in concurrently run control animals (Table 4). The addition of progestins, as provided in the commercially available products used, appeared to have some protective effect, although the thrombus weights were still significantly higher than control with the exception of Norinyl-2 at the low dose. The doses of these commercial contraceptives were given to contain the same estrogen levels on a microgram per kilogram basis as the estrogen-treated animals.

The estrogens elevated the base-line platelet count in relation to the thrombus weight, as a function of dose. The ameliorating effect of the progestins on thrombus weights was similarly accompanied by a diminished increase in platelet count. Bleeding time was decreased by all preparations with the exception of the low dose of Norinyl-2 which did not significantly alter thrombus formation or bleeding time and it induced the smallest increase in base-line platelet count.

As with acetylsalicylic acid and hydroxychloroquine, neither the estrogens nor contraceptives affected blood pressure or flow. Ethynodiol diacetate and norethindrone, the progestins present in Demulen and Norinyl-2, were tested at 40 μg/kg for 3 days. Twenty-four hours after the last dose, thrombus weights, platelet counts, bleeding times, blood pressure, and flow were normal and not significantly different from control.

DISCUSSION

The rabbit extracorporeal shunt is a consistent and statistically reliable assay system for thrombus formation. It provides accurate data on thrombus weights and platelet consumption. It can be used for evaluation of the effects of drugs on thrombus formation and on hemodynamic parameters which could affect thrombus formation.

Acetylsalicylic acid clearly reduced thrombus weights without affecting platelet counts, blood pressure, or blood flow. Its antithrombotic effect was accompanied by related decreases in platelet consumption and increases in bleeding time. Clinical experi-

Table 4. Dose-related effects of estrogens and contraceptive drugs on thrombus formation in the rabbit extracorporeal shunt

Compound	Dose p.o.* as estrogen (μg/kg/day × 3)	Thrombus weight: Mean thrombus wt (mg ± SE)	Thrombus weight: Increase in thrombus wt (%)	Platelet consumption: Initial count cells (× 10^3/mm^3 ± SE)	Platelet consumption: Consumption cells (× 10^3/mm^3 ± SE)	Bleeding time (min, sec ± SE)
	Control	1.87 ± 0.03		248 ± 12	97 ± 7	2′28″ ± 7″
Ethynyl-estradiol	1	2.60 ± 0.06	70	375 ± 14	173 ± 9	1′16″ ± 7″
	3	4.64 ± 0.04	153	483 ± 4	261 ± 16	1′37″ ± 4″
Demulen	1	2.17 ± 0.03	14	357 ± 25	100 ± 35	1′48″ ± 11″
	3	2.77 ± 0.06	50	377 ± 14	175 ± 17	1′01″ ± 5″
Mestranol	2	2.47 ± 0.05	32	395 ± 9	105 ± 8	1′48″ ± 7″
	3	4.83 ± 0.12	160	471 ± 6	250 ± 32	0′48″ ± 4″
Enovid-E	2	2.60 ± 0.01	36	383 ± 17	163 ± 27	0′59″ ± 6″
	3	3.10 ± 0.10	66	391 ± 6	193 ± 4	1′02″ ± 8″
Norinyl-2	2	1.93 ± 0.03	2	310 ± 17	85 ± 12	2′10″ ± 7″
	3	2.20 ± 0.10	36	318 ± 10	87 ± 11	1′26″ ± 3″

	Estrogen	Progestin
Demulen	50 μg ethynyl-estradiol	1 mg ethynodiol diacetate
Enovid-E	100 μg mestranol	2.5 mg norethynodrel
Norinyl-2	100 μg mestranol	2 mg norethindrone

* p.o., per os.

ences with acetylsalicylic acid as an antithrombotic agent have yielded mixed results (Harrison *et al.*, 1971; British Medical Research Council Report, 1972), but some of the available data correlate with our observations in the rabbit. Salzman *et al.* (1971) reported that acetylsalicylic acid, 1.2 g/day, reduced the incidence of postoperative venous thromboembolism but with some increase in hemorrhagic tendency. Harker and Slichter (1970) found acetylsalicylic acid, 1 g/day, to potentiate the inhibition of platelet consumption induced by dipyridamole in patients with prosthetic cardiac valves. Acetylsalicylic acid was ineffective by itself, however.

Hydroxychloroquine was effective in decreasing thrombus weights, without an increase in bleeding time. In man, Carter *et al.* (1971), using clinical signs and phelobography, found hydroxychloroquine to be effective in preventing postoperative deep venous thrombosis and pulmonary embolism, without affecting bleeding or clotting times. The lack of a direct relationship between decrease in thrombus weight and platelet consumption may have been due to an artifact, or to the participation of an antithrombotic mechanism not measured in these studies. Madow (1960) demonstrated the inhibition of red blood cell sludging by hydroxychloroquine and other antimalarials. It cannot be determined from our experiments whether this action is related to the inhibition of thrombus formation but it does appear that hydroxychloroquine may affect formed blood elements other than platelets.

The hemostatic effect of estrogens is well known and was readily apparent in our studies. The dose-related prothrombotic effect of estrogens was similarly anticipated. Inman *et al.* (1970) suggested a relationship between the dose of the estrogen in contraceptive preparations and the risk of pulmonary embolism, deep vein thrombosis, cerebral thrombosis, and coronary thrombosis.

We cannot explain the increased platelet count observed in the estrogen-treated rabbits. Platelet counts in women taking daily doses of 50 μg of mestranol, 1 mg of ethynodiol diacetate, or both combined, did not differ from control values through the course of an entire menstrual cycle (Howie *et al.*, 1970). Because platelet counts were elevated in our estrogen experiments, the increase in thrombus weights may simply reflect the increased number of platelets circulating through the shunt. Alternatively, both the thrombotic and hemostatic effects in our studies may relate to estrogen-induced depression of antithrombin III activity (Peterson *et al.*, 1970; Fagerhol *et al.*, 1970; Howie *et al.*, 1970).

The two progestins studied in the rabbit were without effect on any of the parameters studied but reduced the prothrombotic effect of estrogen, when given as the commercial contraceptive. This suggests a pharmacological antagonism of the estrogen rather than titration of a prothrombotic drug with an antithrombotic agent.

REFERENCES

Bizzozero, J. 1882. Ueber einen neuen Formbestand teil des Blutes und dessen Rolle bei der Thrombose und der Blutgerinnung. Virchows Arch. Pathol. Anat. Physiol. Klin. Med. 90: 261.

British Medical Research Council. 1972. Report of the Steering Committee. Effect of aspirin on postoperative venous thrombosis. Lancet I: 440.

Carter, A. E., Eban, R., and Perrett, R. D. 1971. Prevention of postoperative deep venous thrombosis and pulmonary embolism. Brit. Med. J. 1: 312.

Davidsohn, I. 1962. The blood: methods used in the study of blood, pp. 61–262. *In* J. C. Todd and A. H. Sanford (eds.) Clinical diagnosis by laboratory methods. Saunders, Philadelphia.

Downie, H. G., Murphy, E. A., Rowsell, H. C., and Mustard, J. F. 1963. Extracorporeal circulation: a device for the quantitative study of thrombus formation in flowing blood. Circ. Res. 12: 441.

Eberth, J. C., and Schimmelbusch, C. 1888. Die Thrombose nach Versuchen und Leichenbefunden. Ferdinand Duke, Stuttgart.

Fagerhol, M. K., Abildgaard, V., Bergsjo, P., and Jacobsen, J. H. 1970. Oral contraceptives and low antithrombin III concentration. Lancet II: 1175.

Harker, L. A., and Slichter, S. J. 1970. Studies of platelet and fibrinogen kinetics in patients with prosthetic heart valves. N. Engl. J. Med. 283: 1302.

Harrison, M. J. G., Marshall, J., Meadows, J. C., and Ross Russell, R. W. 1971. Effect of aspirin in amaurosis fugax. Lancet II: 743.

Howie, P. W., Mallinson, A. C., Prentice, C. R. M., Horne, C. H. W., and McNicol, G. P. 1970. Effect of combined oestrogen-progestogen oral contraceptives, oestrogen, and progestogen on antiplasmin and antithrombin activity. Lancet II: 1329.

Inman, W. H. W., Vessey, M. P., Westerholm, B., and Engelund, A. 1970. Thromboembolic disease and the steroidal content of oral contraceptives. A report to the committee on safety of drugs. Brit. Med. J. 2: 203.

Madow, B. P. M. 1960. Use of antimalarial drugs as "desludging" agents in vascular disease processes. J. Amer. Med. Assn. 172: 1630.

Murphy, E. A., Rowsell, H. C., Downie, H. G., Robinson, G. A., and Mustard, J. F. 1962. Encrustation and atherosclerosis: the analogy between early *in vivo* lesions and deposits which occur in extracorporeal circulations. Can. Med. Assn. J. 87: 259.

Mustard, J. F., Glynn, M. F., Nishizawa, E. E., and Packham, M. A. 1967. Platelet surface interactions: relationship to thrombosis and hemostasis. Fed. Proc. 26: 106.

Mustard, J. F., Jorgenson, J., Hovig, T., Glynn, M. F., and Rowsell, H. C. 1966. Role of platelets in thrombosis, pp. 131–158. *In* F. Duckert (ed.) Pathogenesis and treatment of thromboembolic diseases. F. K. Schattauer-Verlag, Stuttgart.

Mustard, J. F., and Packham, M. A. 1970. Factors influencing platelet function: adhesion, release and aggregation. Pharmacol. Rev. 22: 97.

O'Brien, J. R. 1968. Effects of salicylates on human platelets. Lancet I: 779.

Packham, M. A., Nishizawa, E., and Mustard, J. 1968. Response of platelets to tissue injury. Biochem. Pharmacol. 17(suppl.): 171.

Peterson, R. A., Krull, P. E., Finley, P., and Ettinger, M. G. 1970. Changes in antithrombin III and plasminogen induced by oral contraceptives. Amer. J. Clin. Pathol. 53: 478.

Rosenberg, F. J., Gimber-Phillips, P. E., Groblewski, G. E., Davison, C., Phillips, D. K., Goralnick, S. J., and Cahill, E. D. 1971. Acetylsalicylic acid: inhibition of platelet aggregation in the rabbit. J. Pharmacol. Exp. Ther. 179: 410.

Rowntree, L. G., and Shionoya, T. 1927. Studies in experimental extracorporeal thrombosis. I. A method for the direct observation of extracorporeal thrombus formation. J. Exp. Med. 46: 7.

Salzman, E. W., Harris, W. H., and DeSanctis, R. W. 1971. Reduction in venous thromboembolism by agents affecting platelet function. N. Engl. J. Med. 284: 1287.

Weiss, H. J., Aledort, L. M., and Kochwa, S. 1968. The effect of salicylates on the hemostatic properties of platelets in man. J. Clin. Invest. 47: 2169.

Welch, W. H. 1887. The structure of white thrombi. Trans. Pathol. Soc. (Philadelphia) 13: 25.

New Pharmacological Approaches to Inhibition of Platelet Aggregation

Robert D. MacKenzie

This paper deals with methods used in the evaluation of drugs for their effect on platelet aggregation and on other platelet functions. It describes the use of adenosine diphosphate (ADP), collagen, epinephrine, and serotonin as *in vitro* aggregating agents. Other procedures described here include activation by drugs of platelet factor 3 (PF-3), determination of the effects of intravenously administered ADP on platelet counts, and pretreatment of animals with inhibitors of platelet aggregation followed by *in vitro* determination of sensitivity of their platelets to ADP. The pharmacological studies with a series of experimental and standard compounds are used to illustrate the practical application of the methods listed above.

The general physiological approaches to the prevention or treatment of thrombosis have been discussed by many investigators (Alexander, 1962; Hampton, 1966; Hampton, 1967; O'Brien, 1964; Ingram, 1967; Mustard and Packham, 1970; Mershey and Drapkin, 1965). The main aim of anticoagulant therapy is to prevent vascular occlusion. The anticoagulants are not, however, entirely effective in the prevention of arterial thrombosis (Salzman, 1965; Seaman *et al.*, 1964). Therefore, other approaches to the development of antithrombotic drugs were needed. One of them is the control of platelet aggregation. This paper deals with the evaluation of various compounds as *in vitro* inhibitors of platelet aggregation and *in vivo* antithrombotic agents.

METHODS

To obtain platelets, the blood was drawn from a vein or in small animals by heart puncture and was collected in a siliconized centrifuge tube (G. E. Dri-Film, SC-87) containing 1 part of 3.8 per cent sodium citrate to 9 parts of blood. Platelet-rich plasma (PRP) was obtained by centrifuging at 100 $\times$ *g* for 10 min. The platelet-poor plasma (PPP) was obtained from the blood residue centrifuged at 1000 $\times$ *g* for 15 min. For measuring platelet aggregation, an aggregometer (Bryston model, Scarborough, Ontario, or Chronolog model, Broomall, Pa.) was used. Most of our procedures have been previously described (MacKenzie, Henderson, and Steinbach, 1971; MacKenzie, Blohm, and Auxier, 1971; MacKenzie *et al.*, 1971; MacKenzie and Blohm, 1971; MacKenzie, Blohm, and Steinbach, 1972).

Platelet factor 3 (PF-3) activity was measured *in vitro* by a modified Stypven test (MacKenzie, Blohm, and Auxier, 1971).

Two *in vivo* methods were used. One method (MacKenzie, Henderson, and Steinbach, 1971) consisted of cannulation of the right jugular vein and right carotid artery of guinea pigs. ADP was infused into the jugular vein and blood samples were removed from the carotid cannula for platelet counts. Guinea pigs were chosen because their platelets are particularly sensitive to ADP.

The other method involved an *in vivo-in vitro* system. Animals were pretreated with drugs and blood was removed by heart puncture. Citrated PRP was tested *in vitro* in platelet aggregometer (MacKenzie, Blohm, and Steinbach, 1972). ADP was used at two concentrations: 0.45 and 0.8 μg/ml PRP. At least five or six animals were used in each experimental group.

RESULTS

Typical dose-response curves for ADP-induced platelet aggregation in human citrated PRP are shown in Fig. 1. Maximum change in transmittance (ΔT) was plotted against *in vitro* concentration of

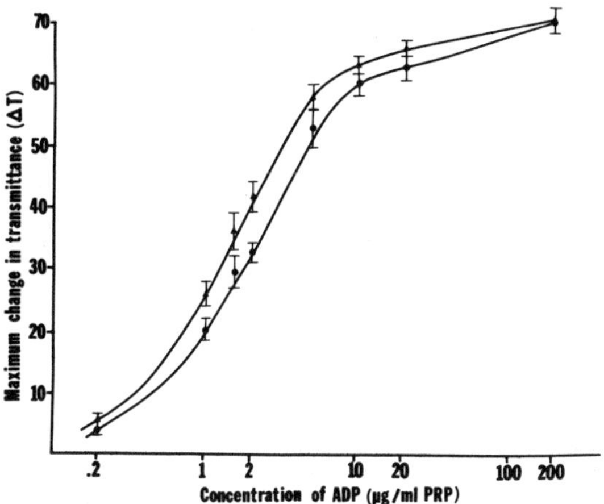

Figure 1. Dose response of ADP-induced platelet aggregation with citrated human platelet-rich plasma. ●, male ± SEM; ▲, female ± SEM (six subjects of each sex determined twice).

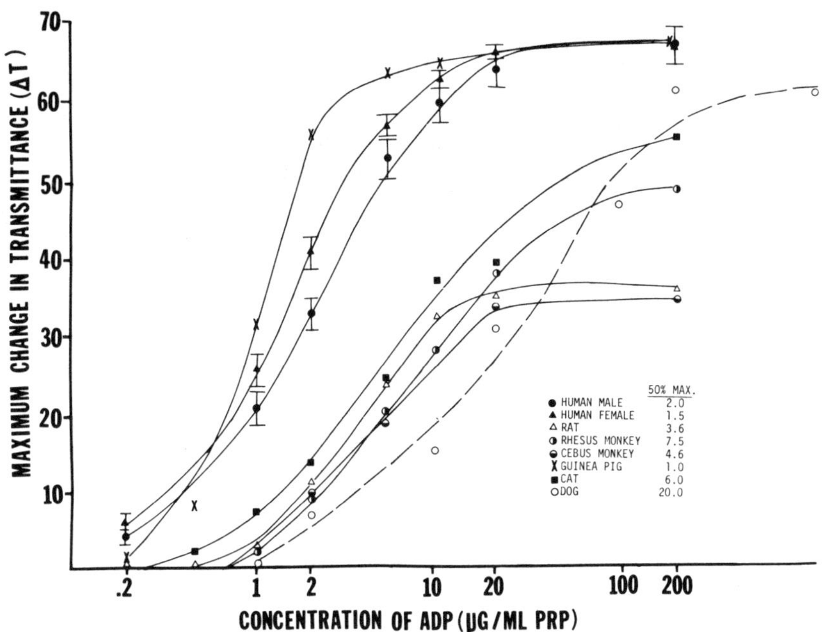

Figure 2. Dose response of ADP-induced platelet aggregation in platelet-rich plasma of human and other animals.

ADP in micrograms per milliliter of PRP. The platelets from female volunteers were found to be slightly more sensitive to ADP than from male volunteers.

In vivo activity of drugs must be first evaluated in an animal model. *In vitro* sensitivity to ADP of platelets from several animal species was therefore determined. It was found that human and guinea pig platelets were considerably more sensitive to ADP than platelets of other species (Fig. 2).

Thrombin at low concentrations (~0.2 unit/ml citrated PRP) caused platelet aggregation which was qualitatively similar to that induced by low concentrations of ADP. As shown in Fig. 3, secondary deaggregation was observed with both aggregating agents. When calcium ion (45–60 per cent optimum for fibrin formation) was added along with 0.08–0.1 unit/ml of thrombin, aggregation became greater and irreversible. This was independent of visible fibrin formation, although such formation helped to stabilize aggregates.

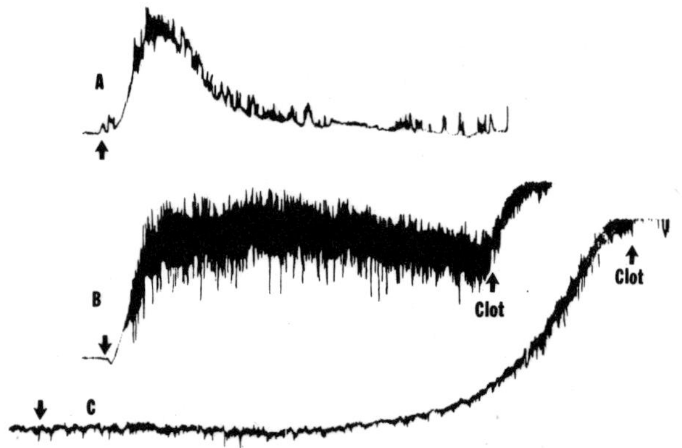

Figure 3. Effects of thrombin and calcium ion on platelet aggregation. A, 0.18 unit of thrombin/ml citrated human platelet-rich plasma. B, 0.10 unit of thrombin + 60 per cent optimum $CaCl_2$ concentrated/ml platelet-rich plasma. C, 100 per cent optimum $CaCl_2$ concentrated/ml platelet-rich plasma.

ADP *in vivo* was found to lower platelet count. Figure 4 shows the response of a control group of guinea pigs in which ADP infusion was adjusted to produce approximately a 50 per cent drop in platelet count and a return to normal in about 30 min. The required dose of ADP was 0.2 mg/kg infused in 1 min.

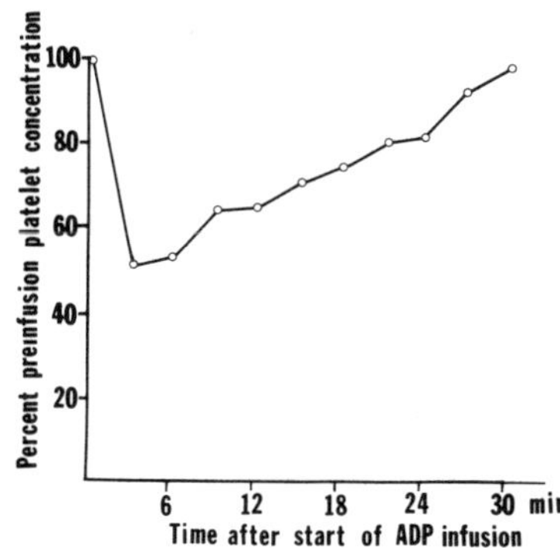

Figure 4. Effect of ADP infusion (0.2 mg/kg over 1 min) on platelet concentration in the guinea pig. Average values for nine determinations.

In the *in vivo-in vitro* system, sensitivity of platelets to ADP was determined. Parameters measured are shown in Fig. 5. They are initial slope, maximum change in transmittance, and total response for 5 min (area under the aggregation curve).

Figure 6 shows the structures and names of the compounds which were evaluated. The results of *in vitro* ADP-induced platelet aggregation on RMI 10,393, RMI 6792, RMI 7822, RMI 10,276, RMI 10,415, benzoazepine derivative, dipyridamole (RA8), RA 433, and PGE_1 are summarized in Fig. 7. PGE_1, RMI 10,276, and RMI 10,415 are relatively more and dipyridamole relatively less potent than other compounds.

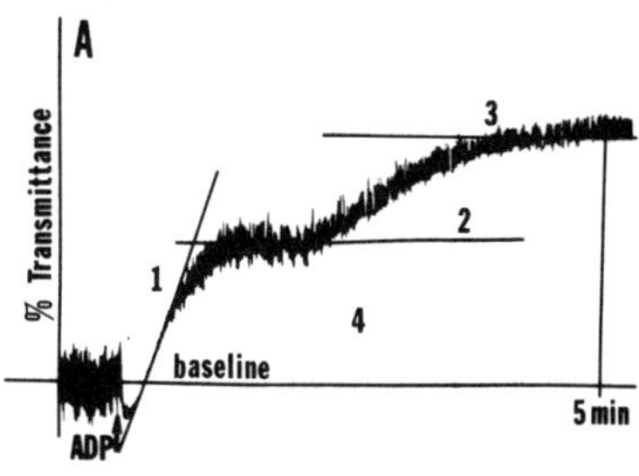

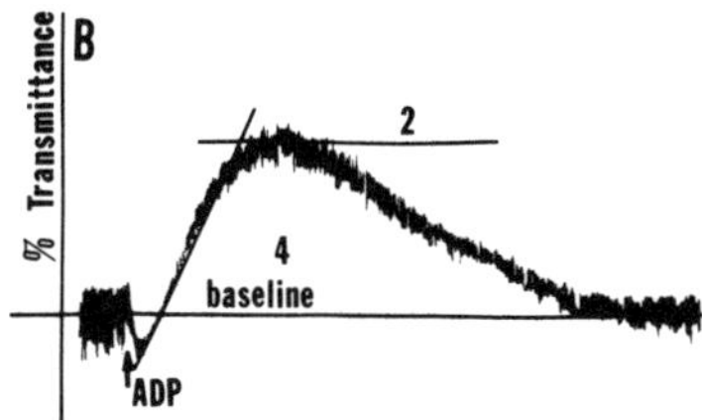

Figure 5. Parameters measured for ADP-induced platelet aggregation. 1, initial slope, the rate of change in percentage of transmittance; 2, initial (primary) ΔT, the amount of the first maximum change in transmittance; 3, secondary ΔT, the second maximum change in percentage of transmittance; 4, the area described by the curve in a given time (5 min).

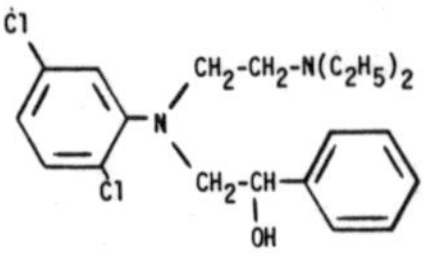

N-(2-DIETHYLAMINOETHYL)-N-(2-HYDROXY-2-PHENYL-ETHYL)-2,5 DICHLOROANILINE
(RMI 6792, AN 162) MW = 381.34
(MacKenzie RD and TR Blohm, 1971)

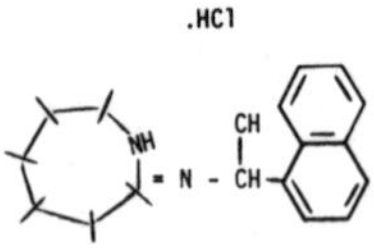

HEXAHYDRO-2-[1-(1-NAPHTHYL)ETHYLIMINO]AZEPINE HYDROCHLORIDE
(RMI 7822A) MW = 302.8
(Roberts EM et al, 1973)

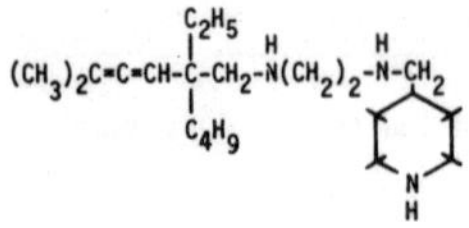

4-[2-(2-BUTYL-2-ETHYL-5-METHYL-3,4-HEXADIENYL-AMINO)ETHYLAMINOMETHYL]-PIPERIDINE
(RMI 10,276) MW = 335.56

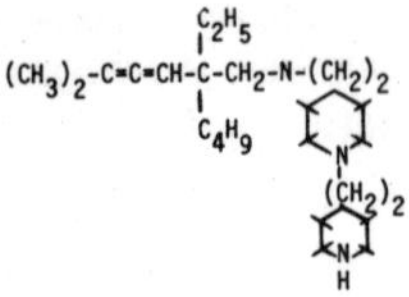

4-[2-(2-BUTYL-2-ETHYL-5-METHYL-3,4-HEXADIENYLAMINO)ETHYL]-1-[2-(4-PIPERIDYL)-ETHYL]PIPERIDINE
(RMI 10,415) MW = 417.7

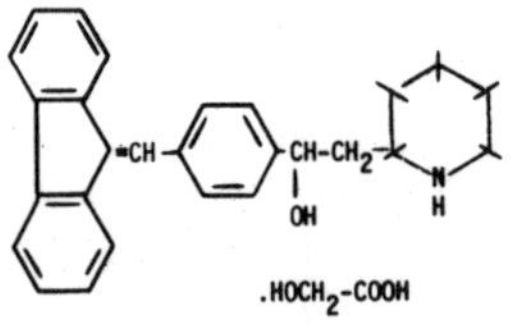

α-[P-(FLUOREN-9-YLIDENEMETHYL)PHENYL)-2-PIPERIDINEENTHANOL
(RMI 10,393) MW glycolate salt = 457.55
(MacKenzie RD et al, 1971, 1972)

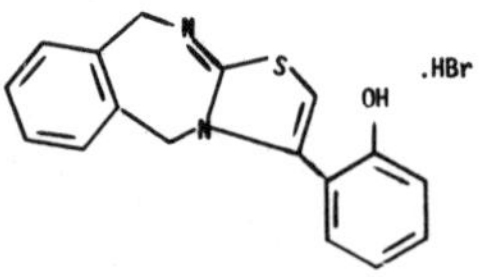

2-(5,10-DIHYDROTHIAZOLO[3,2-b][2,4]-BENZODIAZEPIN-3YL) PHENOL HYDROBROMIDE (Courtesy of E. F. Elslager, Parke-Davis & Co.) MW = 375.3
(Elslager EF, et al, 1971)

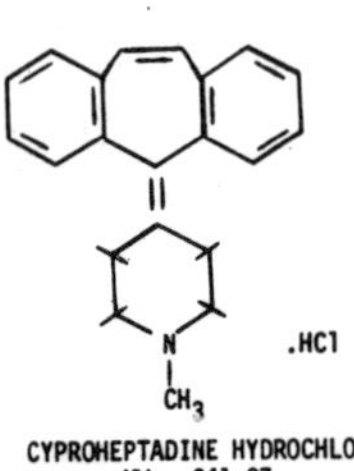

CYPROHEPTADINE HYDROCHLORIDE
MW = 341.87

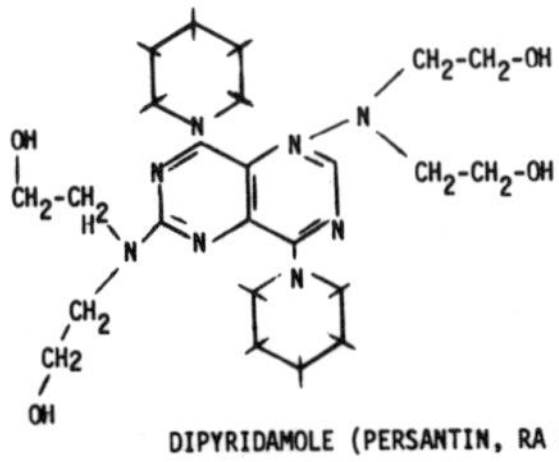

DIPYRIDAMOLE (PERSANTIN, RA 8)
MW = 504.62

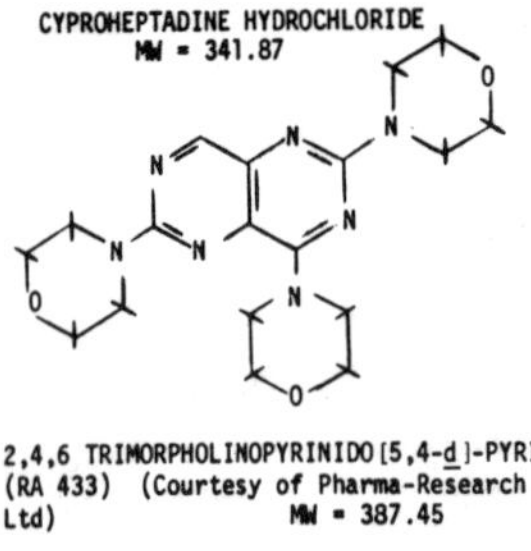

2,4,6 TRIMORPHOLINOPYRINIDO[5,4-d]-PYRIMIDINE
(RA 433) (Courtesy of Pharma-Research Canada Ltd) MW = 387.45

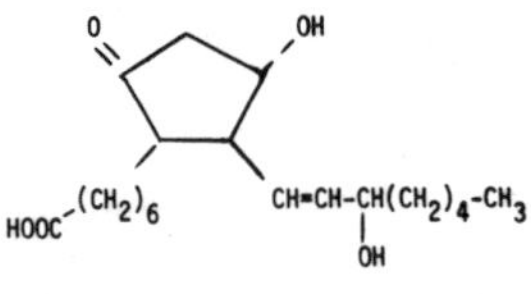

PROSTAGLANDIN E_1 (PGE_1)
MW = 354.49

Figure 6. Structures and names of compounds used in pharmacological studies.

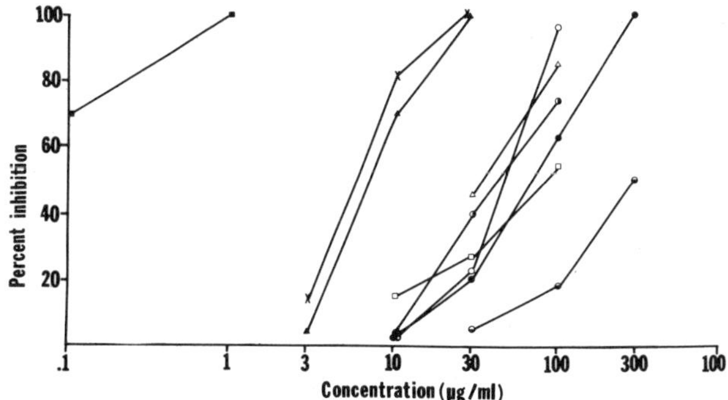

Figure 7. *In vitro* inhibition of ADP-induced platelet aggregation in human citrated platelet-rich plasma by: ○, RMI 10,393; ●, RMI 6792; ◑, RMI 7822; ◒, RA8; □, RA433; ■, PGE_1; △, benzodiazepine derivative; ▲, RMI 10,276; ×, RMI 10,415.

The *in vitro* inhibition of RMI 10,393 of ADP-, thrombin-, collagen-, epinephrine-, and serotonin-induced platelet aggregation is summarized in Fig. 8. RMI 10,393 inhibited platelet aggregation caused by these aggregating agents to approximately the same extent. RMI 7822 and cyproheptadine, however, were found to be highly potent as antagonists of serotonin- but not of ADP-induced platelet aggregation (Fig. 9).

Although these compounds inhibited platelet aggregation, most of them also activated platelet factor 3 (PF-3). This effect is considered undesirable. Results of a comparison between inhibition of platelet aggregation and PF-3 activation of four of these compounds are shown in Fig. 10. RMI 10,415 caused activation of a large amount of PF-3, while RMI 7822 had little effect on PF-3 activation. RMI 6792 and RMI 10,393 were intermediate in re-

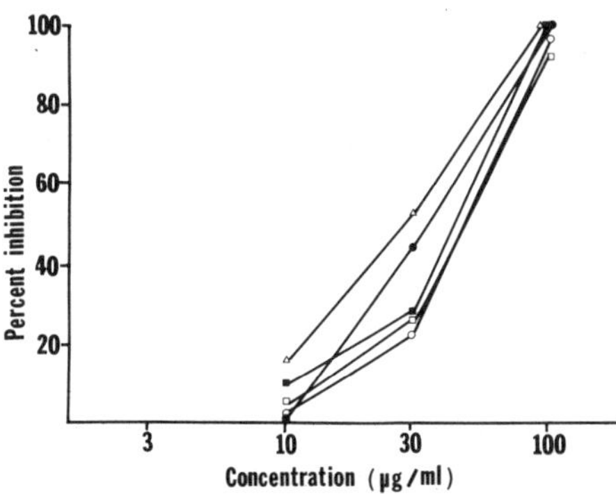

Figure 8. Inhibition by RMI 10,393 of *in vitro* platelet aggregation induced by various aggregating agents. ○, ADP; ●, collagen; □, thrombin; ■, epinephrine; △, serotonin.

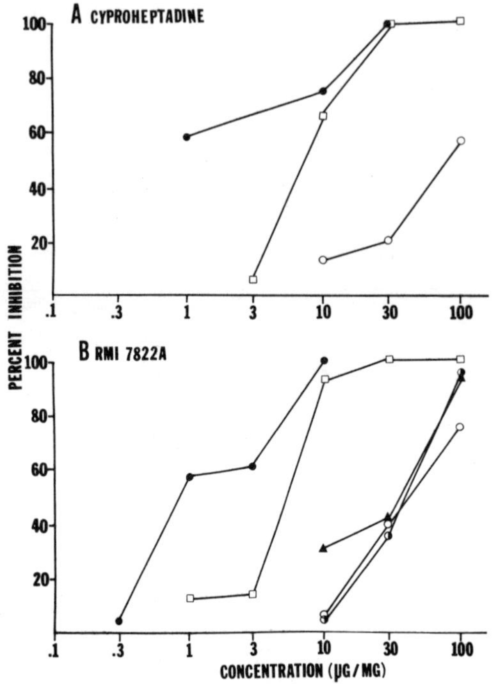

Figure 9. **Comparison of RMI 7822A and cyproheptadine on inhibition of** platelet aggregation in citrated human platelet-rich plasma by various aggregating agents. ○, ADP; □, epinephrine; ●, serotonin; ◑, collagen; ▲, thrombin.

spect to PF-3 activation. A line was drawn at 20 per cent of inhibition of platelet aggregation and at 0.15 per cent PF-3 activation. Only the values above this line were considered as significant.

Clot retraction was inhibited by many of these compounds. The inhibition seemed to correlate well with the activation of PF-3. For example, RMI 10,415 inhibited clot retraction only 5 per cent at 10 μg/ml but 61 per cent at 30 μg/ml, while RMI 7822 did not inhibit clot retraction at concentrations as high as 300 μg/ml.

RMI 6792 or RMI 10,393 were given orally to guinea pigs for 1 or 4 days. They were found to inhibit platelet aggregation as determined by both *in vivo* methods. The dose-response curves for both compounds are shown in Fig. 11. It should be noted that by repeated administration RMI 10,393 was more potent than by single administration and that, in the completely *in vivo* system, RMI 10,393 was active at lower dose levels than in the *in vivo-in vitro* system.

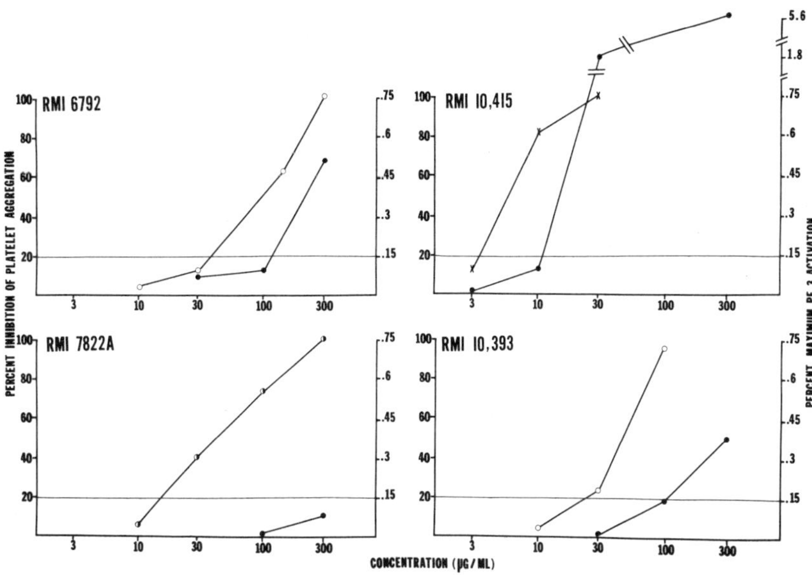

Figure 10. Comparison between inhibition of ADP-induced platelet aggregation and platelet factor 3 activation by RMI 7822, RMI 10,415, RMI 6792, and RMI 10,393 added *in vitro* to citrated human platelet-rich plasma. ●, **platelet factor 3 activation; ○, X, ◑, inhibition of platelet aggregation.**

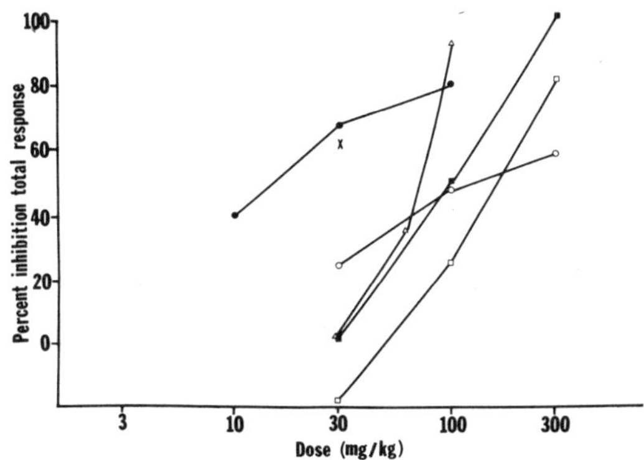

Figure 11. Effect of RMI 10,393 and RMI 6792 on platelet aggregation in the guinea pig. Dose-response curves for a single dose and four daily doses. □, RMI 10,393, single dose, *in vivo-in vitro;* ■, RMI 10,393, multiple dose (4), *in vivo-in vitro;* △, RMI 6792, multiple dose (4), *in vivo-in vitro;* ○, RMI 10,393, single dose, complete *in vivo* system; ●, RMI 10,393 multiple dose, complete *in vivo* system; X, RMI 6792, multiple dose, complete *in vivo* system.

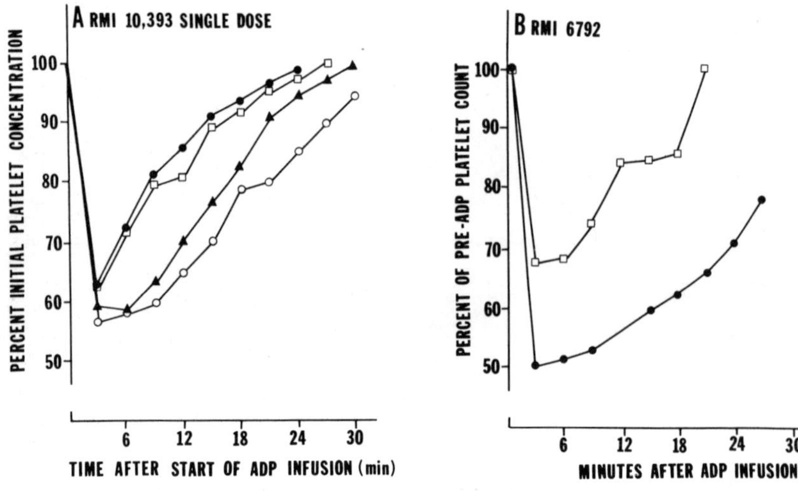

Figure 12. Effect of RMI 10,393 and RMI 6792 on platelet aggregation induced by ADP infusion in the guinea pig. A, RMI 10,393, single dose; ○, control; ▲, 30 mg/kg (average of five determinations); □, 100 mg/kg (average of seven determinations); ●, 300 mg/kg (average of six determinations). B, RMI 6792; ●, control (3); □, test, 30 mg/kg·day, 4 days.

Of interest also was our observation (Fig. 12) that RMI 10,393 had less effect on the maximum reduction in platelet count than on the rate of deaggregation. RMI 6792, however, affected both drop in platelet count and the rate of deaggregation to a similar extent. Such differences may indicate different mechanisms of action for the two compounds.

DISCUSSION

The use of several *in vitro* and *in vivo* methods for evaluation of various compounds that inhibit certain platelet functions, primarily ADP-induced platelet aggregation, was described. Guinea pig platelets were used because of their similarities to human platelets in respect to ADP-induced aggregation. There are, however, also many dissimilarities between human and guinea pig platelets. Adenosine and its derivatives inhibit ADP-induced aggregation of human but not of guinea pig platelets. Serotonin does not aggregate guinea pig platelets.

There are a variety of *in vivo* test systems such as the plastic tube shunt described by Didisheim (1969), the extracorporeal shunt described by Downie *et al.* (1963), the thrombosing test of E. Boyle (unpublished data), platelet aggregation with ADP (MacKenzie, Henderson, and Steinbach, 1971; MacKenzie, Blohm, and Steinbach, 1972), platelet aggregation induced by free fatty acids (Zbinden, 1964), or microcirculation studies with different traumas such as wires, punctures, chemicals such as thrombin and ADP, or laser light. No one test can be considered *the* pertinent one. There is a need for good thrombosis models that more truly reflect the pathophysiological conditions in man. The development of such models is highly improbable. Until better understanding of the conditions that produce thrombosis in man is achieved, a large variety of chemical compounds should be tested in a variety of thrombosis models and other test systems.

Progress in this field has been very rapid over the last decade. New chemicals that inhibit platelet aggregation are the tools that will help us learn more about platelet function and the role of platelets in thrombosis.

ACKNOWLEDGMENTS

I wish to acknowledge the expert technical assistance of Edward M. Auxier, James G. Henderson, Lela M. Lancaster, and John M. Steinbach. I also wish to thank Dr. Thomas R. Blohm for his support and counsel.

REFERENCES

Alexander, B. 1962. Blood coagulation and thrombotic disease. Circulation 25: 872.

Didisheim, P. 1969. Microscopically typical thrombi and hemostatic plugs in Teflon arteriovenous shunts, pp. 64–71. *In* S. A. Johnson and M. M. Guest (eds.) Dynamics of thrombus formation and dissolution. J. B. Lippincott Co., Philadelphia.

Downie, H. G., Murphy, E. A., Rowsell, H. C., and Mustard, J. F. 1963. Extracorporeal circulation: A device for the quantitative study of thrombus formation in flowing blood. Circ. Res. 12: 441.

Elslazer, E. F., McLean, J. F., Perricone, S. C., Perricone, D., Veloso, H., Worth, D. F., and Wheelock, R. H. 1971. Inhibitors of platelet aggregation. I. 5,10-Dihydro-3-(phenyl, thienyl, and furyl)thiazolo[3,2-b][2,4]benzodiazepines and related compounds. J. Med. Chem. 14: 397.

Hampton, J. R. 1967. The study of platelet behavior and its relevance to thrombosis. J. Atheroscler. Res. 7: 729.

Hampton, J. W. 1966. Platelets and coronary thrombosis. J. Okla. State Med. Ass. 59: 529.

Ingram, G. I. C. 1967. Current views on haemostasis. Practitioner 199: 5.

MacKenzie, R. D., and Blohm, T. R. 1971. Effects of N-(2-diethylamino-ethyl)-N-(2-hydroxy-2-phenylethyl)-2,5-dichloraniline (AN 162) on platelet function and blood coagulation. Thromb. Diath. Haemorrh. 26: 577.

MacKenzie, R. D., Blohm, T. R., and Auxier, E. M. 1971. A modified Stypven test for the determination of platelet factor 3. Amer. J. Clin. Pathol. 55: 551.

MacKenzie, R. D., Blohm, T. R., Auxier, E. M., Henderson, J. F., and Steinbach, J. M. 1971. Effects of a-(p-(fluoren-9-ylidenemethyl)phenyl)-2-piperidinethanol (RMI 10,393) on platelet function. Proc. Soc. Exp. Biol. Med. 137: 662.

MacKenzie, R. D., Blohm, T. R., and Steinbach, J. M. 1972. Effects *in vivo* of a(p-(fluoren-9-ylidenemethyl)phenyl)-2-piperidinethanol (RMI 10,393) on platelet aggregation and blood coagulation. Biochem. Pharmacol. 21: 707.

MacKenzie, R. D., Henderson, J. F., and Steinbach, J. M. 1971. The evaluation of a method for adenosine diphosphate induced platelet aggregation in the guinea pig. Thromb. Diath. Haemorrh. 25: 30.

Mershey, C., and Drapkin, A. 1965. Anticoagulant therapy. Blood 25: 567.

Michal, F. 1969. D-Receptor for serotonin on blood platelets. Nature 221: 1253.

Mustard, J. F., and Packham, M. A. 1970. Thromboembolism a manifestation of the response of blood to injury. Circulation 42: 1.

O'Brien, J. R. 1964. The mechanism and prevention of platelet adhesion and aggregation considered in relation to arterial thrombosis. Blood 24: 309.

Salzman, E. W. 1965. The limitations of heparin therapy after arterial reconstruction. Surgery 57: 131.

Seaman, A. J., Griswald, H. E., Reaume, R. B., and Ritzman, L. W. 1964. Prophylactic anticoagulant therapy for coronary artery disease. J. Amer. Med. Ass. 189: 183.

Zbinden, G. 1964. Transient thrombopenia after intravenous injection of certain fatty acids. J. Lipid Res. 5: 378.

Use of the Biolaser in the Evaluation of Antithrombotic Agents

J. S. Fleming, J. O. Buchanan, S. P. King, B. T. Cornish, and M. E. Bierwagen

The rabbit ear chamber-biolaser system provides us with an *in vivo* model of intravascular thrombosis that is proving useful in the evaluation of new antithrombotic agents. Several advantages of this model over those employing other means of inducing thrombosis are apparent. Preparatory surgery is completed long before animals are used experimentally, thus minimizing the stress factor. Conscious animals are employed, thus avoiding the complications of anesthesia. The injury stimulus is highly localized, thus minimizing the involvement of more general physiological responses, and direct observation of the formation and fate of the thrombus adds considerably to the evaluation of the process. The biolaser model has played a major role in our evaluation of the antithrombotic activity of two new synthetic anti-inflammatory agents. It also was employed in extending the *in vivo* implications of our observation of a supra-additive interaction between acetylsalicylic acid and prostaglandin E_1. In view of the fact that absolute correlation is not always observed between various test systems, it is particularly beneficial to have available an *in vivo* model of thrombosis such as the biolaser. However, critical evaluation regarding the relevance of this as well as other test systems to the clinical situation must await feedback from the evaluation of antithrombotic agents in humans.

The search for effective pharmacological agents useful in clinical thrombosis has greatly intensified in recent years. A deeper understanding of the factors involved in arterial thrombosis and the realization that anticoagulant therapy is of limited value have led to investigations of other types of compounds which may have antithrombotic activity, particularly those acting through inhibition of platelet aggregation.

As our knowledge in this area has expanded, new methodology designed for studying platelet function and the role of platelets in thrombosis has appeared in the literature. A major problem that we now face in this regard is that of establishing the relevance of various laboratory models to human pathology and determining which of these test systems are most useful in predicting the potential utility of new antithrombotic agents. The task is especially difficult in view of the limited clinical feedback that we have regarding the efficacy of currently available drugs. Dipyridamole, sulfinpyrazone, and acetylsalicylic acid are the only three compounds which have received any appreciable degree of clinical testing and at this point the results are still inconclusive.

Currently used laboratory methodology ranges from strictly *in vitro* systems, such as platelet adhesiveness to glass surfaces and aggregometry, to rather complex *in vivo* models, such as endotoxin shock, where platelet aggregation is thought to play a role but where the exact mechanisms are not well established.

In view of the fact that thrombosis is a basic clinical problem with which we are concerned, it would seem reasonable that an *in vivo* laboratory model of thrombosis should play an important role in the evaluation of new drugs in this area. The biolaser method of inducing intravascular thrombosis has been used in our laboratory for the past several years. Two studies will be described in which results obtained in this model are compared with those obtained in other systems.

EVALUATION OF THE ANTITHROMBOTIC POTENTIAL OF TWO NEW ANTI-INFLAMMATORY AGENTS

Two new (Bristol Laboratories) synthetic, nonsteroidal anti-inflammatory agents, 1-(4-chlorobenzoyl)-3-(5-tetrazolylmethyl)-indole (BL-R 743) and (−)-5-cyclohexylindan-1-carboxylic acid

(BL-2365), were compared with acetylsalicylic acid (ASA) and phenylbutazone (PBZ) in a variety of laboratory models where platelet aggregation is thought to be involved, including the biolaser (Fleming *et al.*, 1970, 1972).

The optical density method of Born (1962) as modified by Mustard *et al.* (1964) was used to assess the activities of the various compounds in inhibiting collagen-induced platelet aggregation. In strictly *in vitro* studies, employing citrated rabbit platelet-rich plasma (PRP), ASA was the most potent of the four compounds, followed closely by BL-2365 and then by PBZ and BL-R 743. The EC_{50} values calculated on the basis of multiple dose response determinations are summarized in the top row of Table 1. None of these compounds produced a significant inhibition of ADP-induced aggregation up to concentrations of 512 μg/ml. This would imply that all four agents probably exert their effect via inhibition of the platelet release reaction.

When aggregometry studies are extended to the *in vivo-in vitro* situation, the relative efficacy of compounds is not necessarily maintained. This most likely is due to differences in drug absorption, distribution, or metabolism. ASA was still the most potent of the four compounds when the drugs were administered to rabbits via the intraperitoneal route. However, PBZ, which was more potent than BL-R 743 *in vitro*, was less potent in the *in vivo-in vitro* situation. The ED_{50} values for the four compounds tested are summarized in the bottom row of Table 1.

It has been suggested that platelet aggregation plays a role in the shock syndrome (McKay and Margaretten, 1967). It has also been shown that bacterial endotoxins are capable of inducing platelet aggregation and that during endotoxin shock the screen filtration pressure of the blood is elevated, indicating the presence of circulating platelet aggregates (Evans *et al.*, 1969; Fleming *et al.*, 1970).

Table 1. Effect of four synthetic nonsteroidal anti-inflammatory agents on collagen-induced platelet aggregation in rabbit platelet-rich plasma

	ASA	PBZ	BL-2365	BL-R 743
In vitro				
EC_{50} μg/ml	7	50	10	105
In vivo-in vitro				
ED_{50} mg/kg ip	3	45	18	40

While the exact role that platelets play in the shock syndrome is not fully understood, we have found that the nonsteroidal anti-inflammatory agents inhibit the rise in the screen filtration pressure of whole blood and the simultaneous fall in arterial blood pressure associated with the intravenous administration of bacterial endotoxin to dogs (Fleming *et al.*, 1970, 1972). A summary of these studies is presented in Fig. 1. It can be seen that mean arterial blood pressure fell from a pre-endotoxin level of 126 mm Hg to a mean level of 62 mm Hg in saline control experiments following 3 mg/kg of *Salmonella typhosa* endotoxin intravenously. At the same time, screen filtration pressure increased from a mean of 32 mm Hg in the pre-endotoxin period to a mean of 87 mm Hg following endotoxin. All four anti-inflammatory agents, when infused at a rate of 2 mg/kg·min throughout the 35-min experiment, modified these effects of endotoxin, with BL-2365 and PBZ being slightly more effective than ASA or BL-R 743.

In another series of experiments, the four anti-inflammatory agents were evaluated for their ability to prevent lethality due to intravenous endotoxin administration in rats. In this case the compounds were administered orally prior to the endotoxin challenge. BL-2365 and BL-R 743 were the only two compounds found to modify significantly endotoxin lethality in this model.

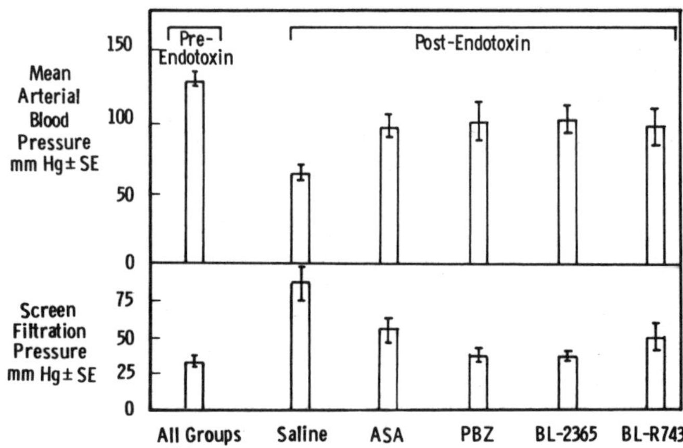

Figure 1. Effect of four anti-inflammatory agents, infused intravenously at the rate of 2 mg/kg·min, on endotoxin-induced fall in arterial blood pressure and rise in whole blood screen filtration pressure in the anesthetized dog. N = 5/group.

The dose response curves are depicted in Fig. 2. The fact that ASA and PBZ in the same study did not enhance survival may indicate a lack of sufficient activity in this very complex and rather severe *in vivo* model or may be a result of species variation in terms of drug absorption and metabolism.

The biolaser equipment and methodology used in our *in vivo* thrombosis model has been described in detail (Kochen and Baez, 1965; Grant and Becker, 1965; Arfors *et al.*, 1968; Fleming *et al.*, 1970). Our particular setup pictured in Fig. 3 consists of a TRG model 513 biolaser unit coupled to a Leitz Ortholux microscope. A Sony CVC 2100A video camera is mounted above the laser head and is connected directly to a Sony monitor, providing continuous observation of the microvasculature at the time of laser firing.

Adult, English half-lop rabbits were used in these experiments. Transparent ear chambers of the type described by Sanders *et al.* (1954) and modified in that they did not have the removable pin were chronically implanted. Approximately 3 weeks following surgery, a film of vascularized tissue had grown into the 40-μ-thick transparent central region of the chamber, permitting visualization of the microcirculation. The rabbits were conditioned to lie quietly in the supine position during the experiment, making anesthesia unnecessary.

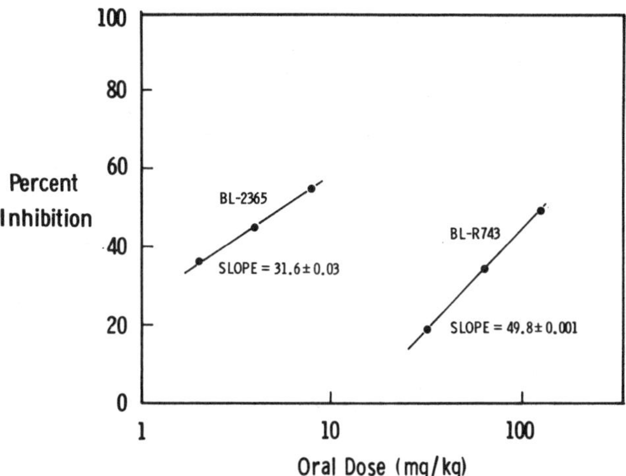

Figure 2. Effect of BL-2365 and BL-R 743 on the lethality of intravenously injected bacterial endotoxin in rats. $N = 20$/dose level.

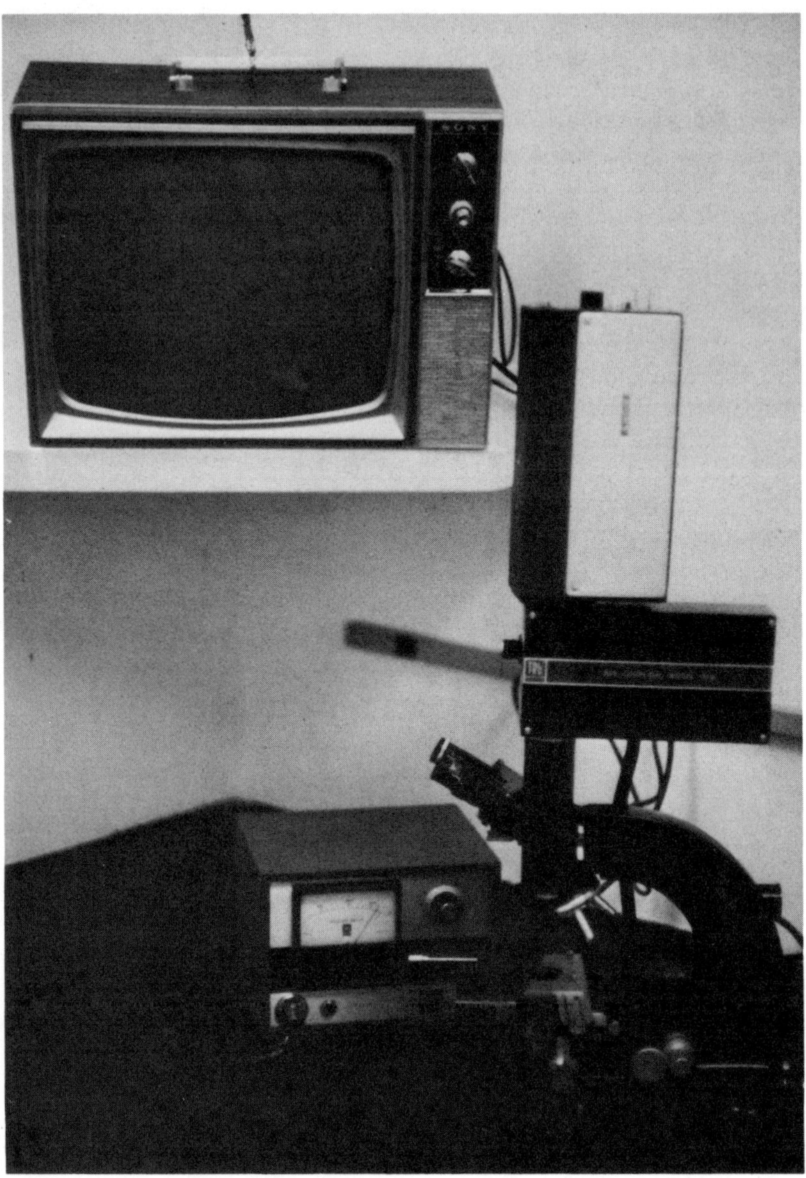

Figure 3. Biolaser system: TRG model 513 biolaser unit coupled to a Leitz Ortholux microscope. Above the laser head is a Sony CVC 2100A video camera. The video monitor and the biolaser power supply unit are also pictured.

A single pulse ruby laser beam focused through the microscope on the interior of a vessel (10–30 μ diameter) is capable of producing a microburn which results in the formation of a small thrombus. In most cases, a damaged red cell forms the central core, which is 7–8 μ in diameter. Platelet material accumulates around this core as the thrombus builds. An example of such a thrombus is seen in Fig. 4. This sequence of events occurs very quickly and is then followed by varying degrees of embolization and rebuilding of the thrombus. Although these thrombi are not entirely stable, one can approximate the thrombus area by determining the length and width with a micrometer eyepiece. Thrombus areas determined at threshold energy levels are fairly consistent from one rabbit to the next. The values average 200 μ^2, of which

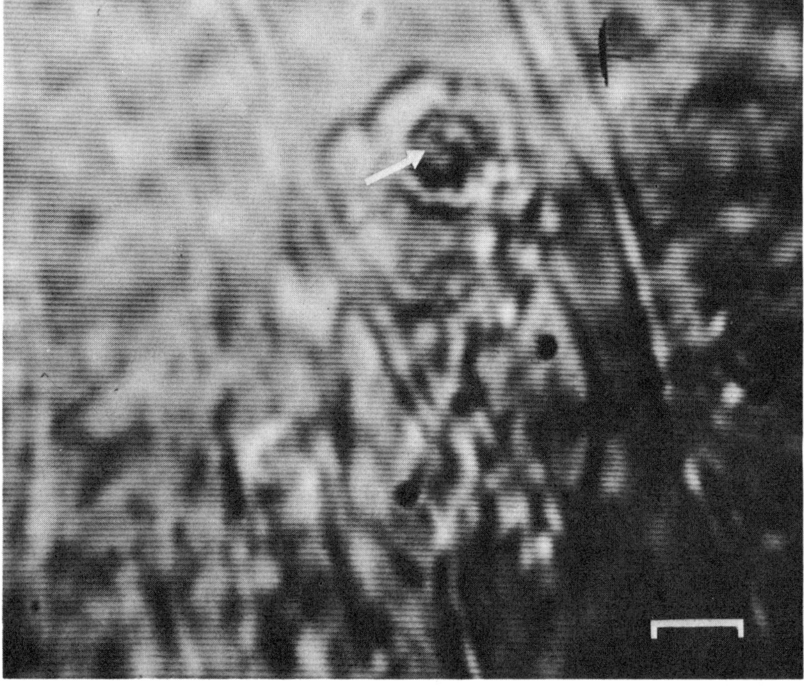

Figure 4. A laser-induced intravascular thrombus formed in a 25-μ vessel located within the rabbit ear chamber. Note the red cell central core indicated by the arrow and the surrounding platelet material. The scale in the lower right-hand corner measures 10 μ in length.

approximately 50 μ^2 represents the central core and 150 μ^2 represents accumulated platelet material.

The nonsteroidal anti-inflammatory agents were tested in this model for their ability to inhibit platelet buildup around the central core. These results are depicted in Fig. 5. Mean thrombus area minus the area of the central core is plotted for untreated and saline-treated animals as well as for those which received ASA, BL-R 743, PBZ, and BL-2365 at three dosage levels each. All compounds were administered as intravenous infusions throughout the course of each 25-min experiment, during which time 10 thrombi were formed and measured. Thrombi areas averaged 142 μ^2 for the untreated group and 166 μ^2 for the saline controls. At a dose of 2 mg/kg·min, the mean thrombi areas obtained were 133 μ^2 with ASA, 76 μ^2 with BL-R 743, 66 μ^2 with PBZ, and 21 μ^2 with BL-2365. The other dose levels employed support a conclusion that BL-2365 was the most effective of the four agents tested in this model.

These results demonstrate the problem that we face in a comparative evaluation of antithrombotic agents, even in the case where they are all of the same pharmacològical category and supposedly acting via a similar mechanism. ASA was found to be the most active agent on the basis of aggregometry results, while in *in vivo* models designed to resemble clinical situations, it was the

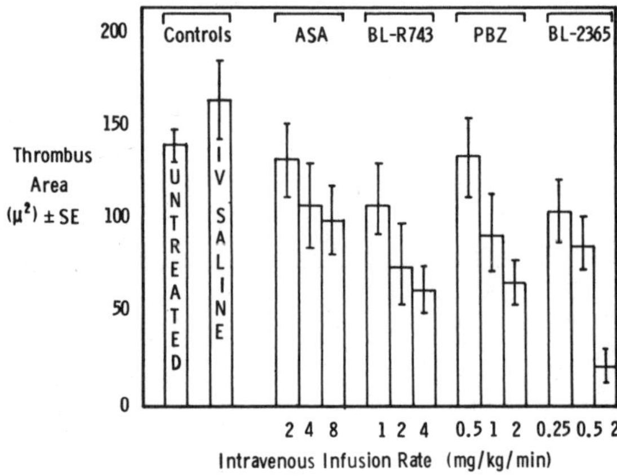

Figure 5. Effect of four anti-inflammatory agents on biolaser-induced thrombus formation in the ear chamber microvasculature of unanesthetized rabbits. $N = 30$ trials in three rabbits/dose.

least active of the four compounds tested. There are a number of possible explanations for this, including species differences, different routes of drug administration, and, perhaps most important, great variability in the complexity of the test systems investigated. Many factors other than platelet aggregation are likely involved in a model as complex as endotoxin shock, and the acute effects of endotoxemia as studied in the dog may be quite different than the delayed effects which influence lethality in the rat.

Our experience with a variety of other *in vivo-in vitro* and *in vivo* models such as extracorporeal shunts, bleeding time from the mouse tail, phenol-induced venous thrombosis, hemorrhagic shock, and ADP-induced thrombocytopenia also support this observation of a lack of consistency in drug activity between various laboratory test systems. However, it should be pointed out that this may reflect the rather weak level of activity associated with the majority of compounds thus far investigated. We have found that consistency between different experimental models improves considerably as the potency of the compounds studied increases, especially when one investigates agents which are potent inhibitors of both collagen- and ADP-induced platelet aggregation.

In any case, the use of a model which more closely approximates a clinical situation in which we are primarily interested, such as the biolaser, should be of major importance in the comparative evaluation of antithrombotic agents. The use of the biolaser to produce intravascular injury and to induce thrombosis appears to have certain advantages over some of the other methods used, such as those employing mechanically, chemically, or electrically induced vascular injury (Berman and Fulton, 1961; Honour *et al.*, 1971; Danese *et al.*, 1971). This model provides the opportunity to observe directly the formation and fate of intravascular thrombi in unanesthetized animals. Surgical preparation for laser studies is completed long before the animals are used. Three to four weeks are required for vascularization after the chambers are implanted. Consequently, the animals are fully recovered at the time of the experiment. The fact that the study can be conducted without the use of anesthesia is of major importance in view of recent reports concerning the effect of both gaseous and barbiturate anesthetics on platelet function (Ueda, 1971; McKenzie *et al.*, 1972). Direct visualization of the thrombotic process is of great advantage, lending the dimension of dynamics to the evaluation of the process itself and to the evaluation of inhibiting agents. The thrombus-producing injury can be pinpointed within a vessel without observable disruption of surrounding tissues; thus, other more general physiological responses are less likely to come into play. The magnitude of the injury stimulus, while not precisely known, can be controlled within relatively narrow limits. A variety of methods is possible for evaluating the thrombotic response to laser injury. While most of these methods are semiquantitative, such as our technique of a two-dimensional area measurement, reproducibility appears to be quite satisfactory and detection of drug activity reasonably sensitive.

EFFECT OF THE COMBINATION OF ACETYLSALICYLIC ACID AND PROSTAGLANDIN E_1 (PGE_1) ON PLATELET AGGREGATION AND THROMBOSIS

PGE_1 has been shown by a number of workers to be a highly effective inhibitor of platelet aggregation *in vitro* (Kloeze, 1966; McKinnon *et al.*, 1969; Hissen *et al.*, 1969). However, owing to its very short biological half-life, *in vivo* activity can be demonstrated only with rather large doses or under rather restricted laboratory conditions (McKinnon *et al.*, 1969; Hissen *et al.*, 1969; Emmons *et al.*, 1967). The possibility that PGE_1 might be clinically useful per se as an antithrombotic agent is, therefore, quite remote.

ASA, as previously described, has been extensively studied for its ability to inhibit the platelet release reaction. However, in view of the fact that ASA does not block primary ADP-induced aggregation and is not particularly effective in *in vivo* laboratory models, its clinical utility as an antithrombotic agent may also be rather limited.

As one approach to the problem of finding a clinically useful means of pharmacologically controlling platelet aggregation, we have studied a number of drugs in combination. Individually, these drugs had shown at least some degree of *in vitro* activity. The interaction of PGE_1 and ASA proved to be most interesting, owing to the supra-additive nature of the effect with the two compounds in combination.

The isobolographic method of Loewe (1959) was used to analyze drug interaction in aggregometry studies. By this method the various concentrations of the two drugs can be predicted which will produce an EC_{50} effect if they are interacting through simple addition of their respective actions. If concentrations actually required are smaller than concentrations predicted by this

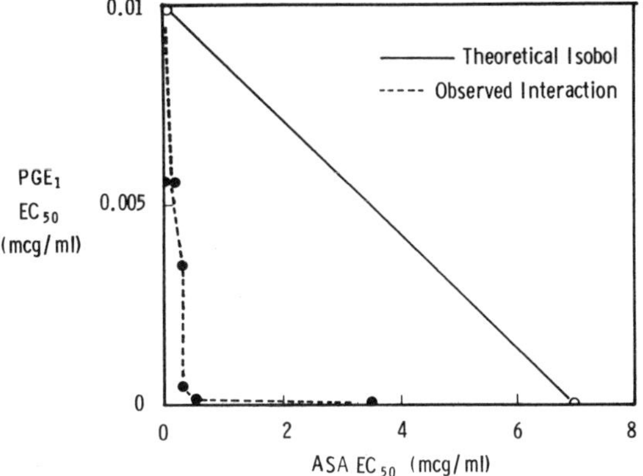

Figure 6. Isobolographic analysis of the interaction of acetylsalicylic acid and PGE_1 *versus* collagen-induced platelet aggregation in rabbit platelet-rich plasma. $N = 5$ determinations/point.

method of analysis, then the combination is said to be supra-additive.

Various combinations of ASA and PGE_1 were studied *in vitro* in the aggregometer by holding one member at a constant concentration and varying the second in a dose response fashion. Each combination studied was evaluated in this manner five times. Dose response curves were then generated, using a least squares regression analysis computer program and a G. E. Mark II time-sharing system.

Figs. 6 and 7 depict the interaction seen in rabbit PRP for PGE_1 and ASA *versus* collagen- and ADP-induced aggregation, respec-

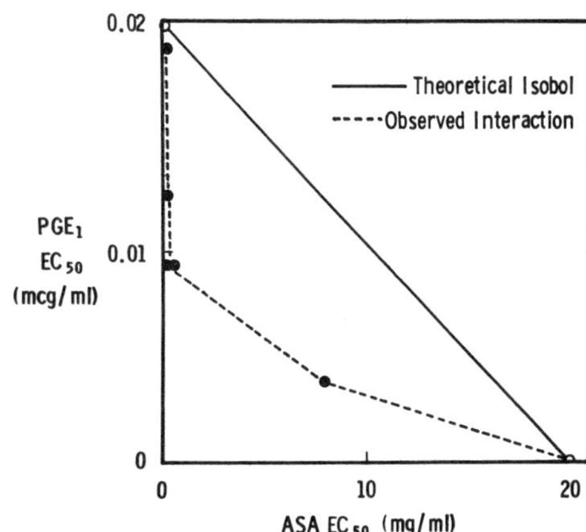

Figure 7. Isobolographic analysis of the interaction of acetylsalicylic acid and PGE_1 *versus* ADP-induced platelet aggregation in rabbit platelet-rich plasma. $N = 5$ determinations/point.

tively. The solid isobol line connects the EC_{50} values for each drug individually and predicts all possible combinations of the two drugs which should produce the EC_{50} effect, assuming simple addition of action. Experimental points falling to the left of the isobol line would imply supra-additive effects (potentiation), while points falling to the right of the line would imply infra-additive effects (antagonism). As can be seen, all eleven combinations of ASA and PGE_1 producing an EC_{50} effect fell well to the left of the isobol lines. Thus, PGE_1 and ASA exhibited marked supra-additive interaction against both collagen- and ADP-induced platelet aggregation *in vitro*.

Two different combinations of PGE_1 and ASA were also studied *in vivo-in vitro*. In this case PRP was obtained before and 2 or 4 hr after the rabbits were dosed with the compounds individually or in combination. ASA was administered intraperitoneally, dissolved in polyethylene glycol-400, while PGE_1 was given subcutaneously in sesame oil. The levels of platelet aggregation induced by ADP and collagen in the post-drug PRP samples were compared with the pre-drug levels. Figure 8 compares the activities of two combinations, ASA (1 mg/kg ip) + PGE_1 (10 μg/kg sc) and ASA (1 mg/kg ip) + PGE_1 (100 μg/kg sc) to the activities of the two compounds used individually. There was definite enhance-

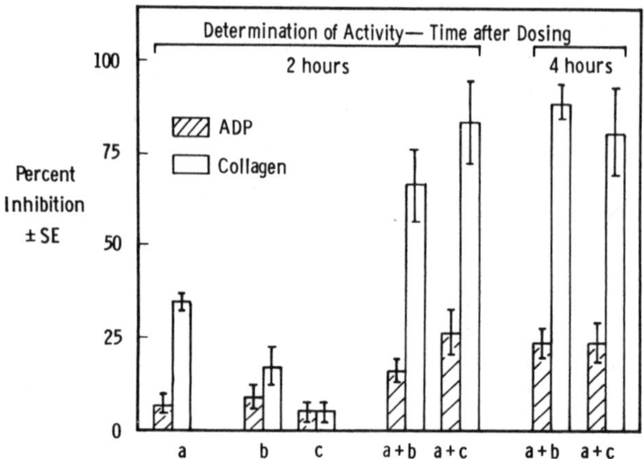

Figure 8. Effect of acetylsalicylic acid and PGE_1 alone and in combination on ADP- and collagen-induced platelet aggregation in rabbit platelet-rich plasma following *in vivo* dosing. a, ASA, 1 mg/kg ip; b, PGE_1, 0.01 mg/kg sc; c, PGE_1, 0.10 mg/kg sc. $N = 5$/group.

ment of activity in both cases, with collagen aggregation being most dramatically affected. Enhanced activity observed 2 hours after dosing was maintained at least through 4 hours.

Biolaser-induced thrombosis was used to evaluate the combination in a strictly *in vivo* system. The effects of ASA and PGE_1 alone and in combination were evaluated on thrombus buildup as previously described. Figure 9 summarizes the results of these experiments. ASA alone at an infusion rate of 4 mg/kg·min iv had only a slight inhibitory effect on thrombus buildup. PGE_1 at a dose of 0.1 mg/kg sc was inactive. However, the combination of PGE_1 at a dose of 0.1 mg/kg sc, followed 2 hr later by ASA infusion at a rate of 4 mg/kg·min iv, produced a marked reduction in thrombus area.

These results suggest the possibility that ASA administered in combination with PGE_1 may be useful in antithrombotic therapy. The fact that the supra-additive effects exhibited by the combination *in vitro* appear to extend to *in vivo* dosing and especially to biolaser-induced intravascular thrombosis is particularly encouraging. Since the biological half-life of PGE_1 is extremely short, it is very difficult to demonstrate significant activity for this substance in *in vivo* systems. It is particularly interesting to note that enhanced *in vivo* activity with the combination appears to persist for at least 4 hr. This indicates that the effect produced on

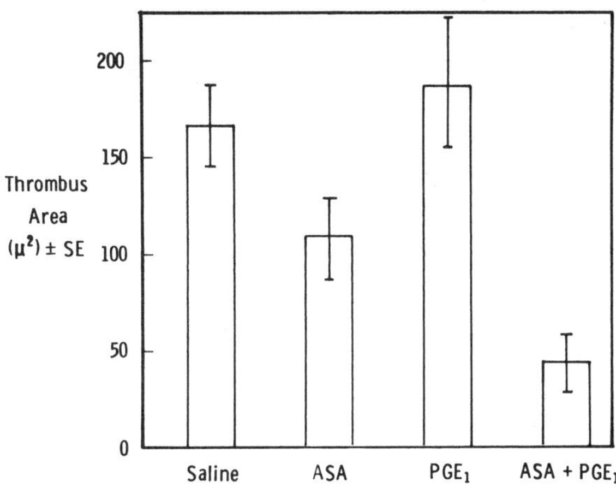

Figure 9. Effect of acetylsalicylic acid and prostaglandin E_1 alone and in combination on biolaser-induced thrombosis in the ear chamber microvasculature of unanesthetized rabbits. $N = 30$ trials in three rabbits/group.

platelets by the combination considerably outlasts the presence of both ASA and PGE_1 in the blood.

Consideration of the possible mechanism of this supra-additive interaction is highly speculative at this point. However, the recent studies of Vane (1971) and Smith and Willis (1971), implicating inhibition of prostaglandin synthesis as a mechanism in the action of ASA, suggest several hypotheses. It is possible that two or more prostaglandins act as a balanced control mechanism of platelet aggregability, one tending to make platelets more responsive and one tending to make platelets less responsive. If ASA has the capacity to inactivate this control system in addition to its other effects on the platelet membrane, the addition of exogenous PGE_1, a prostaglandin tending to make platelets less responsive, would result in an unbalanced system and further reduce platelet aggregability. Such an explanation may be consistent with recent findings regarding the effects of PGE_1 and PGE_2 on platelet adenyl cyclase levels (Salzman, 1972). Another possibility is that ASA may suppress prostaglandin metabolism as well an inhibit prostaglandin synthesis. Such a mechanism would also be consistent with our observation of a prolonged effect, well beyond the expected half-life of PGE_1.

REFERENCES

Arfors, K. E., Dhall, D. P., Engeset, J., Hint, H., Matheson, N. A., and Tangen, O. 1968. Biolaser endothelial trauma as a means of quantifying platelet activity *in vivo.* Nature 218: 887.

Berman, H. J., and Fulton, G. P. 1961. Platelets in the peripheral circulation, pp. 7–20. *In* S. A. Johnson, R. W. Monto, J. W. Rebuck, and R. C. Horn (eds.) Blood platelets. Little, Brown & Co., Boston.

Born, G. V. R. 1962. Quantitative investigations into the aggregation of blood platelets. J. Physiol. (London) 162: 67.

Danese, C. A., Voleti, C. D., and Weiss, H. J. 1971. Protection by aspirin against experimentally induced arterial thrombosis in dogs. Thromb. Diath. Haemorrh. 25: 288.

Emmons, P. R., Hampton, J. R., Harrison, M. J. G., Honour, A. J., and Mitchell, J. R. A. 1967. Effect of prostaglandin E_1 on platelet behavior *in vitro* and *in vivo.* Brit. Med. J. 2:468.

Evans, G., Lewis, A. F., and Mustard, J. F. 1969. The role of platelet aggregation in the development of endotoxin shock. Brit. J. Surg. 56: 624 (abstr.).

Fleming, J. S., Bierwagen, M. E., Losada, M., Campbell, J. A. L., King, S. P., and Pindell, M. H. 1970. The effects of three anti-inflammatory agents on platelet aggregation, *in vitro* and *in vivo.* Arch. Int. Pharmacodyn. Ther. 186: 120.

Fleming, J. S., Bierwagen, M. E., Campbell, J. A. L., and King, S. P. 1972. The effect of a new anti-inflammatory agent (5-cyclohexylindan-1-carboxylic acid (BL-2365)) on platelet aggregation. Arch. Int. Pharmacodyn. Ther. 199: 164.

Grant, L., and Becker, F. F. 1965. Mechanisms of inflammation. 1. Laser-induced thrombosis, a morphologic analysis. Proc. Soc. Exp. Biol. Med. 119: 1123.

Hissen, W., Fleming, J. S., Bierwagen, M. E., and Pindell, M. H. 1969. Effect of prostaglandin E_1 on platelet aggregation *in vitro* and in hemorrhagic shock. Microvasc. Res. 1: 374.

Honour, A. J., Pickering, G. W., and Sheppard, B. L. 1971. Ultrastructure and behavior of platelet thrombi in injured arteries. Brit. J. Exp. Pathol. 52: 482.

Kloeze, J. 1966. Influence of prostaglandins on platelet adhesiveness and platelet aggregation, pp. 241–252. *In* S. Bergstrom and B. Samuelsson (eds.) Nobel Symposium 2, Prostaglandins. Almqvist & Wiksell, Stockholm.

Kochen, J. A., and Baez, S. 1965. Vascular and intravascular effects of a pulsed laser micro-beam. Bibl. Anat. 7: 46.

Loewe, S. 1959. Randbemerkungen zur quantitativen Pharmakologie der Kombinationen. Arzneimittel-Forschung 9: 449.

McKay, D. G., and Margaretten, W. 1967. An electron microscope study of endotoxin shock in rhesus monkeys. Surg. Gynecol. Obstet. Int. Abstr. Surg. 125: 825.

McKenzie, F. N., Svensjo, E., and Arfors, K. E. 1972. Effect of sodium pentobarbital anesthesia on platelet behavior *in vitro* and *in vivo.* Microvasc. Res. 4: 42.

McKinnon, E. L., Tangen, O., and Berman, H. J. 1969. Effects of prostaglandin E_1 on platelet aggregation: an electron microscopic study. Anat. Rec. 163: 315 (abstr.).

Mustard, J. F., Hegardt, B., Rowsell, H. C., and MacMillan, R. L. 1964. Effect of adenosine nucleotides on platelet aggregation and clotting time. J. Lab. Clin. Med. 64: 548.

Salzman, E. W. 1972. Cyclic AMP and platelet function. New Engl. J. Med. 286: 358.

Sanders, A. G., Dodson, L. F., and Florey, H. W. 1954. An improved method for the production of tubercles in a chamber in the rabbit's ear. Brit. J. Exp. Pathol. 35: 331.

Smith, J. B., and Willis, A. L. 1971. Aspirin selectively inhibits prostaglandin production in human platelets. Nature New Biol. 231: 235.

Ueda, I. 1971. The effect of volatile general anesthetics on adenosine diphosphate-induced platelet aggregation. Anesthesiology 34: 405.

Vane, J. R. 1971. Inhibition of prostaglandin synthesis as a mechanism of action for aspirin-like drugs. Nature New Biol. 231: 232.

Use of Inhibitors of Platelet Function in Renal Rejection Phenomena

L. M. Aledort, R. Taub, L. Burrows, E. Leiter, S. Glabman, M. Haimov, G. Nirmul, and S. Berger

Cyproheptadine is known to have antiserotonin and antihistamine properties and to inhibit platelet aggregation. Its effects on rejection of renal transplants were studied in rat and man. Cyproheptadine was found to increase the survival time of rats with renal transplants. In addition, it appeared to reduce the incidence of rejection crises and to alter occlusive patterns of renal rejection phenomena. Cyproheptadine may represent a useful adjunct in transplantation therapy.

As early as 1964 (Porter *et al.*) it was recognized that platelets played a role in canine renal allograft rejection. In addition, renal capillary endothelial damage occurred during rejection (Dempster, 1953). It is now well recognized that renal allograft rejection is associated with a reduction in platelet count and survival, accumulation of platelets in the kidney (Mowbray, 1966), a significant decrease in the platelet count from renal artery to renal vein, and deposition of fibrin in the renal vessels (Porter *et al.*, 1967) leading to microthrombotic occlusions. Renal ischemia creates the typical findings of rejection with decreased renal blood flow and azotemia.

In studying human renal transplant rejections Porter *et al.* (1967) classified them into two groups, reversible and irreversible. The reversible group showed platelet plugging of the renal capillaries. The platelets remained intact without loss of granules but with pseudopod formation. By increasing immunosuppressive therapy (steroids and azathioprine) renal function could be restored. The irreversible group was unamenable to medical management and required removal of the kidney. Here the capillaries revealed platelets which had undergone degranulation and release and had formed a hemostatic plug with fibrin formation.

At present, renal transplantation takes are considerably less than 50 per cent over a 5-year period. The present regimen of steroids and azathioprine is fraught with complications such as steroid-induced peptic ulcer disease, tuberculosis, and the threat of neoplasia in the recipient (Scribner, 1971). Newer approaches to transplantation must therefore be sought.

Platelet-deaggregating agents aspirin, dipyridamole, and dextran (Kincaid-Smith, 1969; MacDonald *et al.*, 1970; Messmer *et al.*, 1971) have been studied as potential adjuncts for transplantation. Cyproheptadine, a potent antiserotonin and antihistamine capable of inhibiting platelet function (Aledort *et al.*, 1973) (Goldman *et al.*, 1971; Berger *et al.*, 1972), has been shown to inhibit successfully platelet sequestration in canine renal allografts and canine-feline heterografts (Burrows *et al.*, 1970; Claes, 1972). The studies to be presented deal with our experience using cyproheptadine in both human and rat renal transplantation.

MATERIALS AND METHODS

Animal Studies

Nephrectomized rats of Lewis strain received renal allografts from LBNF hybrid rats. The only therapy the recipient rats received was cyproheptadine daily (1.5–2 mg/kg intramuscularly). All animals were followed until death.

Human Studies

Twelve prerenal transplant patients, on chronic dialysis, and eight postrenal transplantation patients were studied. The latter were taking steroids, azathioprine and cyproheptadine (32 mg/day by mouth). These patients were studied by measuring their platelet count, IVY bleeding time, clot retraction, clotting time, fibrinogen, platelet factor 3, platelet aggregation, and ^{14}C-serotonin (5-HT) uptake and release. Aggregation and release studies were carried out using adenosine diphosphate (ADP) at a final concentration 2×10^{-6} *M*, epinephrine, 50 μM, and a human connective tissue preparation. All studies were carried out with stirred, citrated, platelet-rich plasma (PRP) with platelet count of 300,000/μl and Chronolog aggregometer at 37°C (Goldman and Aledort, 1972).

Thirteen patients who received renal allografts from either cadaver or living related donors were followed for signs of rejection. All patients were receiving a regimen of: 150 R local irradiation to the graft on postoperative days 1, 3, 5, 7; prednisone, azathioprine, and 32 mg of cyproheptadine orally in four divided doses from the day of transplantation. Rejection was diagnosed when any of the following occurred: increase in BUN and serum creatinine; decrease in urine volume, creatinine clearance, or urine osmolality, or all three; clinical signs such as fever or pain at graft site.

RESULTS

Animal Studies: Rat Transplants

In 12 untreated Lewis recipients the mean survival time was 13.5 ± 2.1 days. The eight treated animals had a mean survival time of 84 ± 9.2 days. The difference in the survival time between the two groups of animals was highly significant statistically ($p = 0.01$). Two treated animals survived more than 100 days. Their survival time was tabulated as 100 days. In the untreated group the BUN rose steadily until death. In contrast the treated group showed a slight rise in BUN at 3 days and a further rise at 14 days with stabilization at 60–80 mg/100 ml. Prior to demise the BUN rose again.

Human Studies: Renal Transplants

The platelet count, clotting time, prothrombin time, partial thromboplastin time, fibrinogen, platelet factor 3, and ^{14}C 5-HT uptake by platelets were all normal in pre- and post-transplantation patients. In the pretransplantation patients, 11 of the 12 had prolonged IVY bleeding times. All had elevated creatinine and BUN levels. Only one patient had a decrease in the release of 5-HT in the presence of ADP (Table 1).

Eight post-transplantation patients who were receiving prednisone, azathioprine, and cyproheptadine revealed some platelet function abnormalities, even at a time when their renal function was relatively normal (Table 1). Four (50 per cent) of the patients had prolonged bleeding times. Only one of these patients had evidence of abnormal renal function. All eight patients showed no impairment in ^{14}C 5-HT uptake or release induced by epinephrine and connective tissue. In six patients (75 per cent) the release of ^{14}C 5-HT induced by ADP was markedly impaired. There were no significant abnormalities in aggregation with these three agents in either group.

Thirteen patients were followed after transplantation and treated with steroids, azathioprine, and cyproheptadine. One patient died of candidiasis without rejection at 71 days. Four patients have had rejection crises at 28–358 days.

Eight patients have had no signs of rejection from 73–797 days. Renal biopsies in four of these patients showed only minimal small vessel disease, either as endothelial thickening or occlusive disease (Table 2).

DISCUSSION

Early studies in our laboratory demonstrated that a platelet-deaggregating agent, cyproheptadine (Goldman *et al.*, 1971), inhibited both the primary and secondary wave of platelet aggregation *in vitro*. This drug interfered with platelet sequestration in canine renal allografts, feline-canine renal xenografts, and inhibited acute renal rejection (Burrows *et al.*, 1970). These studies were further extended by Claes (1972) using canine-renal allografts in sensitized recipients. The monitored parameters were rejection time, renal blood flow, accumulation of ^{51}Cr-marked platelets in the rejecting

Table 1. Comparison of laboratory values in pretransplant and post-transplant groups of patients

Pretransplant patients												
Creatinine, serum (mg/100 ml)	9.7	20	13.6	12.9	2	10.4	10.5	12.4	7.6	9.0	11.2	12.8
Blood urea nitrogen (mg/100 ml)	38	90	49	69	46	70	55	41	38	44	66	63
Bleeding time*	↑	↑	↑	N	↑	↑	↑	↑	↑	↑	↑	↑
5-HT release by ADP (%)	18.0	35	27	0.6	47	61	59	35	32	45	42	37
Post-transplant patients												
Creatinine, serum (mg/100 ml)	1.4	1.2	1.3	2.0	3.5	1.6	2.2	1.5				
Blood urea nitrogen (mg/100 ml)	55	47	29	29	91	21	19	35				
Bleeding time*	N	S1↑	N	N	S1↑	N	↑	↑				
5-HT release by ADP (%)	2.0	6	9	47	0	55	2.0	6.0				

*↑ signifies bleeding time greater than 15 min; S1↑ signifies bleeding time of 8.5–15 min; N signifies bleeding time of 3.5–8.5 min.

Table 2. Cumulative results of renal transplantation with cyproheptadine* as adjunct to immunosuppressive therapy

Patient	Sex	Age	Dx	Donor	(Match)	Rejection crisis	Days since transplant or rejection crisis	Remarks	Azathioprine (Imuran® dose) (mg/kg/day)
P.S.	M	31	CGN†	Brother	(1)	No	379		1.0
E.K.	F	33	CGN	Cad†	(2)	Yes	359	Rejection, reversed with some difficulty	0.5
R.B.	F	25	CGN	Father	(2)	No	386		0.2
R.W.	M	40	CGN	Sister	(2)	No	405		0.5–1.0
D.D.	F	21	CGN	Mother	(4)	Yes	71	Rejection, now on dialysis	
M.C.	F	24	CGN	Cad	(3)	?	28	Minimal rejection, rapid reversal, now > 400 days, no further crises	0.25–0.5

G.B.	F	24	CGN	Father	(2)	No	671	ALG†	0.5
G.K.	M	28	CPN†	Father	(2)	No	73	Died, Candida sepsis	
L.G.	M	41	CGN	Sister	(1)	No	788	ALG	1.0
G.S.	M	17	CGN	Cad	(3)	No	797	2 Tx, CR† 1.2 mg/100ml	0.12–0.25
J.S.	M	24	CGN	Father	(2)	No	255		0.2–0.4
C.T.	M	28	CGN	Brother	(2)	No	295		0.25
A.O.	F	17	CGN	Father	(2)	Yes?	30	CR never > 3.6 mg/100 ml, easily reversed, minimal rejection	0.5

* Cyproheptadine given since 1970.

† CGN, chronic glomerulonephritis; Cad, cadaveric kidney; CPN, chronic pyelonephritis; ALG, antilymphocyte globulin; CR, creatine.

kidney, renal arterial-venous platelet count, and the deposition of ^{125}I-fibrinogen as fibrin. By daily intravenous administration to the recipient animal, 1.2 mg of cyproheptadine significantly prolonged the transplant with preservation of renal blood flow, and without platelet trapping or deposition of fibrin.

In both animal and human renal transplant models, cyproheptadine was capable of prolonging renal takes and decreasing the severity of rejection crises. The rat model is of particular interest since the platelet-deaggregating agent was the only agent used to combat rejection. Rat platelets respond *in vitro* to cyproheptadine in a fashion similar to human platelets. Increasing concentrations of cyproheptadine inhibit both ADP-induced aggregation and 5-HT uptake (Aledort and Berger, unpublished data).

In our human studies the majority of patients receiving 32 mg of cyproheptadine daily following renal transplantation exhibited an abnormality in the ability of their platelets to release 5-HT in the presence of ADP. The prolonged bleeding time in 50 per cent of the cases may represent an effect of cyproheptadine. This is, however, difficult to assess as the patients were also taking steroids and azathioprine. A prospective double blind study is in progress to evaluate the effects of cyproheptadine on platelet function and renal rejection.

Other platelet-deaggregating agents have been used to prolong renal transplant takes. Aspirin (MacDonald *et al.*, 1970) and dipyridamole (Kincaid-Smith, 1969) were shown to modify rejection. Dextran 60 delayed rejection in pig to dog xenografts (Messmer *et al.*, 1971). Claes (1972) using Dextran 70, 100 mg/kg I.V. daily, demonstrated results similar to those obtained by him with cyproheptadine.

Platelet aggregation, either initiated by endothelial damage or by antigen-antibody complexes, plays a significant role in transplantation rejection. Cyproheptadine, a deaggregating agent, has few side effects (Medical Letter, 1971) and is capable of altering the pattern of renal rejection. Platelet-deaggregating agents may represent useful adjuncts to the therapeutic regimen in transplantations.

ACKNOWLEDGMENTS

The authors would like to thank Mrs. Sadie Chu for her technical assistance. This work was supported by a grant from Merck Sharp and Dohme Research Laboratories, Division of Merck and Co., Inc. Part of this work was presented in Transp. Prog. Vol. 5, Page 157: 1973.

REFERENCES

Aledort, L. M., Berger, S., Goldman, B., and Puszkin, E., 1973. Antiserotonin and antihistamine drugs as inhibitors of platelet function. This symposium.

Berger, S., Puszkin, E., and Aledort, L. M. 1972. The effect of antiserotonin and antihistamine drugs on platelet function *in vitro*, p. 168. Abstract, Third Congress of International Society on Thrombosis and Haemostasis, Washington, D.C.

Burrows, L., Haimov, M., Glabman, S., Wong, D., Bauer, J., Aledort, L., Severin, C., and Kark, A. 1970. The obliterative vascular transplant rejection phenomenon: the role of platelet aggregation. Abstracts, Proceedings of the Third International Congress of the Transplantation Society.

Claes, G. 1972. Studies on platelets and fibrin during rejection of canine renal allografts. Scand. J. Urol. Nephr. Suppl. 10: 1.

Dempster, W. J. 1953. Kidney homotransplantation. Brit. J. Surg. 40: 447.

Goldman, B., and Aledort, L. M. 1972. Essential athrombia: a family study. Ann. Intern. Med. 76: 269.

Goldman, B., Aledort, L. M., Puszkin, E., and Burrows, L. 1971. Cyproheptadine, a new platelet deaggregating agent. Circulation 44: 68 (abstr.).

Kincaid-Smith, P. 1969. Modification of the vascular lesions of rejection in cadaveric renal allografts by dipyridamole and anticoagulants. Lancet 2: 920.

MacDonald, A., Bush, G. J., Alexander, J. L., Pheteplace, E. A., Menzoian, J., and Murray, J. E. 1970. Heparin and aspirin in the treatment of hyperacute rejection of renal allografts in presensitized dogs. Transplantation 9: 1.

Medical Letter, 1971. 13: 17.

Messmer, K., Hammer, W., Land, W., Fiedler, L., Klovekorn, W., Holper, K., Lob, G., Merzel, D., and Brendel, W. 1971. Modification of hyperacute xenogeneic kidney rejection. Transpl. Proc. 3: 542.

Mowbray, J. F. 1966. Methods of suppression of immune responses. Excerpta Med. Int. Congr. Ser. 137: 106.

Porter, K. A., Caine, R. Y., and Zukoski, C. F. 1964. Vascular and other changes in 200 canine renal homotransplants treated with immunosuppressive drugs. Lab. Invest. 13: 810.

Porter, K. A., Dossetor, J. B., Marchioro, T. L., Peart, W. S., Rendall, J. M., Starzl, T. E., and Terasaki, P. I. 1967. Human renal transplants. 1. Glomerular changes. Lab. Invest. 16: 153.

Scribner, B. H. 1971. The artificial kidney: emerging interrelationship between kidney transplantation and regular dialysis, pp. 1–9. *In* F. T. Rapaport and J. P. Merril (eds.) Artificial organs and cardiopulmonary support systems. Grune and Stratton, New York.

Defibrinogenation with Arvin in Thrombotic Disorders

William R. Bell*

Arvin, the active fraction from the crude venom of the Malayan pit viper (*Agkistrodon rhodostoma*), is a polypeptide which is a coagulant (*in vitro* and *in vivo*) with proteolytic enzyme properties. When administered to man, Arvin reduces plasma fibrinogen, reduces blood viscosity, and initially induces a state of fibrinolysis indicated by a rise in fibrinogen-fibrin degradation products and a reduction in plasma plasminogen. Arvin reacts with fibrinogen differently from the enzyme thrombin. Arvin in prothrombin-deficient plasma cleaves only the A-fibrinopeptides from fibrinogen to form a friable clot with electrophoretically unique fibrin. The stability of the resultant fibrin is further reduced since Arvin completely degrades the α(A) chain of fibrinogen at sites different from plasmin. Arvin differs from thrombin and reptilase in that it does not activate factor XIII. Unlike thrombin, Arvin does not release potassium, serotonin, ADP, or ATP from platelets but does induce minimal and delayed platelet aggregation. In man, platelet counts, function, and

*Hubert E. & Anne E. Rogers Scholar in Academic Medicine

metabolism are normal and in rabbits and dogs platelet survival is normal when treated with Arvin. Despite a severe degree of hypocoagulability, hemorrhagic tendency has not been observed. Consistent clinical features in patients treated with Arvin are the absence of thrombotic or embolic events during therapy, the absence of fibrinogen rebound, and a low incidence of recurrent thrombosis following discontinuation of the agent. At the present time, because of lack in objective data in most clinical studies employing Arvin, meaningful conclusions cannot be made. Controlled defibrinogenation should be considered as an approach to the therapy of thromboembolic disease.

Few compounds are as complex pharmacologically and biochemically as those found in the crude venom of many snakes. Although a few venoms have been used in the areas of biochemistry and medicine since time immemorial (Fontana, 1787), there has been recent resurgence of interest in these compounds. This has been evidenced by several hundred articles published in the past 5 years (Jimenez-Porras, 1970). The qualitative composition of the crude venoms may vary widely from family to family, species to species, or even within the same genus. Fractionation of some of these crude venoms has yielded components nearly identical in composition with properties of unique specificity (Markland and Davis, 1971; Esnouf and Tunnah, 1967).

One of the most important and most utilized major classes of proteins found in snake venoms is that of the proteolytic enzymes (Lee, 1972; Devi, 1968; Sarkar and Devi, 1968). Within this class can be found enzymes with either coagulant or anticoagulant properties (Rosenfeld *et al.*, 1968). In the discipline of blood coagulation, two venom preparations, because of their specificity, have been widely utilized as diagnostic agents in the laboratory and as hemostatic agents in the clinical setting. The first such agent is Russell's viper venom obtained from the East Indian viper Cobra manil (*Vipera russelli*) and is important because of its capacity to activate factor X selectively. The other agent is derived from the South American pit viper *Bothrops jararарca* (atrox), called Reptilase, which converts fibrinogen to fibrin and also activates factor X and possibly factors II and VII.

In 1963 Reid and his associates made the important observation of incoagulable blood in victims bitten by the Malayan pit viper *Agkistrodon rhodostoma.* Despite the absence of coagulable blood, hemorrhage was not observed in these patients. Laboratory studies of their blood revealed marked hypofibrinogenemia.

The benign nature of this state prompted further investigation for the possible use of this venom as a therapeutic agent for the prevention of clot formation. Incoagulable blood following snake bite is not unique to *A. rhodostoma*, but is found associated with many members of the Crotalidac family (Markland and Davis, 1971). Similar observations in pigeons were recorded by Taylor *et al.* (1935) using the crude venom of *Daboia (Vipera elegans)* and *Echis carinatus*. The active principle of *A. rhodostoma* venom has been purified and separated from the hemorrhagic factor found in the crude venom by a two-stage column chromatographic technique (Esnouf and Tunnah, 1967). This active fraction, designated Arvin[1], is a glycopolypeptide, a coagulant with proteolytic enzyme properties. By the approach-to-equilibrium method it has a molecular weight between 30,000 and 37,000. In solution at pH 7.0, 70 per cent of Arvin exists in the monomeric form and 30 per cent in the dimeric form. By weight approximately 70 per cent is a polypeptide of 17 amino acids and 20 per cent is a carbohydrate moiety.

MECHANISM OF ACTION

Of the many possible actions of this proteolytic enzyme the most widely recognized and best studied is its action on fibrinogen. Arvin releases the A-fibrinopeptides A, AP, AY, but not B-fibrinopeptide, from fibrinogen. Thrombin, the proteolytic enzyme found in blood, cleaves both A- and B-fibrinopeptides from fibrinogen. Also, unlike thrombin this agent splits the released A-fibrinopeptides into smaller subunits (Ewart *et al.*, 1970; Holleman and Coen, 1970). In addition Arvin, as opposed to thrombin, progressively and totally digests the α(A) chain of human fibrinogen. The sites attacked by Arvin appear to be different from those affected by plasmin. The α(A) chain digestion by Arvin is markedly (Mattock and Esnouf, 1971) or completely (Pizzo *et al.*, 1972) inhibited if the α(A) chain has previously been cross-linked by factor XIII. This digestion does not depend on the presence of calcium.

[1] Arvin is the registered trade name for Twyford Laboratories Ltd., T.C.L. (Park Royal) Ltd., Park Royal Brewery, London N.W.10, 7RR, England. This material has been given the nonproprietary name ancrod by the British Pharmacopoeia Commission. In the United States this material is produced by Abbott Laboratories, North Chicago, Ill. 60064 under the name Venacil (Abbott-38414).

The various reactions described above take place in the absence of prothrombin and thrombin (Mattock and Esnouf, 1971) and are not inhibited by heparin, hirudin, and soy bean trypsin inhibitor (Esnouf and Tunnah, 1967).

The fibrin polymer formed by the action of Arvin on fibrinogen contains only end-to-end anastomotic bonding (Kwaan and Barlow, 1971), has a unique pattern of electrophoretic migration, and has a significantly reduced gel tensile strength and elastic modulus as compared with the thrombin-formed fibrin clot. Arvin with the exception of factor I does not alter any of the clotting factors (Bell *et al.*, 1968) and repeated studies have demonstrated that this agent does not activate factor XIII (Bell and Pitney, 1970; Pizzo *et al.*, 1972a; Barlow *et al.*, 1970). These features of a(A) chain digestion, end-to-end anastomotic bonding, and the absence of cross-linking no doubt account for the increased susceptibility to lysis by plasmin and plasminogen-activating agents.

Arvin has esterase activity on basic amino acid esters. It is more active than thrombin in the hydrolysis of *p*-nitrophenyl esters of amino acids. Because of inhibition with diisopropyl phosphofluoridate it appears that Arvin is a serine proteinase. Detailed studies (Exner and Koppel, 1972) have demonstrated that Arvin has methyl esterase specificity limited to esters of L-arginine and the N^x-substitute acyl derivatives of arginine.

ACTION OF ARVIN

The intravenous (also intramuscular and rectal) administration of Arvin to man produces four recognizable alterations in the circulating blood. Within minutes after the intravenous administration of Arvin there is a reduction in plasma fibrinogen and within hours the level of fibrinogen is very low (Fig. 1). Reduction in fibrinogen refers to reduction in clottable protein. It has been observed during the reduction of fibrinogen by Arvin, when techniques not dependent on protein clottability are employed for the measurement of fibrinogen, that higher values are obtained than when a thrombin assay is used (Silberman *et al.*, 1972). It has been postulated that Arvin renders the fibrinogen nonclottable by thrombin or that Arvin promotes the formation of soluble non-thrombin-clottable fibrin complexes (Rodriguez-Erdman *et al.*, 1971). The unlikeliness of such possibilities is shown in Table 1. In this instance these techniques, that do not measure clottable

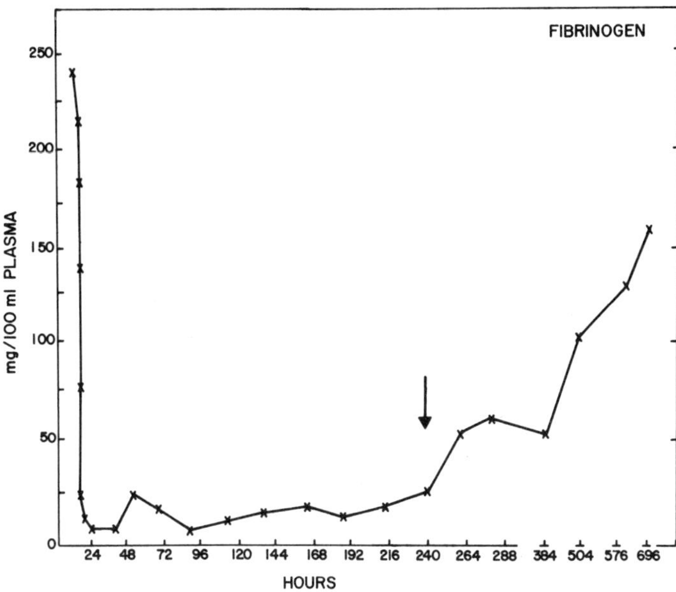

Figure 1. Plasma fibrinogen concentration following the initiation of Arvin therapy at time 0. Arrow indicates discontinuation of Arvin therapy.

protein per se, may be measuring fibrinogen-like compounds, proteins that may be the early breakdown products of fibrinogen or fibrin in addition to fibrinogen (clottable protein). As therapy with this agent continues (Fig. 1) fibrinogen remains at low levels. When the agent is discontinued in patients with normal body metabolism, fibrinogen returns slowly to the normal pretreatment level (Bell *et al.*, 1968). When fever, infection, active underlying disease, or subcutaneous turpentine in animals (Bell and Regoeczi, 1970) are present the fibrinogen may return more rapidly to the pretreatment value. This delay in fibrinogen return has been studied employing radioactively labeled fibrinogen and may in part be explained by an increase in the fractional catabolic rate of fibrinogen (Bell and Regoeczi, 1970). The regeneration phase of the curve in Fig. 1 is not influenced by the administration of specific antivenin (Regoeczi and Bell, 1969). During Arvin administration when the fibrinogen concentration is rapidly falling, there is a striking rise in fibrinogen-fibrin degradation products (FDP-fdp) in the blood (Fig. 2). These FDP-fdp peak in concentration 12–18 hr following the administration of this agent. In patients with normal

Table 1. Action of Arvin on plasma

In vitro	Supernatant*	
	Clottable protein	Immunoreactive fibrinogen FDP-fdp
Plasma	+	+1:4.19 × 10^6
Plasma + Arvin, 25°C, 6 hr	0	0
Plasma + Arvin, 37°C, 6 hr	0	0
Plasma Ca^{++} clot + Arvin, 25°C, 6 hr		0
Plasma Ca^{++} clot + Arvin, 37°C, 6 hr		0
UK + plasma	+	+1:2048 (serum)
SK + plasma	+	+1:4096 (serum)

Results of Arvin incubated with plasma and recalcified plasma at both 25 and 37°C for 6 hr.

* When the supernatant was mixed 1:1 with normal plasma the clotting time was 12 sec. Neat-normal plasma control clotting time was also 12 sec.

metabolic states the FDP-fdp decline to very low levels 36–48 hr after institution of therapy.

Considerable discussion has arisen in speculation about the origin of the FDP-fdp following administration of Arvin. Some have postulated that the action of Arvin per se on fibrinogen gives rise to the FDP-fdp. Another possibility is that the FDP-fdp result from the proteolytic action of the endogenous fibrinolytic system on the abnormal Arvin-fibrin polymer. When Arvin (final concentration 1–20 units/ml) is incubated with normal human plasma at 25 and 37°C for 6 hr a friable clot forms. Examination of the supernatant, following clot removal by centrifugation, reveals the absence of both clottable and immunologically (employing anti-human fibrinogen) recognizable fibrinogen-related protein (Table 1). When this supernatant is mixed with an equal volume of normal plasma there is no prolongation of the control clotting

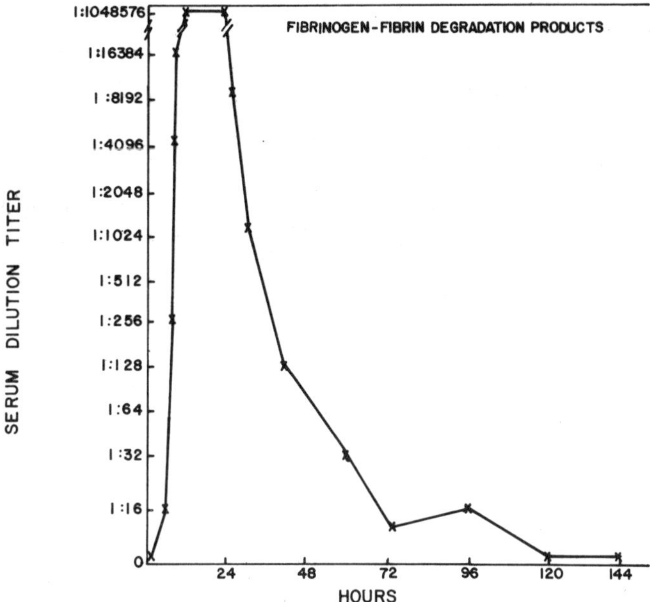

Figure 2. Evolution of fibrinogen-fibrin degradation products in the serum following the institution of Arvin therapy.

time. Arvin (final concentration 1–20 units/ml) incubated at 25 and 37°C with recalcified plasma fails to give rise to any immunologically recognizable fibrinogen- or fibrin-related protein. These *in vitro* findings indicate that Arvin removes fibrinogen (clottable protein) from plasma. Arvin does not produce fibrinogen-like or fibrin-soluble complexes nor does it give rise to an inhibitor of normal coagulation. Arvin per se does not produce immunologically recognizable breakdown products (FDP-fdp) from fibrinogen. These *in vitro* studies suggest that FDP-fdp and "soluble complexes" seen following *in vivo* administration of Arvin are the result of the proteolytic activity of the endogenous plasminogen-plasmin system. In mice pretreated with ϵ-aminocaproic acid followed by intravenously administered Arvin, a marked reduction in the number of FDP-fdp was noted in comparison with mice given Arvin but not ϵ-aminocaproic acid (Silberman *et al.*, 1972). Again, the endogenous fibrinolytic system is suggested as the responsible activity giving rise to these FDP-fdp. Extensive blood clots and death in animals result when the fibrinolytic system is inhibited simultaneously with Arvin administration (Regoeczi *et al.*, 1966).

Characterization of FDP-fdp found in the serum of mice treated with Arvin reveals a paucity of fragment D but normal amounts of fragment E.

Important in the understanding of the appearance and disappearance of FDP-fdp in subjects receiving Arvin is the status of the reticuloendothelial system (RES). In normal healthy rabbits treated with Thorotrast to block their RES there is observed a greater quantity and longer persistence of FDP-fdp than in control animals with normal RES function (Fig. 3). Earlier studies with crude *Agkistrodon* venom demonstrated that the removal of resultant microclots was via the phagocytic ability of the RES (Regoeczi *et al.*, 1966), thereby lending support to the above observation.

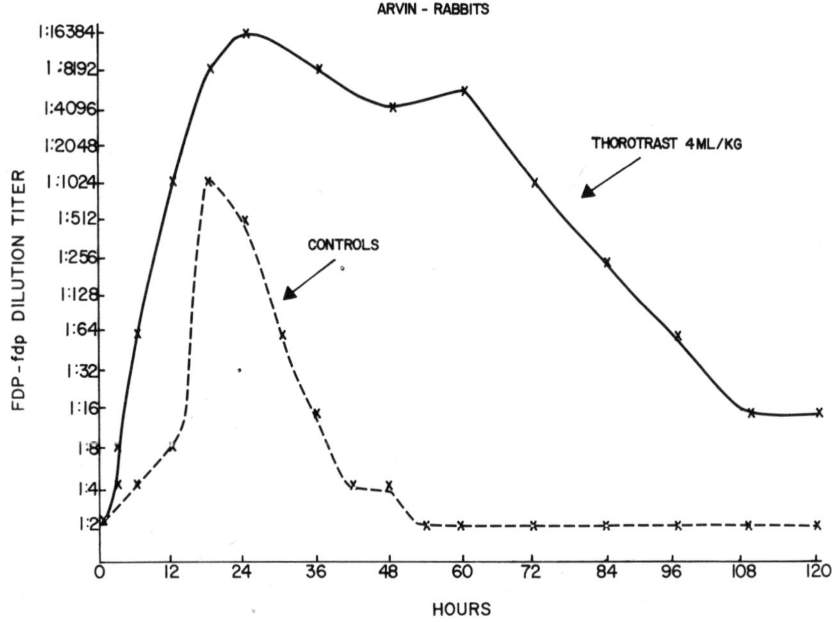

Figure 3. Degradation products appearing in the serum of animals who have been pretreated with Thorotrast to block the RES (X—X) persist for a longer period of time than in animals treated with Arvin who have not received Thorotrast (X- - -X), control animals.

Associated with the administration of Arvin is a fall in plasma plasminogen concentration (Fig. 4). Plasminogen remains low during therapy and returns to normal following discontinuation. *In vitro* the concentration of plasminogen in the supernatant of plasma defibrinogenated by Arvin is normal (Pitney *et al.*, 1969). When Arvin is incubated with purified plasminogen there is no inhibition or loss of plasminogen activity (Pizzo *et al.*, 1972b; Exner and Koppel, 1972).

The presence of FDP-fdp (Fig. 2) and the reduction in plasminogen concentration clearly indicate the presence of fibrinolysis following the administration of this agent. A possible explanation for the reduced level of plasminogen may be its conversion to the active proteolytic enzyme plasmin. When labeled plasminogen was given prior to the administration of Arvin, the disappearance of radioactivity from the blood followed a curve superimposable on that shown in Fig. 4 (personal observation).

Recently it has been demonstrated that the low quantities of plasminogen present during Arvin therapy are exquisitely sensitive

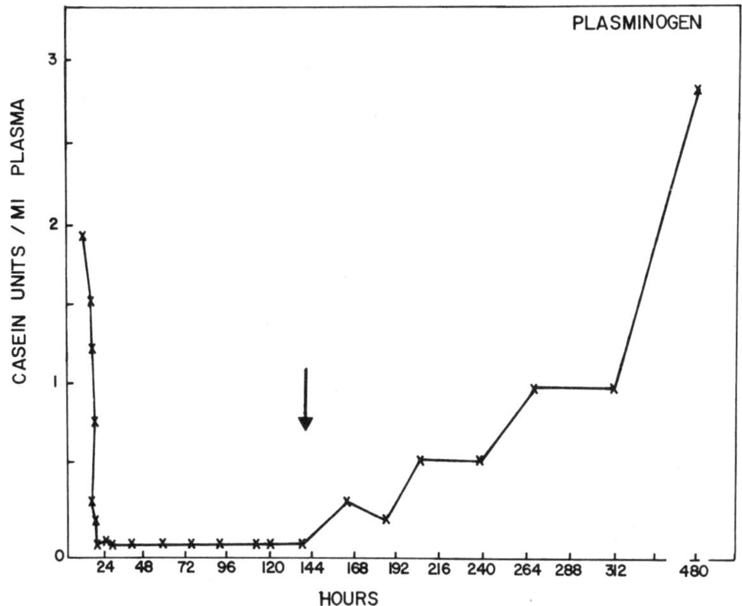

Figure 4. Plasma plasminogen following the institution of Arvin therapy. Arrow indicates discontinuation of Arvin.

to activation either by streptokinase or urokinase (Silberman *et al.*, 1972). In mice 25–50 CTA units of either streptokinase or urokinase activates this plasminogen as opposed to 1500 CTA units required for similar activation of normal non-Arvin-treated mouse plasma. This information suggests the possible use of Arvin prior to or in conjunction with thrombolytic agents to allow a reduction in the dose of urokinase or streptokinase needed to achieve adequate fibrinolysis. Preliminary reports of such studies have appeared (Latallo and Lopaciuk, 1972). It is apparent, however, that one must be cautious with this form of therapy because Arvin reduces plasminogen to low levels and concomitant thrombolytic therapy may deplete plasminogen and thereby remove the natural protection afforded by the fibrinolytic system. If depletion of plasminogen takes place the necessary substrate for both urokinase and streptokinase would be absent and these drugs would be unable to act.

The fourth recognizable effect on the blood following the administration of Arvin to man is a reduction in blood viscosity. Measurements made before and serially during the infusion of the initial dose of Arvin demonstrate a reduction in blood viscosity. As the fibrinogen level falls from a normal pretreatment value the blood changes from its normal non-Newtonian fluidity to a fluid with Newtonian characteristics (Fig. 5). In animal models, when the initial dose of Arvin is given more rapidly than in man, fever, tachycardia, and cyanosis have been reported. These findings have been attributed to "soluble fibrin complexes" which are thought to increase the blood viscosity of these animals (Rodriguez-Erdman *et al.*, 1971) (C. A. Owen, Mayo Clinic, Rochester, Minn., personal communication). For many reasons that will be developed later, the rapid infusion of Arvin into man is not recommended.

Arvin does not alter any of the circulating formed blood elements. Hematocrit, hemoglobin concentration, white blood count, differential, and platelet count are not altered during or following therapy with this agent. Extensive evaluation of red cell morphology during Arvin therapy failed to detect any bizarre or fragmented forms such as those seen in pathological defibrinogenating states. Platelet numbers and metabolism are unaltered in man by Arvin therapy. During the time when FDP-fdp are present in large quantities following institution of Arvin therapy, *in vitro* platelet aggregation to ADP is reduced (Bell, 1968; Prentice *et al.*, 1969). Platelet survival in dogs (Martin *et al.*, 1971) and rabbits

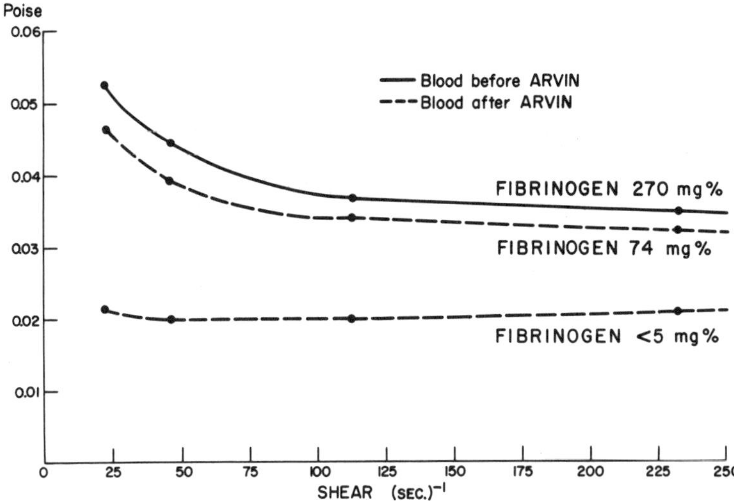

Figure 5. Blood viscosity following the institution of Arvin therapy. The properties of the blood change from the normal non-Newtonian fluid to the characteristics of a Newtonian fluid as fibrinogen is removed progressively.

(Brown *et al.*, 1972) during therapy with Arvin is normal. These studies clearly demonstrate that the process of defibrinogenation by Arvin does not produce a reduction in platelet count.

Detailed *in vitro* studies where Arvin was incubated with washed platelets demonstrated unique properties of this enzyme (Prentice *et al.*, 1969). Arvin, unlike thrombin, does not release potassium, serotonin, ADP, ATP, platelet factor 3, or platelet factor 4 from human platelets. Both Arvin and thrombin clotted platelet fibrinogen. Arvin induced platelet aggregation that was minimal and delayed. Platelets aggregated by Arvin were loose morphologically in network structure, and individual platelets remained discrete and did not undergo fusion with viscous metamorphosis as seen with thrombin. Platelets incubated with Arvin were capable of supporting retraction of thrombin-induced clots. When Arvin was administered to patients whose platelets migrated abnormally in an electrophoretic field, the electrophoretic migration became normal (Turpie *et al.*, 1972). When Arvin was discontinued in the same patients, the platelet electrophoretic migration reverted to the abnormal pattern seen prior to Arvin administration. The precise reason for this phenomenon is not understood.

PHARMACOLOGY

The protein nature of Arvin and its prompt denaturation by gastric acid eliminates the oral route as a route of administration. Arvin is absorbed from the intramuscular (Pitney *et al.*, 1969b), subcutaneous (Gilles *et al.*, 1968), rectal compartments (personal observation), and intraperitoneal route (Ashby *et al.*, 1970). Resistance to Arvin has been detected when the intramuscular (IM) route is used and the mechanism demonstrated (Pitney *et al.*, 1969a; Pitney and Regoeczi, 1970; Ross *et al.*, 1969). When resistance develops following IM injection additional Arvin given intravenously is without effect on the level of circulating fibrinogen. In this instance Arvin appears to be inactivated by forming a complex with a protein that migrates in the γ-globulin region (antibody) on immunoelectrophoresis. When the agent is given by the intravenous route (I.V.), inactivation takes place when the Arvin is formed in a complex by proteins of the a-2 macroglobulin region and a protein that may be anti-thrombin III.

The intravenous route of administration is the most acceptable. When Arvin is injected intravenously it rapidly migrates to extravascular spaces. Studies with ^{131}I-Arvin in man and rabbits indicate that the extra- to intravascular distribution ratio is 1.7 (man) and 2.5 (rabbit). These data indicate the extravascular diffusion volume of Arvin is approximately twice the volume of the intravascular space. The initial disappearance of intravascular ^{131}I-Arvin follows a complex multiple exponential function but after 4 days a single exponential elimination rate of 11.5 days was observed. Arvin appears to be catabolized in the intravascular compartment and is excreted in the urine. Only a small percentage of the administered dose is excreted unchanged in the urine. Catabolism is identical in nephric and anephric man and rabbits (Regoeczi and Bell, 1969). When Arvin is formed in a complex with antivenin, catabolism is markedly reduced. Via the I.V. route resistance is exceedingly rare, but has been reported after prolonged administration (Voss, 1968).

When Arvin is given I.V. the resultant Arvin-fibrin microclots are cleared by the RES (Regoeczi *et al.*, 1966). Detailed study has shown that this agent enhances the clearing activity of the RES which is not seen with the crude venom (Ashford and Bunn, 1970). The RES stimulant effect appears to be due to Arvin since it is present when employing small doses that are without effect on fibrinogen.

Arvin does not alter cardiovascular hemodynamics (Klein *et al.*, 1969) or renal function (Marshall and Esnouf, 1968; Fedor *et al.*, 1971) and is without analgesic effect (Dr. E. J. Fedor, Abbott Laboratories, personal communication). Anti-inflammatory properties of Arvin are minimal (Ashby *et al.*, 1970; Ford *et al.*, 1970) or absent (Dr. E. J. Fedor, personal communication).

The pharmacology of Arvin has also been studied in the dog, cat, mouse, and rat (Ashford *et al.*, 1968).

DOSE ROUTE AND SCHEDULE OF ADMINISTRATION

Arvin clots plasma or solutions of fibrinogen at a rate inversely proportional to its concentration. This has provided the basis for determination of biological potency by an *in vitro* assay. One Arvin unit (2 μg of protein) is that amount of material that will clot a standard solution of fibrinogen at 37°C in the same time as 1 NIH unit of thrombin. Arvin is stable at 4°C in concentrations of 50–100 units/ml in a sodium phosphate-sodium chloride-chlorbutol mixture at pH 6.8 for 36 months and possibly longer.

Although several different routes of administration have been examined the acceptable route is intravenous. Employing this route, tachyphylaxis and variation in dose response from patient to patient or within the same patient from day to day have not been seen. The dose and schedule currently recommended for therapeutic defibrinogenation is as follows: the initial dose is 1–2 units/kg body weight homogeneously mixed in a volume of 50–100 ml of 5 per cent dextrose in water or 0.85 per cent sodium chloride and given I.V. carefully and precisely over 4–6 hr via constant infusion. Subsequent doses of 2–3 units/kg body weight should be given I.V. in 20 ml of 5 per cent dextrose in water or 0.85 per cent sodium chloride over 10–15 min every 12 hr for the duration of therapy. Should therapy be interrupted for a prolonged period of time, a plasma fibrinogen level should be checked before additional doses are administered. Should the fibrinogen level be greater than 75 mg/100 ml, therapy should be continued only after repeating the initial slow infusion and procedure described above.

Following the initial infusion, the employment of a 12-hour intermittent administration schedule offers the advantage of complete mobilization and ambulation of the patient, a very important consideration in the management of thrombotic disorders (The Urokinase Pulmonary Embolism Trial, 1972).

Rarely, adequate hypofibrinogenemia will not be easily maintained by intermittent therapy because a nonspecific stimulus for the synthesis of fibrinogen such as high fever, infection, malignancy, etc., may be present. In such a situation, following administration of the second dose as outlined above, subsequent doses can be given by continuous intravenous infusion using 2–3 units/kg body weight in 250–500 ml of 5 per cent dextrose in water or 0.85 per cent sodium chloride, and infused constantly over 12–24 hr. With this technique hypofibrinogenemia can be maintained satisfactorily.

LABORATORY MONITORING

The most important item to follow before and at frequent intervals during treatment with Arvin is plasma fibrinogen concentration. This is best accomplished simply and rapidly in a very few minutes by the semiquantitative thrombin-fibrinogen titer (Sharp *et al.*, 1958) or more accurately by a modified thrombin-clotting time (Clauss, 1957). A more precise method is that described by Ratnoff and Menzie (1951). The latter method should be performed at 3- to 4-day intervals during therapy to make accurate assessment of the thrombin-clottable protein in the blood. Routine base-line and infrequent measurement of the hematocrit, white blood count, differential, platelet, urine, and stool for occult blood are suggested. The measurements of coagulation factors, hepatic, renal, and pancreatic function are probably unnecessary since a large clinical experience has repeatedly demonstrated that these studies do remain normal during Arvin therapy. The determination of blood viscosity, plasminogen, plasmin, and FDP-fdp are of interest but are not critical in clinical management.

During administration of Arvin, should the need arise for prompt reversal of hypofibrinogenemia, such as urgent surgery or massive bleeding, this can be accomplished in the following way. First, Arvin should be immediately discontinued. Then the specific anti-Arvin venin (Lewis *et al.*, 1971) should be given to neutralize any circulating Arvin. Prior to or simultaneous with the antivenin, washed packed red blood cells can be quickly given (personal observation). Following the anti-Arvin venin, replacement therapy with plasma, whole blood, or fibrinogen may be safely given. With such a technique the plasma fibrinogen can be restored to normal in a short period of time.

PRECLINICAL STUDIES

Studies with Arvin in animals have been carried out to evaluate the efficacy of this agent in thrombotic disease and also to obtain information on the role of fibrinogen and fibrin in the pathogenesis of various diseases. Studies with sheep (personal observation), horses (Archer *et al.*, 1969), rabbits, mice, cats, rats (Ashford *et al.*, 1968), dogs (Marshall and Esnouf, 1968; Ashford *et al.*, 1968; Esnouf and Marshall, 1968), calves (Singh *et al.*, 1970), monkeys, pigs, goats (Martin *et al.*, 1971; Abbott Laboratories, 1971), and guinea pigs (Ross *et al.*, 1969) have demonstrated these animals to be sensitive (reduction in fibrinogen) to small doses (0.1–1 unit/kg) of Arvin. In the rat large doses (90 units/kg) of Arvin are required to achieve a moderate reduction in fibrinogen (Ashford *et al.*, 1968). The golden hamster can tolerate 670 units/kg without a reduction in plasma fibrinogen (D. S. Wood, Merck Institute; Rahway, N.J.)

Venous thrombosis, experimentally produced by a variety of techniques and then treated with Arvin, has been studied by several investigators (Van Der Zeil *et al.*, 1970; Rahimtoola *et al.*, 1970; Kwaan and Fedor, 1969; Chan, 1969). Results indicate that if Arvin is given promptly after the thrombus is formed there is restoration of vessel patency and blood flow. However, if therapy is delayed, allowing the thrombus to age and retract, Arvin is ineffective in restoration of blood flow. In the same experiment there was prompt return of blood flow when thrombolytic therapy was employed. In the study of pulmonary embolism in dogs (Sharma *et al.*, 1972) and rabbits (Olsen and Pitney, 1969) greater resolution of blood clots was observed in the animals treated with Arvin as compared with heparin-treated and control animals.

Because blood clotting and fibrin deposition have been incriminated as possible trigger mechanisms in hyperacute renal allograft rejection, immune arthritis, and the generalized Shwartzman reaction (GSR), removal of fibrinogen by Arvin was performed. Although pretreatment with Arvin removed the circulating fibrinogen from recipient dogs, the transplanted renal allografts and sheep-to-dog xenografts rejected over the same time as the control animals (MacDonald *et al.*, 1972). Histological studies of the rejected kidneys revealed extensive cellular invasion and vascular damage in the absence of any fibrin or fibrinogen deposition. Similarly, in rabbits the removal of fibrinogen failed to protect against the development of immune arthritis (Ford *et al.*, 1970). However, Arvin-induced hypofibrinogenemia of 30-hr duration, prior to Thorotrast and endotoxin administration, prevented the classic lesions of the GSR (Bell *et al.*, 1972). These results suggest that alterations of the coagulation system are secondary events in renal transplant rejection and immune arthritis, but such alterations may play a primary role in the GSR.

Selective studies have defined activation of the clotting mechanism and thrombus formation around tumor cells as the main features of the early phase of metastasis formation (Wood, 1961, 1971). Specific studies in rabbits (Hilgard and Wood, in press) and mice (Austin and Glaser, 1969), designed to test the role of fibrin strands in tumor metastasis, revealed a reduction in metastatic deposits in animals made hypofibrinogenic by Arvin when compared with control animals. Similar studies in two strains of inbred mice revealed only minor alteration in metastasis patterns (Hagmar, 1972). Failure of reduction in the number of lesions in this last study may be explained in part by the relative resistance to defibrinogenation by Arvin in the mice.

Arvin has been successfully employed in the prevention of thrombus formation on artificial devices placed in the vascular system, such as prosthetic heart valves (Singh *et al.*, 1970) and fiber optic lens systems (personal observation).

Some snake venoms are known to alter lipids, but Arvin given I.V. in rabbits was without effect on plasma-free fatty acids, triglycerides, or cholesterol (Barboriak, 1971).

CLINICAL STUDIES-THERAPEUTIC RESULTS

Since introduction of Arvin in 1967 into organized clinical trial for the treatment of deep venous thrombosis, numerous studies have been performed (Bell, 1971). Most of these studies have been performed in England, Ireland, Switzerland, West Germany, and the United States. Interpretation of these studies is particularly difficult because of lack of precise diagnostic criteria and appropriate studies, appropriate controls and proper comparative studies.

Table 2. Disease categories: clinical study

Deep vein thrombosis with or without pulmonary embolism
Pulmonary hypertension: thromboembolic etiology
Myocardial infarction
Embolism from prosthetic cardiac valves
Peripheral arterial thrombosis
Central retinal vein thrombosis
Extracorporeal hemodialysis
Priapism
Sickle cell anemia
Cerebral thrombosis
Rheumatoid arthritis
Metastasis formation in malignancy
Renal transplant rejection
Prevention clot formation membrane oxygenator and fiberoptic lens catheter
Generalized Shwartzman reaction

The conditions listed are currently being studied during treatment with Arvin.

An additional difficulty in making an accurate assessment of this agent is that many of the disorders, where this agent is indicated, are either self-limited or so rapidly fatal that time does not permit adequate study.

As experience with this agent has grown the possible therapeutic scope has widened. Several different diseases under study with respect to the efficacy of Arvin are listed in Table 2. In one study where firm diagnostic criteria and accurate post-therapy studies were performed (Kakkar *et al.*, 1969) it appears that Arvin is not a thrombolytic agent. The *in vitro* studies mentioned earlier support this finding.

In general the clinical therapeutic response, *i.e.* disappearance of the thrombotic process, has been more rapid than observed in similar conditions treated with conventional anticoagulants. Once therapy with Arvin has been instituted, no new thrombotic or embolic events have been observed during therapy. Although clinical responses remain encouraging, more thorough and well organized studies employing methods to generate objective data must be carried out. Such a study involving several medical institutions is in progress in the United States (Dr. J. F. Donahoe, Abbott Laboratories, personal communication).

UNTOWARD SIDE EFFECTS

Complications associated with Arvin have been few. When this agent has been employed in an indicated setting and properly administered with appropriate laboratory monitoring, undesirable effects have been very rare. The most commonly reported complication has been bleeding (Pitney, 1971) and the incidence was 5 per cent or less. In these patients the bleeding was minimal and not of sufficient magnitude to discontinue the Arvin therapy. In most instances of bleeding that have been reported explicable causes such as salicylate ingestion and gastritis, intestinal ulceration, and uremia were present. Arvin has been administered to several patients concomitant with menstrual flow and no increased bleeding or prolonged flow was observed. In two reports (Kakkar *et al.*, 1969; Pitney, 1971) the incidence of bleeding was significantly less than seen in patients concomitantly treated with heparin. The presence of headache has been mentioned by approximately 1 per cent of patients treated with Arvin. This has been difficult to evaluate particularly because a long history of migraine was present in most patients with this complaint. Delayed wound healing has been reported in experimental animals associated with Arvin administration (Holt *et al.*, 1970; Silberman and Kwaan, 1971). Clinical observations have not confirmed these findings in patients treated with Arvin after surgery (Pitney, 1971; Sharp, 1971).

Although red cell fragmentation (Rubenberg *et al.*, 1967), cyanosis, tachycardia, and fever (Rodriguez-Erdmann *et al.*, 1971) have been reported in animals rapidly given large doses of Arvin (Rubenberg *et al.*, 1968), despite searching for such effects, these have not been observed in man (Bell *et al.*, 1968).

The problem with the development of resistance to Arvin has been mentioned above. Should this be suspected, one can confirm this suspicion by performing a precipitin reaction (Pitney *et al.*, 1969b).

CONTRAINDICATIONS

Contraindications for the use of Arvin in humans are those that apply for the use of conventional anticoagulants. The most obvious absolute contraindication for using this agent is the presence of active hemorrhage or recent extensive soft tissue trauma. Arvin probably should not be instituted earlier than 72 hr following surgery (Sharp, 1971). Although it has been shown that Arvin does not cross the placenta (Martin *et al.*, 1971), Arvin must not be administered during pregnancy because of such potential problems as placental separation, hemorrhage, abortion, and teratogenic effects (Penn *et al.*, 1971) on the fetus.

Absolutely contraindicated during therapy with Arvin is the administration of agents that inhibit the fibrinolytic system, cause dysfunction of the RES, disturb platelet function, or contain fibrinogen. Arvin should not be considered safe in severe thrombocytopenia or illness where the fibrinolytic system is incapable of being activated (Mohler *et al.*, 1967; Kwaan *et al.*, 1959).

LABORATORY USE OF ARVIN

Because of the unique properties of this agent, it has become a useful laboratory tool. One of the most practical uses for this agent in the coagulation laboratory is for carrying out studies on samples that may contain heparin. The action of Arvin is not inhibited by even substantial concentrations of heparin. When one is forced to work with heparinized blood one can substitute Arvin for thrombin in performing the thrombin time. Likewise, Arvin can be used instead of thrombin in clotting and removing fibrinogen from plasma for the determination of fibrinogen-fibrin degradation products. Arvin does not quantitatively alter any degradation products that are present (personal observation). Degradation products do not appear to inhibit the action of Arvin on fibrinogen (personal observation). In view of the fact that this agent does not activate factor XIII, one can study factor XIII in serum separate from factor XIII in the plasma associated with fibrinogen. Arvin has been employed to prepare a multifold purification of factor VIII from plasma (Green, 1971). As additional studies are carried out it is very likely that this agent will have more and more use in the laboratory because of its relative unique specificity.

DISCUSSION

Owing to the large number of preclinical and clinical studies that have been carried out in the laboratory by several investigators, it seems reasonable to conclude that the use of this agent is safe in man. Untoward side effects have been exceedingly few. Critically important in the employment of this agent is the requirement that the first dose be given very precisely, slowly, and constantly over a period of 4–6 hr. Because this agent is a coagulant, if the initial dose is administered too rapidly it has the potential of forming large thrombi in the body and possibly overwhelming the capacity of the body to handle these thrombi or resultant fibrinogen-fibrin degradation products. One must never fail to remember that this agent is a coagulant. It is a coagulant both *in vitro* and *in vivo*. By the appropriate *in vivo* administration of this agent its coagulant action results in incoagulable blood. The rationale for employing this agent in disorders of thrombotic disease is that it has the ability to reduce predictably the concentration of circulating plasma fibrinogen. The safety of this agent is further supported by the fact that it does not alter body temperature, blood pressure, heart rate, cardiac dynamics, glucose tolerance, or hepatic, renal, or pancreatic function.

Particularly interesting is the hypofibrinogenemic state that results following the administration of Arvin. In contrast to the hypofibrinogenemia seen in disseminated intravascular coagulopathy, experimentally induced hypofibrinogenemia by the use of thrombin or tissue thromboplastin, Arvin is not associated with a reduction in platelet count, red cell fragmentation, anemia, hemorrhagic diathesis, reduction in cardiac output or organ perfusion, cyanosis, or shock-like state. The precise reasons for these differences are not known. One may speculate that such differences are due to the rather unique biochemical action of Arvin on plasma fibrinogen. The resultant fibrin polymer formed by Arvin is different not only in its content but also in its structure. One may thus expect that the by-products of additional reactions in which this Arvin-fibrin polymer participates may also be different than those seen with endogenous coagulant enzymes. Additional studies are needed to examine the details of these biochemical interactions.

Although this agent appears to be safe, its therapeutic efficacy has not been established. At this time one cannot meaningfully interpret the results of the majority of published reports. In those reports where good diagnostic criteria and studies were employed, and where Arvin was studied in a comparative manner under identical conditions with heparin and thrombolytic therapy along with the appropriate controls, it appears reasonable to conclude that Arvin is not lytic with respect to the preformed blood clot.

At the present time in the United States a well designed, large, multicenter clinical trial with this agent is being carried out. Hopefully similar studies will be started in other geographic locations.

With the advent of this agent and its use in man the new concept of therapeutic defibrinogenation has arisen. This concept is theoretically reasonable and sound. Hopefully sufficient interest has been generated to stimulate thorough exploration of the possible merits of this therapeutic modality.

ACKNOWLEDGMENT

This work was supported in part by Research Grant HL01601 from the National Heart and Lung Institute. The author expresses gratitude to Prof. F. A. Robinson, Ph.D., Twyford Laboratories, and Prof. J. F. Goodwin, Royal Post Graduate Medical School, London, for their continued interest and encouragement.

REFERENCES

Abbott Laboratories. 1971. FDA-required studies on A-38414. Abbott Laboratories, North Chicago, Ill.

Archer, R. K., Close, M., and Ashford, A. 1969. A new therapeutic anticoagulant. Vet. Rec. 84: 150.

Ashby, E. C., James, D. C. O., and Ellis, H. 1970. The effect of intraperitoneal Malayan pit-viper venom on adhesion formation and peritoneal healing. Brit. J. Surg. 57: 863.

Ashford, A., and Bunn, D. R. G. 1970. The effect of Arvin on reticuloendothelial activity in rabbits. Brit. J. Pharmacol. 40: 37.

Ashford, A., Ross, J. W., and Southgate, P. 1968. Pharmacology and toxicology of a defibrinating substance from Malayan pit-viper venom. Lancet 1: 486.

Austin, J. P., and Glaser, E. M. 1969. Inhibition of experimental tumors by defibrinogenation. Clin. Sci. 37: 878 (abstr.).

Barboriak, J. J. 1971. The effect of Arvin on plasma lipids of the rabbit. Proc. Soc. Exp. Biol. Med. 136: 313.

Barlow, G. H., Holleman, W. H., and Lorand, L. 1970. The action of Arvin on fibrin stabilizing factor (factor XIII). Res. Commun. Chem. Pathol. Pharmacol. 1:39.

Bell, W. R. 1968. Further experience in the treatment of thrombotic disorders by therapeutic defibrination. Quart. J. Med. 37: 658.

Bell, W. R. 1971. Current status of therapy with Arvin. Thromb. Diath. Haemorrh. Suppl. 47: 371.

Bell, W. R., Bolton, G., and Pitney, W. R. 1968. The effect of Arvin on blood coagulation factors. Brit. J. Haematol. 15: 589.

Bell, W. R., Miller, R., and Levin, J. 1972. Inhibition of the generalized Shwartzman reaction by hypofibrinogenemia. Blood 40: 697.

Bell, W. R., and Pitney, W. R. 1970. The concept of therapeutic defibrination. Thromb. Diath. Haemorrh. Suppl. 39: 285.

Bell, W. R., Pitney, W. R., and Goodwin, J. F. 1968. Therapeutic defibrination in the treatment of thrombotic disease. Lancet 1: 490.

Bell, W. R., and Regoeczi, E. 1970. Isotopic studies of therapeutic anticoagulation with a coagulating enzyme. J. Clin. Invest. 49: 1872.

Brown, C. H., Bell, W. R., Shreiner, D. P., and Jackson, D. P. 1972. Effects of Arvin on blood platelets. *In vitro* and *in vivo* studies. J. Lab. Clin. Med. 79: 758.

Chan, K. E. 1969. The comparison of antithrombotic action on the thrombin-like fraction of Malayan pit-viper venom and heparin. Cardiovasc. Res. 3: 171.

Clauss, A. 1957. Gerinnungsphysiologische Schnellmethode zur Bestimmung des Fibrinogens. Acta Haematol. (Basel) 17: 237.

Devi, A. 1968. *In* W. Bucherl, E. E. Buckley, and V. Deulofeu (eds.) Venomous animals and their venoms, Vol. I, p. 119. Academic Press, New York.

Esnouf, M. P., and Marshall, R. 1968. The effect of blockade of the RES and of hypotension on the response of dogs to *Ancistrodon rhodostoma* venom. Clin. Sci. 35: 261.

Esnouf, M. P., and Tunnah, G. W. 1967. Thrombin-like activity from *Ancistrodon rhodostoma* venom. Brit. J. Haematol. 13: 581.

Ewart, M. R., Hatton, M. W. C., Basford, J. M., and Dodgson, R. S. 1970. The proteolytic action of Arvin on human fibrinogen. Biochem. J. 118: 603.

Exner, T., and Koppel, J. L. 1972. Observations concerning the substrate specificity of Arvin. Biochim. Biophys. Acta 258: 825.

Fedor, E. J., Brondyk, H. D., Wiemeler, L. H., and Hwang, K. 1971. Effect of Abbott-38414 (ancrod) on renal blood flow and clearance, coronary sinus flow, pO_2 and femoral arterial blood flow. Fed. Proc. 30: 422.

Fontana, F. 1787. Treatise on the venom of the viper, Vol. I and II, J. Murray Co., London.

Ford, P. M., Bell, W. R., Bluestone, R., Gumpel, J. M., and Webb, F. W. S. 1970. The effect of Arvin on experimental immune arthritis in rabbits. Brit. J. Exp. Pathol. 51: 81.

Gilles, H. M., Reid, H. A., Odutola, A., Ransome-Kuti, O., and Ransome-Kuti, S. 1968. Arvin treatment for sickle-cell crisis. Lancet 2: 542.

Green, D. 1971. A simple method for the purification of factor VIII (AHG) employing snake venom. J. Lab. Clin. Med. 77: 153.

Hagmar, B. 1972. Defibrination and metastasis formation: Effects of Arvin on experimental metastases in mice. Eur. J. Cancer 8: 17.

Hilgard, P., and Wood, S. Arvin induced hypofibrinogenemia and early metastasis formation. J. Clin. Pathol., in press.

Holleman, W. H., and Coen, L. J. 1970. Characterization of peptides released from human fibrinogen by Arvin. Biochim. Biophys. Acta 200: 587.

Holt, P. J. L., Holloway, V., Raghupati, N., and Calnan, J. S. 1970. The effect of a fibrinolytic agent (Arvin) on wound healing and collagen formation. Clin. Sci. 38: 9P.

Jimenez-Porras, J. M. 1970. Biochemistry of snake venoms. Clin. Toxicol. 3: 389.

Kakkar, V. V., Flanc, C., Howe, C. T., O'Shea, M., and Flute, P. 1969. Treatment of deep venous thrombosis: A trial of heparin, streptokinase and Arvin. Brit. Med. J. 1: 806.

Klein, M. D., Bell, W. R., Nasser, N., and Lown, B. 1969. The effect of Arvin upon cardiac function. Proc. Soc. Exp. Biol. Med. 132: 1123.

Kwaan, H. C., and Barlow, G. H. 1971. The mechanism of action of a coagulant fraction of Malayan pit-viper venom Arvin and reptilase. Thromb. Diath. Haemorrh. Suppl. 45: 63.

Kwaan, H. C., and Fedor, E. J. 1969. Anticoagulant and thrombolytic effects of a polypeptide extracted from Malayan viper venom. J. Clin. Invest. 48: 47 (abstr.).

Kwaan, H. C., Lo, R., and McFadzean, A. J. S. 1959. Antifibrinolytic activity in primary carcinoma of the liver. Clin. Sci. 18: 251.

Latallo, Z. S., and Lopaciuk, S. 1972. A combined treatment with streptokinase and defibrase. A new approach to therapy of thromboembolic states. Third Congress of International Society on Thrombosis and Haemostosis, p. 432. Abstract, Washington, D.C.

Lee, C. Y. 1972. Chemistry and pharmacology of polypeptide toxins in snake venoms. Annu. Rev. Pharmacol. 12: 265.

Lewis, L. J., Martin, D. L., Buckner, S., Finley, R., Lazer, L., and Fedor, E. J. 1971. Studies on type specific immunity to the whole venom and a fraction of *Agkistrodon rhodostoma.* Res. Commun. Pathol. Pharmacol. 2: 649.

MacDonald, A. S., Bell, W. R., Busch, G. J., Ghose, T., Chan, C. C., Falvey, C. F., and Merrill, J. P. 1972. A comparison of hyperacute canine renal allograft and sheep-to-dog xenograft rejection. Transplantation 13: 146.

Markland, F. S., and Davis, P. S. 1971. Purification and properties of a thrombin-like enzyme from the venom of *Crotalus adamanteus*. J. Biol. Chem. 246: 6460.

Marshall, R., and Esnouf, M. P. 1968. The effect of crude and purified *Ancistrodon rhodostoma* venom in the dog. Clin. Sci. 35: 251.

Martin, D. L., Hollinger, R. E., Suwanwela, N., and Fedor, E. J. 1971. Experimental defibrination produced by Abbott-38414 (Ancrod) and associated effects on some other factors of the hemostatic system. Fed. Proc. 30: 424 (abstr.).

Mattock, P., and Esnouf, M. P. 1971. Differences in the subunit structure on human fibrin formed by the action of Arvin, reptilase and thrombin. Nature New Biol. 233: 277.

Mohler, E. R., Kennedy, J. N., and Brakman, P. 1967. Blood coagulation and fibrinolysis in multiple myeloma. Amer. J. Med. Sci. 253: 325.

Olsen, E. G. J., and Pitney, W. R. 1969. The effect of Arvin on experimental pulmonary embolism in the rabbit. Brit. J. Haematol. 17: 425.

Penn, G. B., Ross, J. W., and Ashford, A. 1971. The effects of Arvin on pregnancy in the mouse and the rabbit. Toxicol. Appl. Pharmacol. 20: 460.

Pitney, W. R. 1971. An appraisal of therapeutic defibrination. Thromb. Diath. Haemorrh. Suppl. 45: 43.

Pitney, W. R., Holt, P. J. L., Bray, C., and Bolton, G. 1969a. Acquired resistance to treatment with Arvin. Lancet 1: 79.

Pitney, W. R., Bell, W. R., and Bolton, G. 1969b. Blood fibrinolytic activity during Arvin therapy. Brit. J. Haematol. 16: 165.

Pitney, W. R., and Regoeczi, E. 1970. Inactivation of Arvin by plasma proteins. Brit. J. Haematol. 19: 67.

Pizzo, S. V., Schwartz, M. L., Hill, R. L., and McKee, P. A. 1972a. Mechanism of ancrod anticoagulation. A direct proteolytic effect on fibrin. J. Clin. Invest. 51: 2841.

Pizzo, S. V., Schwartz, M. L., Hill, R. L., and McKee, P. A. 1972b. Fibrin destruction by Arvin. The mechanism of Arvin anticoagulation. Clin. Res. 20: 46 (abstr.).

Prentice, C. R. M., Hassanein, A. A., Turpie, A. G. G., McNicol, G. P., and Douglas, A. S. 1969. Changes in platelet behavior during Arvin therapy. Lancet 1: 644.

Rahimtoola, S. H., Raphael, M. J., Pitney, W. R., Olsen, E. G. J., and Webb-Peploe, M. 1970. Therapeutic defibrination and heparin therapy in the prevention and resolution of experimental venous thrombosis. Circulation 42: 729.

Ratnoff, O. D., and Menzie, C. 1951. A new method for the determination of fibrinogen in small samples of plasma. J. Lab. Clin. Med. 37: 316.

Regoeczi, E., and Bell, W. R. 1969. *In vivo* behavior of the coagulant enzyme from *Agkistrodon rhodostoma* venom: Studies using ^{131}I-Arvin. Brit. J. Haematol. 16: 573.

Regoeczi, E., Gergely, J., and McFarlane, A. S. 1966. *In vivo* effects of *Agkistrodon rhodostoma* venom. Studies with fibrinogen-^{131}I. J. Clin. Invest. 45: 1202.

Reid, H. A., Chan, K. E., and Thean, P. C. 1963. Prolonged coagulation defect (defibrination syndrome) in Malayan viper bite. Lancet 1: 621.

Rodriguez-Erdmann, F., Carpenter, C. B., and Galvanek, E. G. 1971. Experimental dysfibrinogenemia. *In vivo* studies with Arvin. Blood 37: 664.

Rosenfeld, G., Nahas, L., and Kelen, E. M. A. 1968. *In* W. Bucherl, E. E. Buckley, and V. Deulofeu (eds.) Venomous animals and their venoms, pp. 229–273, Vol. I, Academic Press, New York.

Ross, J. W., Bunn, D. G. R., and Ashford, A. 1969. Antigenicity of Arvin. Lancet 1: 130.

Rubenberg, M. L., Bull, B. S., Regoeczi, E., Dacie, J. V., and Brain, M. C. 1967. Experimental production of microangiopathic hemolytic anemia *in vivo.* Lancet 2: 1121.

Rubenberg, M. L., Regoeczi, E., Bull, B. S., Dacie, J. V., and Brain, M. C. 1968. Microangiopathic haemolytic anemia: The experimental production of haemolysis and red-cell fragmentation *in vivo.* Brit. J. Haematol. 14: 627.

Sarkar, N. K., and Devi, A. 1968. *In* W. Bucherl, E. E. Buckley, and V. Deulofeu (eds.) Venomous animals and their venoms, pp. 167–216, Vol. I, Academic Press, New York.

Sharma, G. W. R. K., Godin, P., Belko, J., Sasahara, A. A., and Bell, W. R. 1973. Effects of Arvin on experimental pulmonary embolism. Amer. Heart J. 85: 727.

Sharp, A. A. 1971. Clinical use of Arvin. Thromb. Diath. Haemorrh. Suppl. 45: 69.

Sharp, A. A., Howie, B., Biggs, R., and Methuen, D. T. 1958. Defibrination syndrome in pregnancy: Value of various diagnostic tests. Lancet 2: 1309.

Silberman, S., Bernik, M. B., Potter, E. V., and Kwaan, H. C. 1973. Effects of ancrod (Arvin) in mice. Brit. J. Haematol. 24: 101.

Silberman, S., and Kwaan, H. C. 1971. The effect of Arvin on wound healing in the rat. Fed. Proc. 30: 424.

Singh, M. P., Bentall, H. H., Bell, W. R., Olsen, E. G. J., and Allwork, S. P. 1970. The use of Arvin in prevention of thrombosis on prosthetic heart valves. Thorax 25: 472.

Taylor, J., Mallick, S. M. K., and Ahuja, M. L. 1935. The coagulant action on blood of *Daboia* and *Echis* venoms and its neutralization. Indian J. Med. Res. 23: 131.

Turpie, A. G., McNicol, G. P., and Douglas, A. S. 1972. Platelet electrophoresis: Effect of defibrination by Ancrod (Arvin). Cardiovasc. Res. 6: 101.

The Urokinase Pulmonary-Embolism Trial. 1973. A national cooperative study. Circulation Suppl. II 47: II-81.

Van Der Ziel, C., Joison, J., Siso, H., Saravis, C., and Slapak, M. 1970. The effect of Arvin on blood coagulation and patency of venovenous shunts in the dog. Brit. J. Surg. 57: 856 (abstr.).

Voss, D. 1968. Therapeutic defibrination: A new concept in anticoagulant therapy. Internist 9: 389.

Wood, S. 1961. Mechanisms of metastases production by blood-borne cancer cells. Canad. Cancer Conf. 4: 167.

Wood, S. 1971. Mechanisms of establishment of tumor metastasis, pp. 281–308. *In* H. L. Ioachim (ed.) Pathobiology annual.

Kinetics of Human Prothrombin and Fibrinogen in Patients with Thrombocytosis Secondary to Myeloproliferative Syndromes

Jose Martinez, Sandor S. Shapiro, and Ruth R. Holburn

Simultaneous studies of the metabolism of ^{125}I-prothrombin and ^{131}I-fibrinogen were performed in 10 patients with thrombocytosis secondary to myeloproliferative syndromes. The mean fractional catabolic rate (FCR) of prothrombin was 61.9 per cent, significantly higher than the normal mean of 42.5 per cent ($p < 0.01$). Similarly, the mean FCR of fibrinogen was 34.0 per cent, differing significantly from the normal mean of 23.0 per cent ($p < 0.01$). Excellent correlation was found between the increased FCRs of prothrombin and fibrinogen, but not between these FCRs and the platelet level. Therapeutic reduction of platelet counts to the normal range was associated with a normalization of FCRs as well.

Patients suffering from one of the diseases in the group known as the myeloproliferative syndromes often show elevations of platelet count, together with the paradoxical presence of thrombotic as well as hemorrhagic manifestations. This combination of findings is particularly common in the entity "primary hemorrhagic thrombocythemia" (Ozer *et al.*, 1960; Gunz, 1960). The pathophysiology of these thrombohemorrhagic episodes is poorly understood. The bleeding disorder has been related to the presence of functionally abnormal platelets (McClure *et al.*, 1966; Spaet *et al.*, 1969; Hardisty and Wolff, 1955), while others believe that high platelet concentrations promote thrombosis in small blood vessels with subsequent infarction and hemorrhage (Soulier *et al.*, 1957). The platelet functional abnormalities reported in the former studies consisted of decreased adhesion, decreased aggregation, especially with epinephrine, and impairment of platelet factor 3 release. These abnormalities were variable and showed poor correlation with the number of platelets circulating or the patient's clinical manifestations.

METHODS

Patient Material and Hemostatic Studies

Ten patients with thrombocytosis due to myeloproliferative syndromes, five with primary thrombocythemia, two with myeloid metaplasia, and three with polycythemia vera, were studied. Platelet counts were performed by the method of Brecher and Cronkite (1950). Prothrombin was measured by the method of Ware and Seegers (1949) and fibrinogen by the method of Ellis and Stransky (1961). Factor VIII concentration was measured by the one-stage PTT method, using congenitally deficient plasma as substrate. The platelet factor 3 was assayed by the thromboplastin generation time (Miale and Garrett, 1967) and by the Russell viper venom (Horowitz *et al.*, 1967) methods, and results expressed as per cent of normal. The results of these coagulation parameters in our 10 patients are shown in Table 1. In patient D.S., fibrinogen, prothrombin, and factor VIII concentrations were low and the fibrinogen-fibrin split products in his serum were increased, suggesting intravascular coagulation. A second patient also had a low factor VIII level. These abnormalities were corrected after the platelet count was reduced to a normal level by treating these patients with Busulfan.

Metabolic Studies

In the presence of normal concentrations of coagulation factors, information regarding the activity of the coagulation mechanism has been obtained by measuring the catabolism of fibrinogen.

Table 1. Coagulation data

Patient	Diagnosis	Platelets (thousands/mm^3)	Fibrinogen (mg/100 ml)	Prothrombin (units/ml)	Factor VIII (%)	Platelet factor 3	
						T.G.T.* (%)	Stypven time (%)
D.S.	Primary thrombocythemia	2150	140	238	40	50	52
E.P.	Primary thrombocythemia	2500	261	259	48	100	100
G.M.	Primary thrombocythemia	1600	290	397	110	50	65
E.L.	Primary thrombocythemia	1200	430	324	63	25	68
H.R.	Primary thrombocythemia	1000	217	298	66	100	82
A.A.	Myeloid metaplasia	760	262	274	100	100	120
B.R.	Myeloid metaplasia	3100	500	230	138	3	40
M.J.	Polycythemia vera	580	380	265	208	100	130
J.M.	Polycythemia vera	1100	229	260	63	50	80
A.K.	Polycythemia vera	650	345	273	73	100	
Normal		150–380	232–444	260–330	48–152	75–125	79–121

* T.G.T., Thromboplastin generation test.

Thus, radioactive fibrinogen has been shown to be metabolized faster than normal in experimental animals given endotoxin (Lerner *et al.*, 1968), in patients with microangiopathic hemolytic anemia (Baker *et al.*, 1968), and in some patients with myeloproliferative diseases (Brodsky *et al.*, 1972; Tytgat *et al.*, 1972). A drawback in these studies is that both intravascular coagulation and fibrinolysis can increase fibrinogen metabolism. To avoid this drawback, use was made of radioactive prothrombin injected simultaneously with fibrinogen. This study provided information regarding (*a*) the catabolic rate of these proteins in patients with thrombocytosis due to myeloproliferative syndromes, (*b*) relation of the catabolic rate with the level of platelet count, and (*c*) relationship between prothrombin and fibrinogen catabolism.

Preparation of Labeled Proteins

Prothrombin was purified by the method of Shapiro and Waugh (1966). Fibrinogen was prepared by the glycine precipitation method of Kazal and associates (1963). Both proteins were prepared from plasma obtained from healthy, Australian-antigen-negative donors. Prothrombin was labeled with ^{125}I and fibrinogen with ^{131}I by the iodine monochloride method of McFarlane (1958), as previously described (Shapiro and Martinez, 1969). Unbound iodine was removed by passage of each protein through an Amberlite MB-1 column, 1.5 × 3 cm. Other impurities were removed by gel filtration of the iodinated proteins on a Sephadex G-100 column, 2 × 90 cm, equilibrated with sterile, pyrogen-free buffer consisting of 0.25 *M* NaCl-0.01 *M* sodium citrate, pH 7.0. The labeled proteins were free of unbound iodine and each protein contained an average of less than one-half atom iodine per molecule. Specific activities ranged between 2 and 10 μCi/mg protein. Fibrinogen clottability, performed by the method of Regoeczi (1967), ranged between 92 and 96 per cent. Immediately prior to injection, the labeled proteins were passed separately through G2, 0.22 μ Millipore filters. Ten to fifteen microcurie of each protein were injected through separate syringes and 5-ml blood samples were drawn 20 min and 12 hr later, and then once daily for the remaining 6–7 days of the study. Blood was drawn into one-ninth volume of 3.2 per cent trisodium citrate, and 2-ml aliquots of platelet-free plasma were counted for radioactivity. Corrections were made for overlap of ^{131}I counts into the ^{125}I window, based on prior experiments with isotope mixtures. Residual radioactivity adsorbed to blood cells (including platelets) was found to be less than 2.5 per cent of the total radioactivity of any blood sample.

In Vivo Studies

Catabolic and synthetic rates as well as intra-extravascular distribution of prothrombin and fibrinogen were calculated from plasma radioactivity disappearance curves by the method of Matthews (1957). Fractional catabolic rates were also calculated from 24-hr urinary excretion of radioactivity. Patients received 10 drops of saturated potassium iodide solution orally twice daily for 1–2 days before, and once daily during, the study. Hematocrits, platelet counts, and prothrombin and fibrinogen concentrations were measured and found to be stable throughout each study. Patients were afebrile and were not taking any medication during, and for at least 2 weeks prior to, the study.

RESULTS AND DISCUSSION

The prothrombin metabolic parameters obtained in nine patients are shown in Table 2. The mean prothrombin half-life for this group was 2.2 days, significantly shorter than the 2.8 days obtained in normal subjects. The fractional catabolic rate (FCR) was greater than the normal mean in all nine patients, the increase exceeding one standard deviation in eight. The mean fractional catabolic rate for prothrombin in this group of nine patients was highly significantly increased above normal ($p < 0.01$). Results

Table 2. Prothrombin turnover data in nine patients with thrombocytosis due to myeloproliferative syndromes

		FCR data derived from:		
	Half-life (days)	Plasma (% plasma pool/day)	Urine	Fibrinogen synthesis rate (mg/kg/day)
Mean	2.22	61.9	59.8	3.87
Normal	2.81	42.5	45.4	2.43
± SD	±0.25	±6.2	±5.6	±0.38

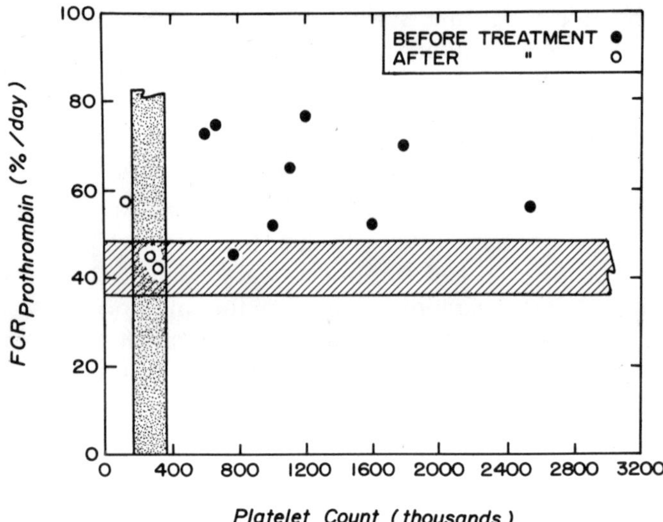

Figure 1. Relationship of platelet concentration and fractional catabolic rate of prothrombin. Hatched area represents mean ± SD.

from plasma and urine data were in excellent agreement. The prothrombin synthesis rate was increased, and this would explain the normal plasma prothrombin concentration found in the majority of these patients.

The lack of relationship between the platelet count and prothrombin FCR is shown in Fig. 1. The solid circles represent the FCR, elevated in eight patients with no relation to platelet count. The open circles represent the FCR in three patients on whom these studies were repeated after their platelet count returned to a normal level. The FCR fell to a normal level in two patients and decreased toward normal in a third patient.

As shown in Table 3 and Fig. 2, the mean fibrinogen half-life in these nine patients was shorter than normal. The mean fractional catabolic rate was greatly increased above normal ($p < 0.01$). Again, the FCR of fibrinogen fell in the three patients whose platelet count had returned to normal after treatment. A very high degree of correlation was found (Fig. 3) between the fractional catabolic rates of prothrombin and fibrinogen, expressed in terms of the respective normal mean values.

The mechanism responsible for the activation of the coagulation system in this group of patients is unknown. It has been shown

Table 3. Fibrinogen turnover data in nine patients with thrombocytosis due to myeloproliferative syndromes

	Half-life (days)	FCR data derived from: Plasma	Urine	Fibrinogen synthesis rate (mg/kg/day)
		(% plasma pool/day)		
Mean	3.05	34.0	38.2	57.9
Normal ±SD	3.79 ±0.26	23.9 ±3.7	21.2 ±1.1	24.8 ±5.2

that the injection of platelet factor 3 under cer ain conditions can induce intravascular coagulation with a rapid turnover of fibrinogen (Evensen and Jeremic, 1970). It is possible that a release of intracellular proteases from leukocytes (Niemetz, 1972; Janoff, 1970) or platelets (Nachman and Ferris, 1968) might cause an increase in the catabolic rate of some coagulation proteins. If this is the case, it would appear to be mediated by activation of the coagulation system, since heparin administration normalizes the increased fibrinogen catabolism in these patients (Tytgat *et al.*, 1972).

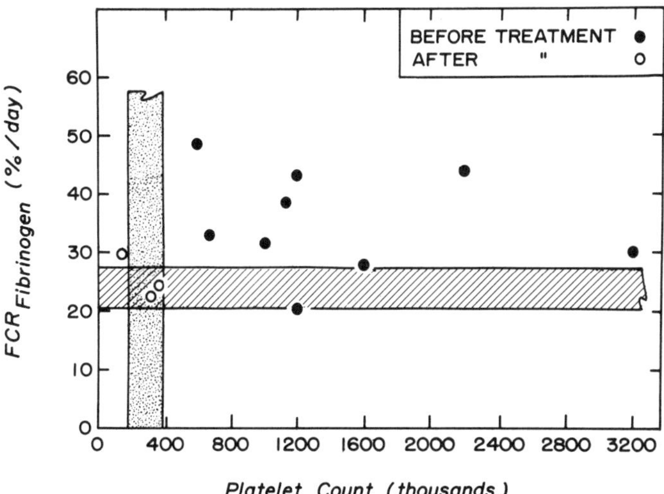

Figure 2. Relationship of platelet concentration and fractional catabolic rate of fibrinogen. Hatched area represents mean ± SD.

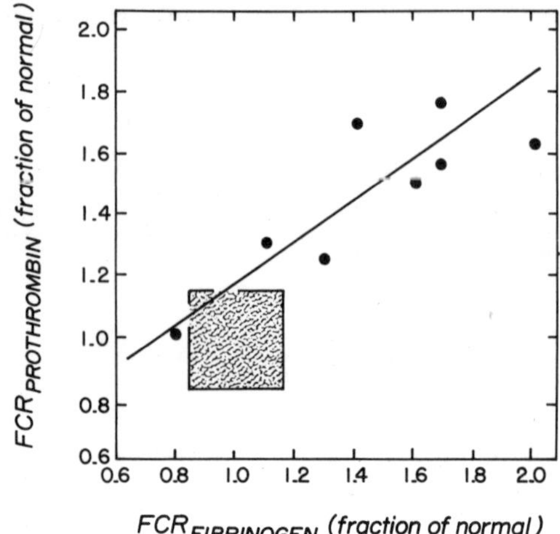

Figure 3. Correlation between the fractional catabolic rates of prothrombin and fibrinogen.

That the thrombocytosis per se is responsible for the hypercatabolism of prothrombin and fibrinogen is suggested by the fact that in three patients in whom these studies were repeated after platelet counts had normalized (Table 4), prothrombin and fibrinogen metabolic parameters returned toward normal. As can be seen, prothrombin concentrations increased after treatment and

Table 4. Effect of therapy on prothrombin and fibrinogen metabolism in nine patients

	Prothrombin		
	Mean concentration (units/ml)	Mean half-life (days)	Mean FCR (%/day)
Before	254	2.20	63.9
After	299	2.43	48.1
	Fibrinogen		
	Mean concentration (mg/100 ml)	Mean half-life (days)	Mean FCR (%/day)
Before	260	2.41	45.1
After	320	3.38	26.7

the prothrombin half-life increased from 2.2 days before, to 2.4 after, they were treated. The FCR fell from a mean of 63.9 per cent before, to 48.1 per cent after, treatment. Similar findings are shown for fibrinogen.

Our studies strongly suggest that thrombocytosis in patients with myeloproliferative disorders is accompanied by a hypercoagulable state, as defined by large increases in the rate of catabolism of prothrombin and fibrinogen. It appears that effective treatment of the thrombocytosis is able to correct the metabolic abnormalities as well. The measurement of radioactive prothrombin turnover seems a useful technique for investigating this problem in myeloproliferative disorders as well as in other conditions.

ACKNOWLEDGMENTS

This work was supported in part by Grants HE-09163 and HE-13695 from the National Institutes of Health.

This study was presented in part at the annual meeting of the Southern Section, American Federation for Clinical Research, New Orleans, January 1971, and at the annual meeting of the American College of Physicians, Denver, March 1971.

REFERENCES

Baker, L. R. I., Rubenberg, M. L., Dacie, J. V., and Brain, M. C. 1968. Fibrinogen catabolism in microangiopathic hemolytic anemia. Brit. J. Haematol. 14: 617.

Brecher, G., and Cronkite, E. P. 1950. Morphology and enumeration of human blood platelets. J. Appl. Physiol. 3: 365.

Brodsky, I., Ross, E. M., Petkov, G., and Kahn, S. B. 1972. Platelet and fibrinogen kinetics with ^{75}Se-selenomethionine in patients with myeloproliferative disorders. Brit. J. Haematol. 22: 179.

Ellis, B. C., and Stransky, A. 1961. A quick and accurate method for the determination of fibrinogen in plasma. J. Lab. Clin. Med. 58: 477.

Evensen, S. A., and Jeremic, M. 1970. Platelets and the triggering mechanism of intravascular coagulation. Brit. J. Haematol. 19: 33.

Gunz, F. W. 1960. Hemorrhagic thrombocythemia: A critical review. Blood 15: 706.

Hardisty, B. M., and Wolff, H. H. 1955. Hemorrhagic thrombocythemia. A clinical and laboratory study. Brit. J. Haematol. 1: 390.

Horowitz, H. I., Cohen, B. D., Martinez, P., and Papayoanou, M. F. 1967. Defective ADP-induced platelet factor 3 activation in uremia. Blood 30: 331.

Janoff, A. 1970. Mediators of tissue damage in human polymorphonuclear neutrophils. Ser. Haematol. 3: 96.

Kazal, L. A., Amsel, S., Miller, O. P., and Tocantins, L. M. 1963. The preparation and some properties of fibrinogen precipitated from human plasma by glycine. Proc. Soc. Exp. Biol. Med. 113: 989.

Lerner, R. G., Rappaport, S. I., Siemsen, J. K., and Spitzer, J. K. 1968. Disappearance of ^{131}I-fibrinogen after endotoxin: effects of a first and second injection. Amer. J. Physiol. 214: 532.

Matthews, C. M. 1957. The theory of tracer experiments with ^{131}I-labelled plasma proteins. Phys. Med. Biol. 2: 36.

McClure, P. D., Ingram, G. I. C., Stacey, R. S., Glass, U. H., and Matchett, M. O. 1966. Platelet function tests in thrombocythaemia and thrombocytosis. Brit. J. Haematol. 12: 478.

McFarlane, A. S. 1958. Efficient trace-labelling of proteins with iodine. Nature 182: 53.

Miale, J. B., and Garrett, V. 1957. Studies on the thromboplastin generation test. III. The effects of dilution, storage and concentration of platelets. Amer. J. Clin. Pathol. 27: 701.

Nachman, R. L., and Ferris, B. 1968. Studies on human platelet protease activity. J. Clin. Invest. 47: 2530.

Niemetz, J. 1972. Coagulant activity of leukocytes. Tissue factor activity. J. Clin. Invest. 51: 307.

Ozer, F. L., Truax, W. E., Miesch, D. C., and Levin, W. C. 1960. Primary hemorrhagic thrombocythemia. Amer. J. Med. 28: 807.

Regoeczi, E. 1967. Measuring the coagulability of fibrinogen in plasma by isotopic means: Methods and principles of its use for *in vivo* studies. Thromb. Diath. Haemorrh. 18: 276.

Shapiro, S. S., and Waugh, D. F. 1966. The purification of human prothrombin. Thromb. Diath. Haemorrh. 16: 469.

Shapiro, S. S., and Martinez, J. 1969. Human prothrombin metabolism in normal man and in hypocoagulable subjects. J. Clin. Invest. 48: 1292.

Soulier, J. P., Flagille, D., and Larriue, M. J. 1957. Etude physiopathologique des hemorrhagies des thrombocythemies. Le Sang 28: 277.

Spaet, T. J., Lejnieks, I., Gaynor, E., and Goldstein, M. L. 1969. Defective platelets in essential thrombocythemia. Arch. Int. Med. 124: 135.

Tytgat, G. N., Collen, D., and Vermylen, J. 1972. Metabolism and distribution of fibrinogen. II. Fibrinogen turnover in polycythemia, thrombocytosis, haemophilia A, congenital afibrinogenaemia and during streptokinase therapy. Brit. J. Haematol. 22: 701.

Ware, A. G., and Seegers, W. H. 1949. Two-stage procedure for the quantitative determination of prothrombin concentration. Amer. J. Clin. Pathol. 19: 471.

Index

F

G

H

R

S

U

V